THE SOCIOLOGY
AND
SOCIAL PSYCHOLOGY
OF DISABILITY
AND REHABILITATION

THE SOCIOLOGY
AND
SOCIAL PSYCHOLOGY
OF DISABILITY
AND REHABILITATION

Constantina Safilios-Rothschild
The Merrill-Palmer Institute

Random House New York

Manufactured in the United States of America
by The Haddon Craftsmen Inc., Scranton, Pa.

First Printing

To My Mother

The Sociologist and the Disabled:
An Invitation and a Challenge for Involvement

Despite the impressive growth that has taken place in the field of medical sociology within the past decade or so, there surprisingly has been only relatively limited sociological research into the problems of patient adjustment and reaction to physical illness per se. For the most part, sociological interest in the field of health has tended to focus on the organizational and demographic aspects of medical care rather than on patient behavior and the treatment process itself. In part, we suspect, the reluctance of many of our professional colleagues to come to grips with the world of the physically ill may be as much a function of their own personal inclination and aversion to illness as it is the limitation of our theory and methods, considerable as the latter may be. Direct involvement with persons who are sick or bedridden, after all, is not always a pleasant experience, nor are such situations particularly receptive to outside intrusion. Similarly, many investigators are neither emotionally equipped nor desire to become so involved. Moreover, the exigencies of human behavior in a time of illness often do not easily lend themselves to neat mathematical models or to laboratory simulation and experimentation. Finally, the sociologist may experience considerable confusion over the perception of his role within the therapeutic setting. In some cases, for instance, his presence and the value of his contributions may engender considerable skepticism and restraint on the part of the treatment staff, whereas in others he may embarrassingly find himself unequivocally endorsed as the primary source from which all behavioral science knowledge flows.

But for whatever the reason, sociological inquiry into the behavioral aspects of physical illness and the therapeutic process has generally been extremely limited.* For the most part, much of the activity to date has tended to be more theoretical and descriptive in nature than empirical and analytical. As a result, much of our knowledge, understanding, and conceptualization of the behavior and response of the physically ill has unfortunately been borrowed or stimulated by the contributions of other social science disciplines. This has been especially true of the area of chronic disease and physical rehabilitation.

The impact of a rather sudden, often unexpected physical disability, for example, a stroke, poliomyelitis or spinal cord injury, may necessitate not only considerable personal adjustment, but social adjustment as well on the part of both the individual involved and those with whom he normally interacts. In addition to coming face to face with the realistic limitations imposed on him by his condition —that is, acts formerly performed in an unthinking, almost automatic fashion soon represent new challenges to functionless nerve patterns and unresponsive joints and muscles—the disabled may be forced to

* For an extensive review of the literature to date on the sociopsychological aspects of disease, see: Gerald Gordon, Odin Anderson, Henry Brehm, and Sue Marquis' excellent, *Disease, the Individual and Society* (New Haven: College and University Press, 1968), as well as Theodor Litman, *Bibliography on the Sociology of Medicine and Medical Care—The First Fifty Years* (Berkeley: Glendessary Press, in press).

modify his concept of self as well. For in a society such as our own, in which the body whole and the body beautiful have been ascribed high social value, the physically impaired may often be regarded by themselves and others as less than normal. Thus, confronted by the need for self-esteem and social acceptance, the disabled may feel shame, inferiority, and even worthlessness over the transformation in his physical state. His subsequent adjustment and reaction to his condition tends to be a function of his own conception of himself and that of his non-injured fellows.

While the goals attained may vary with each individual case, the success of any rehabilitation program thus ultimately rests upon a remarkably intriguing interplay of the biogenic, sociogenic, and psychogenic components of human behavior. Yet despite its rather natural amenability to sociological analysis, behavioral research in the area of long-term chronic illness and physical disability has tended to be preempted by the efforts of other disciplines, notably psychiatry and social work in general, and the brilliant work of the Lewinian social psychologists—Barker, Wright, and Dembo in particular.

Like much of the field of medical sociology itself, the sociology— or perhaps better, the social psychology—of physical disability and rehabilitation comprises an amalgam of a number of theoretical approaches, rather than a single cohesive whole. While each of the respective disciplines involved, for example, sociology, psychiatry, psychology, and social work, conceive the problems of the disabled in terms of their own specific points of view, diffusion of information and interaction between the various fields has generally been infrequent, if not totally nonexistent. Publication of the findings and results of most relevant empirical investigations, for instance, have tended to be relegated to a limited number of special journals peculiar to a specific field. Moreover, few investigators have been either able or willing to take the time to keep abreast of the contributions made by those outside their own academic discipline. As a result, as Barry and Malinovsky have noted, concepts and methods long recognized and utilized in one field are often rediscovered and proposed in another as something "new" and/or "revolutionary," when in fact they are hardly either at all.*

* John R. Barry and Michael R. Malinovsky, *Client Motivation for Rehabilitation: A Review*, University of Florida Rehabilitation Research Monograph Series, No. 1 (February 1965).

In general, however, with the notable exception of the pioneering studies of Kelman and his associates on after-care, Sussman and Slater on family response and reaction to chronic illness, and Krause on post-hospital performance, as well as Roth's critical exposition of the "timetables" in the life of the institutionalized tuberculosis patient, Nagi's research on vocational rehabilitation and low back pain, and our own work on the influence of social and psychological factors on the rehabilitation of the orthopedically disabled, sociologists have been rather slow to recognize and come to grips with the theoretical and methodological implications of physical disability and rehabilitation. Parson's classic conceptualization of the sick role, for instance, virtually ignores the consequences of long-term chronic illness. In fact, role expectations, predicated on an assumption of the temporary nature of illness, for example, "get well soon," "don't worry, you'll be back on your feet in a few days, just as well as new," may not only be quite inappropriate in the case of physical disability, but completely unrealistic as well, and pose a serious threat to successful rehabilitation. Similarly, the situation may be further exacerbated by the inability of most of us to either *take the role* of the disabled when well or *play the role* at onset. That is, not only are few of us really able to fully understand the problems of the physically disabled, but the disabled themselves are in large measure neither prepared for nor aware of the ramifications of their impairment, of the limitations, implications, and potential for recovery, prior to being stricken.

But if the applicability of Parson's conceptualization of the sick ' role may be found wanting as far as chronic disease and disability may be concerned, so too are our traditional approaches to hospital and medical care. In contrast to the often dramatic, rather immediate response patterns usually found in normal medical practice, physical rehabilitation is generally long-term, tedious, terribly frustrating, and frequently only moderately successful at best. Rather than in days or hours, accomplishments may often be measured in terms of months or perhaps years. Even the practitioner's traditional orientation and involvement with the patient and his professional reward system may require considerable restructuring as treatment extends not only temporally, but sociopsychologically as well.

Similarly, as Wessen has noted, the classic hospital model with its emphasis on short-term, acute, emergency care, centered on diagnosis and therapeutic procedure, for the care of a basically passive and dependent patient population, must give way to that of rehabilitation, predicated on the notion of long-term chronic illness, and oriented toward restoration of normal function, prognosis, adjustment, and retraining. Thus, rather than being passive recipients *to whom* and *for whom* things are to be done, candidates for rehabilitation are persons whose motivation to master their disabilities must be mobilized as a joint endeavor on the part of both patient and staff.* The resulting disparity in goal orientation and philosophy may even be reflected in the patient's differential perception of the role of the therapeutic and nursing staff themselves. Whereas the therapist may be conceived as a means of fulfilling one's hopes and desires to return to normality, the nurse and hospital ward stand as a constant reminder of the disabled's complete helplessness and dependency upon others. These feelings may be further heightened when the communication channels are restricted and/or the patient is treated indifferently by aids and orderlies. Thus, in view of their custodial, housekeeping role and constant exposure to the patient's daily irritations and frustrations, it is little wonder that the members of the nursing service, justifiably or not, are frequently the butt of the bulk of the disabled's criticism.

In addition, as in many other areas of health care, the conceptual confusion that has arisen over the role of the disabled and their organizational modes of care tends to be further aggravated by the incorporation of two seemingly antithetical themes into government programs on their behalf. While traditionally couched in humanitarian-service terms, such efforts, at all levels, have consistently been tied to a utilitarian, dependency-productivity model predicated upon the entrepreneurial goal of employability. As a result, a sizable segment of the disabled population, the so-called nonemployables, essentially housewives, the aged and children, have been systematically excluded from consideration or service. Such programatic myopia would seem to constitute not only a serious perversion of the nature and intent of the rehabilitation process, but a challenge to its viability as well.

The potential value of sociological analysis to the field of physical

* Albert Wessen, "The Apparatus of Rehabilitation: An Organizational Analysis," in Marvin B. Sussman (ed.), *Sociology and Rehabilitation* (Washington, D.C.: American Sociological Association, 1965), pp. 148–78.

rehabilitation and vice versa perhaps did not attain full recognition until the so-called Carmel Conference, held in 1965 under the joint auspices of the American Sociological Association and the Vocational Rehabilitation Administration. Although most of the participants were generally better known for their distinctive contributions to empirical research, sociological knowledge, and social theory than for their knowledge and experience in rehabilitation, the symposium provided a highly illuminating exploration of the value and applicability of current sociological theory and research to the field of rehabilitation. Unfortunately, while the conference seemed to bring a number of analytically stimulating insights to bear upon what hitherto had been a relatively untapped area of sociological inquiry, the proceedings were generally marred by extensive interdisciplinary parochialism, a distressing lack of familiarity with the rehabilitation literature, and a rather naive understanding of the rehabilitation process itself.*

More recently, a number of sociologists interested in the field of disability joined together under the leadership of Richard T. Smith and Lawrence Haber to form a discussion group to foster and facilitate the dissemination of information, stimulate research, and develop avenues for the expression of these interests through program sessions and workshop conferences. The initial meeting of the group was held in Boston in 1968 during the annual convention of the American Sociological Association, and an Ad Hoc Committee on Disability was established. As a result of the interest and enthusiasm shown at that meeting, arrangements were made with the ASA's section on medical sociology to sponsor a special session on the "Sociology of Disability" as part of the official program of the Association's 1969 meetings in San Francisco. In addition, a workshop was held in June, 1969, in San Juan, Puerto Rico, under the joint auspices of the Committee on Disability and the Institute Psicologico de Puerto Rico. Over twenty participants were able to attend the three-day session. Among the topics examined were: disability and agencies of social control, sociopsychological aspects of disability, methodology and measurement, and research coordination in disability. In view of the success of this initial venture, future workshops and other related activities are being planned.

* Marvin B. Sussman, ed., *Sociology and Rehabilitation*, American Sociological Association, 1965.

Although their efforts continue to pale beside the contributions of other behavioral scientists, sociologists have increasingly begun to demonstrate a greater awareness of the theoretical and empirical implications physical disability and rehabilitation pose to their field. In this, the first major, comprehensive sociological exploration of the world of the disabled, Constantina Safilios-Rothschild presents a highly provocative yet compassionate exposition of the organizational and behavioral manifestations of physical disability and notes the challenges they pose to sociological inquiry. In so doing, she has managed to attain closure and avoid the unnecessary theoretical parochialism and conceptual duplication that have plagued previous efforts of this kind by an imaginative synthesis of the contributions of other disciplines into an integrated whole. Her efforts, indeed, seem destined to join those of Beatrice Wright* as a classic in the field of physical rehabilitation and medical care. *The Sociology and Social Psychology of Disability and Rehabilitation,* however, is just a beginning, much remains to be done. The opportunities for involvement are great, and the prospects stimulating and promising. The only question is whether we as sociologists are willing to accept the challenge Constantina Safilios-Rothschild has so ably laid down for us.

Theodor J. Litman
University of Minnesota

October 1969

* Beatrice Wright, *Physical Disability: A Social Psychological Approach* (New York: Harper & Row, 1960).

Preface

Had rehabilitation always been a part of medical care, there would be no need to write a separate book on the sociology and social psychology of disability and rehabilitation; the subject could have been adequately treated within a chapter of a book on medical sociology. Because, however, rehabilitation has only recently become the so-called third stage of medicine—its integration with medicine is still far from perfect—and because many of the organizational features as well as the philosophy of rehabilitation are distinctly different (or at least they were meant to be different) from those pervading medical practice, a separate book is necessary. Rehabilitation is in a sense the institution that makes up for the deficiencies of medical care in terms of its lack of comprehensiveness in services rendered and its limited responsibility to the patient. Utilizing a wide range of practitioners, rehabilitation has as a goal the maximization of ability in all areas of those who at the termination of medical care have residual disabilities that interfere with or inhibit their "normal" functioning. Because it is a social institution established on humanitarian and idealistic as well as utilitarian premises, financed most often by the federal and state governments and staffed with medical and paramedical personnel trained in a manner not always congruent with rehabilitation ideals, rehabilitation may be defined in a variety of ways with different consequences.

The dynamics and the results of the rehabilitation process as it takes place under the influence of a number of institutional, practical, and ideological motives and contradicting realities will be one of the central themes of this book. The book will deal primarily with the sociological and sociopsychological aspects of physical disability and physical rehabilitation; however, most of the theories, hypotheses, and conclusions could apply to mental disability and psychiatric rehabilitation as well.

Despite the fact that the nature and degree of the disability as well as the age at onset (congenital, or occurring at childhood, at adulthood, or at old age) have serious consequences for the afflicted individual's adjustment, degree of rehabilitation, and degree of handicapping, an effort will be made to examine disability in general, since there are some common elements in all disabilities regardless of their nature and degree. Only through the examination of these common elements can some conclusions be drawn and some attempts to look into theoretical implications be made. Occasionally, however, the differentiation of disabilities into typologies will be fruitful for theoretical purposes.

Thus, it should be clarified at this point that throughout the book, unless a specific disability is mentioned or a distinction made between chronic illness and other types of physical disability or between visible and nonvisible disabilities, the discussion refers to physical disability in general. The terms "physically disabled" or "disabled" refer to all those who have been afflicted with at least some degree of residual physical disability; they are the most generic terms. Whether or not this physical disability represents or becomes a social or vocational handicap depends on a number of sociopsychological factors; only in those cases where the disability is viewed as some kind of handicap by the individuals involved will the term "handicapped" be employed, and then it will usually be qualified as "socially" or "vocationally" handicapped.

In the first chapter on "Societal Response to Disability," we shall examine the status of the sick and disabled historically and cross-culturally and the way in which societies have coped with this problem in the past and in the present. We shall see why rehabilitation emerged as the answer to the social problem of the disabled and to what extent different types of disability programs permit or facilitate rehabilitation, as well as how adequately the present rehabilitation efforts cover the social problem created by disability.

In Chapter 2, "The Career of the Disabled," the entire process by which a person may go from a state of relative health to illness and then to disability is studied, as well as the variety of behavioral alternatives that are open to him at all points of his career from health to disability. The cultural, social, and sociopsychological factors influencing the individual's choice of alternatives at each stage will be examined, as well as the consequences of the different choices for his eventual rehabilitation outcome.

Chapters 3 and 4 deal with the theoretical aspects of disability and rehabilitation. Despite the fact that there is a great degree of interrelationship and interinfluence between, for example, a disabled's reaction to his disability and his motivational level for rehabilitation, or between the nondisabled's attitudes toward the disabled and the mode of interaction between the two groups, disability and rehabilitation have been separated as much as possible to facilitate the conceptual analysis. Chapter 3, "The Sociology and Social Psychology of Disability," examines disability at three analytical levels: personality, social system, and culture. That is, it includes the examination of how different types of disability affect the disabled's self-concept, of the interpersonal relationships between disabled and nondisabled, of the relationship of the social system of the disabled with other social systems, as well as of the cultural and psychological bases of discrimination and prejudice. Chapter 4, "The Sociology and Social Psychology of Rehabilitation," examines rehabilitation at the personality, social system and culture levels of analysis—that is, the disabled's motivation to become rehabilitated, rehabilitation as a social institution, the rehabilitation professions and the rehabilitation social system, and finally, the cultural ideals reflected in rehabilitation and rehabilitation viewed as a social movement.

Chapter 5 on "Work and Disability" explores the meaning of work and its relevance for the identity of individuals in different occupational categories, the implications of these different meanings of work for definitions of illness, disability, and vocational handicaps and for the afflicted persons' rehabilitation outcome as well.

Chapter 6, "The Successful Rehabilitant," examines the medical, demographic, sociopsychological, and vocational factors found to be related to rehabilitation success in the physical as well as in the vocational area. The significance of these findings is examined in terms of the meaningfulness of the criteria used to measure rehabilitation success. The analytical focus of the discussion centers mainly around the meaningfulness and relevance of rehabilitation results for the "rehabilitated" individual rather than for the rehabilitation personnel or administration.

Chapter 7, "After Rehabilitation," examines the fate of the rehabilitated patients after they leave (or are discharged from) a rehabilitation facility and their state of alienation as they find themselves under the influence of a multitude of often incongruent opinions and advice. The different points of view of the several agents who often have an important "say" about the rehabilitants' degree of reintegration into different social systems (familial, medical, legal, vocational, friendship network) are analyzed, as well as the possible consequences of divergent opinions and pressures upon the long-range rehabilitation outcome of the disabled.

Chapter 8 on "Recommendations and Projections About Disability and Rehabilitation in the Future" focuses on the nature of the shortcomings of present rehabilitation schemes and suggests some ways in which these schemes could be improved. Such improvements can come about through good research programs that will provide the information necessary to change policies in the desirable direction. Probable future societal changes and their implications for redefinitions of disabilities and adjustments in rehabilitation programs are also examined.

I have attempted to write a book on the multidisciplinary social institution of rehabilitation by utilizing multidisciplinary information (contributions of social scientists, as well as medical and paramedical scientists) and analyzing it within a sociological and sociopsychological theoretical framework. Thus, students in such fields as sociology, social psychology, counseling psychology, social work, medicine, nursing, and occupational and physical therapy might profitably use it when studying disability and rehabilitation. This book will aid them in understanding disability and the dynamics of rehabilitation so that they may become more effective teachers, researchers, or practitioners in fields dealing with disability and rehabilitation. Students in medicine, nursing, and occupational and physical therapy will be able to use this book after either an introductory course in sociology or an adequate explanation by the instructor of the terms and concepts used. But practitioners such as lawyers specializing in workmen's compensation, physicians interested in problems of disability and compensation, and insurance people will also find it a helpful reference book.

My earliest intellectual debt must go to Ray A. Mangus, who interested me in social psychiatry and medical sociology when I was a student at Ohio State University. Later on, he and Saad Z. Nagi guided me while I wrote my doctoral dissertation on "The Reactions to Disability in Rehabilitation." In writing this book, my sincere thanks for their help and advice are gratefully given to four people who took time from their very busy academic schedules to read and react extensively to at least one draft of the entire manuscript: Jacques Dofny, Theodor J. Litman, Julius A. Roth, and Mayer N. Zald. I would also like to thank David Mechanic, Hyman Rodman, and David Kallen, who read and reacted to individual chapters. The comments of all these readers greatly improved the quality of the book by indicating new ways of seeing and evaluating facts and ideas, but any inaccuracies or inconsistencies remaining are entirely the author's responsibility.

Since English is not my native language, this book owes its present state of clarity and correctness to Mrs. Judith Goldner, who most carefully edited the final draft. Without her loving attention, many of my ideas would have been irretrievably lost in long "Greek-English" sentences. Finally, I wish to express my sincere thanks to Mrs. Irene Zak, who persevered in typing the endless drafts despite the inevitable stresses and frustrations.

Contents

THE SOCIOLOGY
AND
SOCIAL PSYCHOLOGY
OF DISABILITY
AND REHABILITATION

CHAPTER 1

Societal Response to Disability

In this chapter we shall examine disability along its time and space dimensions. We shall see first how disability has been defined in different societies throughout history and what factors have influenced the way the disabled have been viewed and treated by the nondisabled. In particular, we shall analyze in some detail the societal and cultural changes that brought about organized societal responses to the problem of disability and the evolutional process that led to the present legislative and welfare approach in the United States and abroad. Finally, we shall assess the overall qualitative and quantitative effectiveness of the rehabilitation offered to the disabled by different existing programs.

The Status of the Sick and the Disabled
Historically and Cross-culturally

Throughout history, discriminatory practices against the sick and the disabled have varied greatly from country to country and from century to century; they have ranged from complete rejection and ostracism to semideification and the according of special privileges and honors. Thus, in no time and place in the past—and perhaps in the future as well—have the disabled not been either positively or negatively discriminated against in one or more areas.[1] In the militaristic society of ancient Sparta, all malformed babies were thrown off a precipice. In other societies, the presence of such symptoms as hallucinations or epileptic episodes was often considered proof of ability to communicate with supernatural powers. For example, in some segments of the Brazilian population and in some African tribes, those evidencing these symptoms qualify for the most prestigious social role of all, that of the witch-doctor or medium. In modern industrialized societies, discrimination is subtly disguised, and veiled by "civilized" humanitarian efforts and rationalizations. We shall see, however, that even today, in the more developed countries, there persist two basic types of discrimination: the unwillingness to permit the disabled to engage in the entire range of possible jobs and the refusal to grant them "normal" social interaction that would allow them to become integrated into the "normal" society.

In general, the direction and degree of prejudice directed toward the sick and the disabled seems to be influenced by a number of interrelated factors including: (1) the degree of a country's socioeconomic development and its rate of unemployment; (2) the prevailing notions about the orgins of poverty and unemployment and sociopolitical beliefs concerning the proper role of the government in alleviating social problems; (3) the prevailing notions about the etiology of illness and the degree of individual "responsibility" involved in falling ill and remaining disabled; (4) the cultural values or stigmata attached to different physical conditions or characteristics; (5) illness- or disability-connected factors, such as (a) the degree of visibility of the illness or disability, (b) whether or not the incapacitating illness is contagious, (c) the part of the body afflicted, (d) the nature of the illness (physical or mental) and the assumed "pervasive-ness" of the disability, and (e) the severity of functional impairment and the degree of predictability of its course; (6) the effectiveness of the public relations groups representing the interests of a specific dis-ability and the dramatic-sensational image attached to a particular illness (for example, polio); and (7) the degree of importance for the nation's welfare economy and security of such high-disability-risk undertakings as modern warfare and industrial work.

Let us now examine in somewhat more detail each of the factors that influence the intensity and the type of discrimination practiced by the nondisabled toward the disabled. In developing countries, where medical facilities are scarce and large numbers of able-bodied persons are unemployed, the disabled—unless they have inherited wealth or are taken care of by their families—are usually reduced to begging or dependence on other types of philanthropy. Whenever poverty has been considered a result of and closely related to immorality, laziness, and "unworthiness," depending upon how the role of the government has been defined, the disabled have been either left free but unaided or have been compulsorily assembled and then confined to hospitals and workhouses. The latter trend was especially prevalent in the seventeenth and a good part of the eighteenth century in most European countries and in England. These confinement places served mostly as punitive, reformative institutions for the poor, the sick, the infirm, and the insane, as well as for the criminal and the misfit. Through forced labor and punishment, this conglomeration of un-desirables was to be reformed so as to become worthy, moral, and work-loving. In the special case of the insane, even those from good families could not easily escape compulsory confinement.[2]

Throughout history, prevailing notions about the etiology of illness or disability have greatly influenced the degree as well as the nature of social prejudice directed toward the afflicted. When the sick individual has been personally held responsible for his illness, as in the ancient Hebrew culture where illness and physical defects were associated with sin,[3] the social stigma attached to such afflictions is quite strong. The folk belief that blindness is a punishment for sins committed has been prevalent over many cultures and centuries and has had as a consequence the social isolation of the blind. But the Christian religion defined charity and the care of the sick as a major duty of all believers and attempted to combat prejudice by preaching the "dignity and essential worth of human life and the equality of all men in the eyes of God."[4] Also, according to Christian doctrine, suffering was traditionally viewed as a means of purification and of gaining spiritual merit. However, Christian teaching did not have a consistent and long-range impact upon all people nor did it improve the chances of the disabled being accepted by the "normal" society. Its major contribution was to the development of a system for the custodial and moral care of some sick and disabled who could not be cared for by their families. Later on, because of the many surviving superstitions and the mysticism surrounding religion which permeated all areas of social life during the Middle Ages, crippled, malformed and visibly ill individuals were said to be either cursed by the Devil or possessed by him. As such, they were feared, hated, and often persecuted and tortured as collaborators of the Evil One and bringers of all kinds of misfortune to their towns and their fellow-men.

At the present time, some types of diseases, accidents, and disabilities are viewed "scientifically" as the result of amoral natural conditions beyond the will or control of the afflicted individual. For those afflicted with such an illness or disability, it is, theoretically at least, easier to escape some types of social stigma and discriminatory practices. This "scientific" view tends to be more prevalent among medically sophisticated and highly educated persons, although even they may be influenced to some extent by vestiges of other views of illness and disability. Most people, however, seem to be influenced by all four views: the Hebrew, the old Greek notion which associated illness and physical defects with social inferiority, the Christian doctrine, and the scientific view.[5] It is interesting to note that we do not exactly know the effect on society's perception of the sick and the disabled of such recent notions about illness as (a) the increasing recognition of the role played by emotional and sociopsychological factors in the etiology, course, and outcome of illness, as well as in determining the degree of handicap that ensues; and (b) the realization that illness may sometimes represent a handy conscious or unconscious escape from stressful or undesirable social responsibilities, so that in some cases the individual may be held partially responsible for his illness or disability. The current conceptualization of illness as a form of deviant behavior[6] may sometimes result in a questioning of the validity of the disabled's professed inability to perform certain functional activities, to fulfill social responsibilities, and to cooperate in rehabilitation efforts, his behavior being interpreted instead as possible "malingering" or "emotional overlay." Indeed, this current notion of illness may be leading to a new kind of "sophisticated" social prejudice that should be further investigated.

Even among the sick and the disabled, discriminatory practices have not been equally distributed, for some have been much more stigmatized and isolated than others. Visible disabilities in general consistently generate a greater amount of discrimination, both positive and negative. Wright has explained how through the "spread" phenomenon of perceptional association, overall negative and inferior or positive impressions are created about the individual, all emanating from the stimulus of the visible disability.[7] Facial disfigurements, despite the fact that they do not necessarily impair people functionally, set the afflicted apart and bring about negative discriminatory practices, probably because they provoke fear and disgust. And such discrimination has been extreme in all times and cultures. In the case of nonvisible disabilities, it is the knowledge of their existence certified by a doctor's official diagnosis which triggers discrimination and intolerance. As long as the nonvisible disability is not known and the disabled person can pass for normal, he is accepted as such. But usually he cannot pass as normal in all situations or for a very long time despite his having developed a wide range of concealing techniques and tricks, which in themselves may often be painful, stressful or humiliating to him. Once his true identity is uncovered, the seriousness of the discrimination depends upon the nature and the assumed "pervasiveness" of the disability, whether or not it is contagious or considered hereditary, as well as upon the degree and severity of the social stigma attached to it in the particular country in which he is living. For example, in contemporary Greece and Canada the psychiatric diagnosis of mental disorder renders previously tolerated deviant behavior no longer acceptable within the family.[8]

The severity of an illness or disability and the degree to which its course can be predicted and controlled also seems to influence whether or not the afflicted individual will be helped and accepted or confined and isolated. Even in our time, those who are severely disabled or afflicted with multiple disabilities are often excluded from rehabilitation services, refused employment, and placed in complete social isolation. Here Strauss' generalization that throughout time "... only the victims of problems for which remedies were known or anticipated have been treated sympathetically"[9] is relevant and can be amended to include the proposition that only when vocational and medical rehabilitation has a good probability of success are disabled people ordinarily granted rehabilitation services.

In some categories of disability, the disabled have had effective spokesmen and public relations people who have "protected" and "advanced" their interests and succeeded in obtaining special privileges for them. Examples of this kind of humanitarian lobbying are the blind and the war veterans, although the consequences for the two have been somewhat different. In the case of the blind, the sensational nature of their disability coupled with effective lobbying resulted in the passing of legislation granting them such special privileges as tax exemptions, newsstands in government buildings, and the operation of vending machines, as well as sheltered workshops. However, these privileges have not helped them to become integrated into normal society or to become independent and may, on the contrary, have contributed to their apartness by singling them out as unable to compete on an equal footing with others. Thus, every special privilege granted to them contributed also to their social labeling as helpless and diminished their chance for real independence and societal integration. This is a common dilemma for other disabled and minority groups as well, for they must forego most, if not all, of the preferential treatment they now receive if they wish to compete equally with all others and be accepted as equals.[10]

In the case of the war veterans, their organizations have been quite successful not only in getting special privileges for them, but also in helping them integrate more or less successfully into normal society, probably because of the moral connotations of disability incurred while protecting national honor and integrity. Special privileges are therefore granted quite easily as an indication of national gratitude for personal sacrifice; legislators need no other justification, such as their helplessness. For the same reasons, probably, their societal integration is also easier.

Except for the fact that a variety of factors more or less determine people's attitudes toward the disabled, prejudice is a multidimensional variable. Therefore, discriminatory practices may reflect degrees of intolerance for disabled people which may vary from the point at which people do not wish the disabled (especially the visibly disabled) to be present in public places to unwillingness to rent them apartments, let them stay in hotels, give them loans, insurance policies, and drivers' licenses, or admit them to "normal" schools and universities. A person might be tolerant in all the above areas but be unwilling to employ a disabled person (or at least some types of disabled). Or he might be willing to employ the disabled but be reluctant to interact socially with them beyond "fictional" acceptance. This last type of prejudice, which we could call "social" or "affective," is probably the most deeply rooted one and for this reason cannot be touched or modified by legislation.

Attempts have been made to modify several types of discriminatory practices, especially those affecting the employment of the disabled. Several countries have in recent years passed protective legislation to combat this type of discrimination, although not with great success. For example, in some developing countries where most people work in small family businesses or are self-employed, quota legislation favoring the disabled would be meaningless. And if people, including employers, are prejudiced against the disabled as potential workers, quota legislation may be circumvented through technicalities in the definition of a "disabled" person. Thus, many people who would not be thought of as disabled and who would be working "normally" would tend to become stigmatized as disabled and would then have work problems. Employers would tend to count these people as disabled to fulfill the quota requirements, and no progress would have been made in the employment of the truly disabled. Generally, it seems that legislation by itself is powerless unless prevailing values and beliefs concerning the disabled are changed. Otherwise techniques will be developed to get around the law so that the "undesirables" can still be discriminated against.

Another type of protective legislation is being passed very slowly and only in highly industrialized countries. It concerns the modification of architectural barriers in public buildings and private housing that de facto discriminate against several categories of disabled and prohibit their successful integration into society.[11] Unless special care is taken, however, there may be a tendency to create disabled "neighborhoods" and thus a new kind of ghetto. Experience with this legislation is similar to that with employment legislation; only government buildings tend to abide consistently by the regulations.

Some countries have tried to aid the acceptance of the disabled through educational campaigns, but again with no great success. An ever-present danger in protective legislation, fund-raising, or educational campaigns is the possibility of stimulating undesirable side effects which may create almost as much discrimination as they help to eradicate. For example, as we saw earlier, protective employment legislation may make employers more sensitive in differentiating the disabled from the nondisabled and cause them to lower their level of tolerance for deviations from the so-called "normal" physique. Or, educational campaigns informing a population about the nature of an illness or a disability and describing specific symptoms may unintentionally bring about a greater intolerance of mildly disabled persons who might have "passed" as normals. This becomes a serious problem particularly because a negative correlation seems to exist between the potency of social stigma (and ensuing consequences) attached to a disabling illness and the degree of tolerance of a range of symptoms that holds cross-culturally. Thus in a country like Greece, where a wide range of mentally deviant symptoms are usually tolerated without the individual being labeled mentally ill and stigmatized for life, educational programs and campaigns which would sensitize the public about the meaning of symptoms could bring about an intolerance for a whole range of presently "normalized" symptoms and the stigmatization of a much larger number of mildly disturbed persons as a result.

Probably the most serious discriminatory practices are the social and affective ones which refer to unwillingness (or inability) to interact normally with a disabled person and to accept him as an equal, that is, a person one can have as a friend, lover, or spouse. And it is because this "hard-core" discrimination cannot be affected by legislation or educational campaigns that all modern societies have failed to either eradicate or modify it. This type of discrimination reflects a deep-rooted prejudice which in turn reflects a profound and perpetual fear and anxiety about losing one's physical integrity and becoming disabled.[12] The nondisabled feel repulsion and disgust for the disabled—in different degrees of intensity and about different types of disability—a)\d then usually guilt because of these "unaccept-able" feelings.[13] Because of this emotional conflict, the nondisabled either avoid coming into contact with the disabled altogether, or when they do have to interact with them, do not allow themselves to get angry with or to insult the disabled person regardless of how irritating his personality or offensive his behavior. Since the non-disabled have to watch their every gesture and word so closely in order not to make a negative slip or show their aversion—probably because they are also afraid that such behavior might "magically" visit the affliction upon themselves—and since the norms regulating disabled-nondisabled social interaction are quite ambiguous for both parties, such interactions are usually uncomfortable rigid and strained.[14] However, unless societies can find a way to influence social and affective prejudices and the discriminatory practices which result from them, disabled people will never be accepted and reacted to as people and will never succeed in becoming integrated into normal society.

It is undeniably very difficult to intervene and alter such prej-udices, but not all possible intervention techniques have been tried. For instance, a potentially promising technique might be the use of regular entertainment rather than educational channels (such as television, movies, stories in popular magazines, cartoons and chil-dren's stories) to change the image of the disabled and the stereotyped beliefs that are held about them.[15] The mass media and particularly television are increasingly playing a crucial role in the formation of the values of children as well as of adults. By presenting the disabled hero (or a secondary personage) as not basically different from the nondisabled—that is, as neither a hateful, distorted person, a gangster or a murderer, nor an exceptionally gifted or kind and understanding one, but as an individual who performs his social and familial roles with all the ordinary passion, fear, courage, and weakness of all human beings—we may be successful in breaking down the thick crust of social and affective prejudice. Unless modern societies are successful in altering social and affective prejudices in such a way that the dis-abled are accepted as "people with a disability," in the same way that people with green eyes or blond hair are accepted, we will not have moved very far from the prejudices and discriminatory practices of the Middle Ages.[16] Except that now we are more subtle, and there--

fore probably more effective, in segregating the disabled under the cover of humanitarianism and social welfare. We try to give them some kind of employment, we encourage them to live by themselves, to socialize among themselves and even to marry among themselves— since in this way they will be happiest—just as long as they do not demand "real" integration into society. And so it seems that: *Plus ça change et plus ça reste la même chose*.

Society Meets the Challenge of Disability: The Creation of Disability Programs

Besides being discriminated against in one or another way, the sick and the disabled have always been "problematical" for all societies throughout history, since they could not usually perform their social responsibilities satisfactorily and became dependent on the productive able-bodied. This social problem has been handled in a variety of ways, and the societal responses have always varied for differently disabled groups of people. Even in more recent times, the trends observed in most countries indicate that usually the greatest initial societal interest and concern is directed toward disabled veterans, the blind, handicapped children (especially by poliomyelitis), industrial workers, the deaf, and the orthopedically disabled.[17] This differential concern, however, seems to apply mostly when no overall government health policies exist and voluntary and special interest agencies have evolved for the protection of certain groups of disabled. Once comprehensive governmental health policies are established or legislation is passed for war veterans and industrial workers, however, the ground is laid for similar legislation for all the disabled. The lapse of time before comprehensive health legislation for all disabled is passed varies with a country's stage of socioeconomic development. And the type of health legislation passed in each country depends upon the social and political system and the prevailing system of medical care administration.

Because protective legislation covering war veterans and industrial workers was passed without much time lapse in most Western countries, the one aiding the passing of the other, it is rather difficult to examine separately the process through which each evolved. At some point they intertwined and the result was favorable for both groups. In some Western countries such as England and Germany, workmen's compensation programs were enacted before World War I. In others like the United States, the end of World War I brought legislation for both war veterans and industrial workers. We shall examine in some detail the evolution of societal responses to industrial disabilities in two countries—England and the United States—and in less detail, legislation enacted in other European countries.

Before the so-called Industrial Revolution, most people lived by farming, fishing, by selling and trading merchandise, or by using their skill in some kind of small-scale (often family-run) home industry. Although all the usual occupations of the pre-industrial centuries did involve a certain amount of risk, it was quite negligible in comparison to the mortal risk involved in obligatory participation in war. During the Middle Ages the peasants exchanged labor for the protection afforded by the fortifications and the professional soldiers of a king, prince, or lord. Ideologically, fate was the master. Since the environment could not be controlled, accidents, fire, illnesses, and disasters were due either to the whim of fate or to God's wrath, and the consequences for the individual were seen as strokes of bad luck for which society had no responsibility. The extended family and friends took care of the sick or disabled person and often supported him throughout life. In addition, the same often held true when there was a close relationship between employer and employee, such as that between craftsman and apprentices. If there was an accident, local public opinion often made help to the employee mandatory.

Of course, there have always been dangerous occupations and modes of life. The slaves working on the Egyptian pyramids or the road builders of the Roman Empire were exposed to great occupational risks, but few of them had any choice of occupation. When dangerous occupations (excepting the army, which has always managed to attract restless or adventuresome individuals despite the great risks involved)[18] increased in number and people were by no means compelled to follow them, some kind of crude protective legislation concerning the health of these people was sooner or later enacted. It is not clear, however, whether the need for protective health legislation was given recognition because of the spread of the Industrial Revolution or if other factors contributed. Some writers even doubt that the accident rate was greater once factories were established than when improvised and badly run mills were operated in the early 1800s in England.[19] Structural differentiations and social changes, some related to (or even resulting from) the development of factories, and others concomitant with this development, accentuated or probably even created the need for protective health legislation for factory workers.

According to Smelser's brilliant analysis of social change at the advent of the Industrial Revolution in England and throughout the greater part of the eighteenth century, the setting for industrial production was the home and the entire family took part in the different phases of production.[20] As demands for greater production were made and some machinery was used, people outside the family were employed as additional helpers or placed under subcontracts. Central control, however, still remained within the family. Even when the presence of a great number of machines and the desire to control and regulate production led to the establishment of factories in the beginning of the nineteenth century, entire families, or at least fathers and sons (or mothers and sons) still worked together for factory owners who knew them personally and felt responsible for them in case of illness or distress. As the factory system spread and started operating on a more rational and impersonal basis in terms of the hiring as well as the treatment of employees, the composition of the work force changed. Families were no longer employed by the same firm, sometimes purposely and sometimes accidentally, because it was easier to hire whoever was readily available.

And because the hiring base changed, the nature of the relationship between employer and worker underwent a radical change from a personal to an impersonal one. Employers then no longer felt personally responsible for helping their workers in case of illness or misfortune. Simultaneously, trade unions underwent structural differentiations which eventually turned them from benevolent societies into bargaining tools geared to defend the workers' interests. As this transition was also gradual, the unions were to retain some of the characteristics of the benevolent society, such as diffuse welfare benefits in case of illness, accident, or old age, throughout the first half of the nineteenth century. However, after 1850 and the depersonalization of the factories, the unions had to undergo greater differentiation and specialization so that all their activities could be focused on improving working conditions and helping workers in periods of unemployment. They did not, however, extend their activities to cover the worker and his family in the face of illness, accident, or death of the breadwinner.

It seems, then, that it was a combination of such factors as (1) the establishment of "efficient" factories ultilizing increasingly complicated machinery, (2) the depersonalization of the factories and the employer-employee relationship and (3) the structural differentiation of the trade unions which led them to relinquish their function of providing welfare benefits to workers in case of sickness or accident that was responsible for society's newly felt need to provide protective health legislation for the worker. It has been pointed out that an additional factor contributed significantly to this new public attitude, namely, the fact that with the advent of Mercantilism in Europe, industrial laborers were now defined as one of the most important factors of production, "as an essential element in the generation of national wealth."[21] There is an analogy here to the end of the sixteenth century in England, when a hospital was established for seamen, an occupational group deemed extremely important to national prestige and defense as well as to the economy.[22]

In the nineteenth century, because of the spread and the economic importance of industries, national health policies tended to concentrate on industrial workers. At that point the crucial question was raised: Who is to blame for an injury or disease incurred by an employee at work, and who, therefore, must assume financial responsibility for the afflicted worker? Up to that time, according to the common law of most European countries and of the United States, injured workers could always sue their employers for damages; however, the legal defenses available to employers were so numerous that the injured worker or his survivors had very little chance of winning the case. English common law specified that employers were liable for injuries to others only when the employer had neglected his basic duties toward his employees (General Law of Negligence). These duties were: the provision of reasonably safe working conditions, tools and appliances; reasonably careful selection of competent agents and workers; provision of suitable and reasonable work instructions; and "the duty to warn and instruct youthful and inexperienced workers as to the dangers of the employment."[23] Only when the employer had failed to perform the above duties was he liable for injuries suffered by his employees.

Furthermore, the employer had at his disposition three very powerful legal defenses: (a) *The defense of contributory negligence.* According to this defense, if the injured worker had even slightly contributed to his injury through a minor negligence of his own (even when the employer's negligence was great), he could not recover for his injury. (b) *The fellow servant rule.* According to this rule, an employer was not liable for an injury sustained because of the negligence or carelessness of a fellow servant. (c) *The defense of assumption of risk.* This was based on the general rule that the employee assumed the ordinary risks of the employment in which he engaged.[24] The courts, however, extended the assumption of risk rule to include abnormal risks, and the worker could not recover for his injury if he had continued to work after having become aware of potential dangers. The crucial question relating to this defense was whether or not an employee who obeyed the orders of a foreman requiring him to perform a potentially dangerous assignment should be recompensed for injury because he had assumed the risk. The courts usually ruled that under such circumstances he could not recover for injury, and thus the employee who could not quit his job every time he was aware of danger usually worked under dangerous conditions, knowing full well that if he should sustain an injury, no recovery would be made.[25]

Despite the fact that the courts were traditionally on the side of the employers, the plight of the employee was so serious that the courts of some American states adopted exceptions to the employers' defenses. One was the vice principal exception, according to which a foreman or a supervisor was considered to be a vice principal of the master and the master was liable for the vice principal's negligence as well as for his own. Another was the adoption of the rule of comparative negligence. But the partial remedies offered by a few courts could not solve the problem. In England, the Employers' Liability Act of 1800, which contained a rule similar to the vice principal rule adopted by the American courts, could not adequately protect the workers as informal supports and obligations wore thinner and gradually disappeared.[26] After a considerable lapse of time and much controversy, the British Workmen's Compensation Act of 1897 was passed making the insurance of industries with nonprofit government organizations voluntary and not compulsory. At that time the decision was made that it was more just for the industry to carry the financial burden of industrial illness and accident than for the afflicted worker and his family to do so.

The first workmen's insurance programs were enacted earlier in Germany than in England despite the fact that the latter first experienced the changes brought about by the Industrial Revolution. The reason for Germany's pioneering laws was probably the strong tradition of state paternalism reinforced by the social and political ideology of nineteenth-century philosophers, writers, politicians, and scholars which contrasted strongly with English ideas of freedom and independence and the prevailing economic and philosophical doctrine of laissez faire.[27] As early as 1838, a Prussian law made the railroad companies responsible for injuries to passengers and employees, except when the accident was the injured person's fault or an "act of God." Nevertheless, even in Germany ideas were not translated into action until the Socialist movement became noticeable. Then, in the 1880s Bismarck, wishing to satisfy the masses by showing his paternalistic interest in their welfare, adopted the first social insurance programs providing "compensation for all accidents occurring in industrial establishments without regard to whether they were attributable to the negligence of the employer or of the injured worker, or to risks inherent in the business." The German laws, in contrast to the British Workmen's Compensation Act of 1897, made the insurance of industries with nonprofit government organizations compulsory rather than voluntary. Other European countries followed with similar acts influenced almost equally by those of the Germans and the British; legislation in the United States was influenced mainly by the British model.[28]

In the United States, federal interest in the health of the population was quite slow to develop. In 1798, Congress established a marine hospital fund similar to that of the British and based upon the same rationale. Starting at the end of the eighteenth century, several other "deserving" groups, such as members of the armed forces, American Indians, emancipated Negroes, veterans, victims of leprosy, drug addicts, federal prisoners, disabled persons, and rural farm families were gradually granted (or had forced upon them) special provisions for medical care. In the early nineteenth century voluntary movements for the "deserving" poor and the disabled flourished in America, but they usually helped "innocent victims of circumstance, such as orphans, deformed persons and the blind," and always excluded the able-bodied poor.[29] Whatever the humanitarian contribution of these voluntary movements, the puritanical values that prevailed have left an indelible stamp of morality on all subsequent forms of welfare.

The United States, as in many other areas of social legislation, was quite slow in enacting workmen's compensation laws. Some of the reasons for this tardiness were:

1. The prevailing laissez-faire ideologies, incorporating a social philosophy based upon the biological principle of the survival of the fittest, which were very attractive and profitable to the large industrialists and had become popular due to the influence of the English.[30] This ideological orientation contributed to the virtual societal abandonment of the weaker, poorer, and disabled segment of the population, leaving it to its own inadequate devices while permitting American employers to remain free of responsibility toward their employees. Furthermore, the employers were the "strongest and the fittest" not only to survive but to make the maximum profit by not taking safety precautions, by not compensating employees who suffered occupational accidents or diseases, and by being able to replace disabled workers with an ever-ready supply of able-bodied ones provided by the continuous influx of immigrants to America.

2. The availability of abundant and cheap labor provided by the steadily increasing numbers of European immigrants who could barely speak the language, much less understand or attempt to protect their rights. Because of this influx of cheap immigrant labor, a "double standard" resulted which seriously affected early attitudes toward safety and hygiene as well as toward a feeling of responsibility for one's employees when these employees were not "proper Americans," but only some "poor foreigners."[31]

3. The sometimes almost "blind" belief in the equality of rights held by all citizens whether employers or employees, including the right to hire and fire, to quit a job, to sue an employer for sustained injuries or to protect one's industrial enterprise from fraudulent or unjustified suits. This ideological belief was poorly matched with reality in the case of most workers, who had hardly any possibility of making use of their "rights" and were therefore often exploited and maltreated in the name of the

"justice" and "freedom" which existed only for the employers.[32]

4. The reluctance of American businessmen to take the risk of increasing industrial costs through compensation to disabled workers coupled with a political network that created a similar reluctance in state legislators to enact laws which could lessen the industrial productivity of their own state by increasing industrial costs in relation to operating costs in other states.[33]

5. The ever-present rejection of the appropriateness of federal intervention in state matters, a concern which was much broader than the content of the contemplated health bills. Federal legislation was usually seen as a threat to the autonomy of each state and as an undesirable imposition by the central government.[34]

It was only at the beginning of the twentieth century that a number of influential individuals became interested in workmen's compensation, among them President Theodore Roosevelt, who on January 31, 1908, in a message to Congress laid down a general pattern for workmen's compensation legislation.[35] Acting upon the President's recommendation, Congress enacted the Civil Employees Act in 1908 and later on the Federal Employers' Liability Act to cover employees of "common carriers." The federal law was not quite satisfactory in that it was still necessary for the injured worker to prove the fault of the employer, but it influenced state legislatures to adopt similar laws.

The years between 1911 and 1920 were very productive; workmen's compensation laws were adopted by all but eight states, and covered two-thirds of the American workers.[36] Because of medical and surgical progress, more disabled workers had survived World War I than any other war in the country's history, and as the nation was brought face to face with an acute shortage of skilled labor, there was considerable interest in the potential usefulness and purposefulness of vocational rehabilitation.[37] Mainly because of national manpower needs, the sacrifice of a soldier's health in the line of duty and the resulting disability could no longer be defined as merely an individual (or familial) misfortune; it was rather an economic liability affecting the welfare of the entire society and requiring restorative federal policies. The Smith-Sears Act for the vocational rehabilitation of disabled veterans passed in 1916 represents an essential change in the role of the federal government in that for the first time it assumed responsibility for the vocational training of the disabled.

In 1920, the first Vocational Rehabilitation Act was passed providing matched funds on a fifty-fifty basis to those states which established rehabilitation programs. During the Depression, however, progress and interest in rehabilitation almost stopped, for during those years employment for even the able-bodied was quite problematic.[38] Only World War II revived an interest in vocational rehabilitation. By the end of this war, pharmaceutical and surgical progress (especially orthopedic surgery and neurosurgery), as well as the development of physical and occupational therapy as effective restorative disciplines (a development which in turn led to the establishment of physical medicine as a new medical specialty), could successfully meet the challenge of many types of serious injuries. Anything but the full use of these everyday medical "miracles" for the physical and vocational restoration of the returned veterans would have been regarded as a great waste of human energy and potential. Similarly, the development of workmen's compensation laws slowed down in the 1920s. In 1930 three-fourths of the workers were covered, but it was not until 1948 that Mississippi, the last state, passed similar legislation.[39] However, even at present, it is estimated that no more than 80 percent of today's workers are covered.

Probably the most important feature of workmen's compensation is the new economic and legal principle on which it is based: *liability without fault*.[40] According to this doctrine, it does not matter who is at fault; the cost of industrial accidents must not be borne by those who can least afford them, the injured workers, but must be assumed instead by the employer, "who in running his enterprise can make provision for them and can also distribute them among the beneficiaries of the enterprise."[41] For the first time industrial accidents are considered to be inevitable hazards of modern industry and the costs involved in such accidents and compensation thereof a part of the legitimate cost of production.[42] Workmen's compensation, then, is a kind of insurance, and as such it aims to provide sure and prompt benefits (usually in the form of weekly payments) to replace at least a considerable part of the normal expected wages of injured workmen. This approach contributed greatly to the fact that for a long time cash indemnity had priority over medical care, which was considered only a supplementary benefit.[43]

Several social changes precipitated the passing of rehabilitation and other welfare laws in the 1940s, some of the most important being the gradual transformation of the nation from a predominantly rural to a predominantly urban society; industrialization, which brought about a higher standard of living; and a burgeoning economy incongruent with the abandonment of handicapped persons to a charity roll subsistence.[44] A concomitant social change was the alteration in family structure which accentuated even more the need of the handicapped for special services. The nuclear family replaced the traditional extended family, and the multiple functions of the latter were relegated to specialized social institutions. Thus, disabled family members were often confined to asylums, hospitals, or to custodial care so that life in the nuclear family would not be disrupted through day-to-day care of the physically disabled.[45]

Furthermore, in an era in which the prevailing social climate concerning welfare was such that the vocationally disabled would have to be provided for by society (that is, by the taxpayer) throughout life, the economic argument for expanding and strengthening vocational rehabilitation was quite persuasive, since it claimed a potentially considerable cut in required welfare money if only a small part of it was utilized for vocational rehabilitation.[46] From the time that vocational rehabilitation could be advanced and defended in Congress on an economic basis, a series of laws followed which gradually increased the amount of responsibility and financial aid extended by the federal government for different kinds of disabilities and segments of the population, but always with *vocational* rehabilitation as the basic aim. This legislation therefore covered only the disabled of working age and the potential working population. The exaggerated emphasis upon vocational rehabilitation has only recently been challenged, for it has been repeatedly argued that employable persons should not be the sole recipients of federal help for rehabilitation in a nation in which there is no longer a shortage of manpower and in which the level of the economy leaves ample margin for the rehabilitation of all disabled people.[47] Interestingly, when this point was presented in Congress, the soundness of a federal rehabilitation program covering all the disabled was again based mainly upon the freeing of the time of healthy, employable family members and upon the adverse, depressing psychological affect a dependent disabled person may have upon the healthy family members.[48]

In 1965 some very promising legislation was passed, according

22   DISABILITY AND REHABILITATION

to which vocational rehabilitation efforts were to be concentrated on severely handicapped persons (even when old or not employable) and evaluation services extended up to six months. The latter provision will favor the disabled who are often rejected from rehabilitation programs, since they will be able to benefit from at least some rehabilitation services during the evaluation period. Currently there is also a movement toward the definition of poverty and its correlates as a chronic disability, a change that would help reach the hard core of unrehabilitated people with both social and physical disabilities.[49]

Let us now take a brief look at the range of disability programs operating in the United States today other than workmen's compensation and vocational rehabilitation. Some of these programs are federal or state and compulsory; others are private and voluntary; some of them cover the general population, others are specific to some population(s); some provide mainly income in case of illness or accident, while others include or even require that the beneficiary undergo rehabilitation. The main programs are:[50]

1. *Social Security Administration Disability Insurance.* This program provides cash disability benefits regardless of age and includes dependents of beneficiaries. All claimants must be considered for vocational rehabilitation services and a trial work period of one year is permitted during which the benefits are continued. These two regulations are designed to encourage and promote the claimants' return to work.[51]

2. *Commercial Insurance Programs.* At the end of 1963 about 900 insurance companies offered policyholders a fixed sum of payments for anatomical loss and loss of time or wages from work incurred through accident or disease. Furthermore, in recent years several large insurance companies have included rehabilitation in the benefits offered. The Liberty Mutual Insurance Company of Boston has led this movement. In 1943, Liberty Mutual founded its own Rehabilitation Center in Boston and in 1951 established a second one in Chicago. These centers offer comprehensive services to policyholders and boast very high success statistics; namely, more than 85 percent of the admitted disabled adults benefit from the treatment and of these more than 80 percent return to full-time productive employment. Other companies such as Employers' Mutual of Wausau and the Nationwide Mutual Insurance Company of Columbus, Ohio, have in recent years incorporated rehabilitation into the benefits, the latter advancing payments for medicine and rehabilitation

to those seriously hurt by a policyholder (when the policyholder is fully responsible for the accident). And since the publicized statistics of these innovating companies show great savings, similar policies including rehabilitation may be increasingly adopted by all health and accident insurance companies.[52]

3. *The Veterans Administration.* This organization provides indemnity compensation and vocational rehabilitation for service-connected disabilities and life insurance with optional disability features.

4. *Civil Service Retirement.* This is a federal program (equivalent programs exist at the state and local civil service level) providing a retirement annuity for those employees who after at least five years of service are so disabled as not to perform satisfactorily at their usual job.[53]

5. *The Railroad Retirement Board.* This program offers two types of disability retirement benefits to disabled railroad workers depending upon the severity of the disablity and the length of service in the industry. A minimum of ten years' railroad service is necessary, however, in order to qualify for any type of disability benefit.

6. *Armed Forces Disability Retirement.* This provides a disability pension based either upon the extent of disability or length of service (whichever is more advantageous to the disabled person) to regular or reserve officers and enlisted men on active duty.

7. *Employer-Employee Union Health Plans.* These programs protect employees with temporary disability insurance in the event of wage loss and provide hospital, surgical and medical care for the employee and in some cases also for his dependents.

8. *State Temporary Disability Insurance.* Laws setting up this compulsory program have been enacted in Rhode Island, California, New Jersey, and New York. Under this program workers receive a "cash sickness compensation" when they cannot work because of nonoccupational illnesses or injuries; in California, they also receive limited hospital benefits.

9. *Welfare Programs.* These provide financial assistance and services to the permanently and totally disabled and the blind as well as rehabilitation services for some of the beneficiaries.

In all these programs, it is a physician who determines the presence and the extent of the disability, although the status of this physician may vary from staff doctor (as in the case of the Veterans Administration) to general practitioner or to consulting specialists whose opinion is asked in addition to the staff physicians' reports.

Probably the greatest difference among these programs is the manner in which they are adjudicated. Each public program has an administrative authority that makes policy and can rule on individual cases, but the claimant has the right to appeal to the courts after the administrative hearing.[54] The only exception to this is the Veterans Administration decisions, which cannot be reviewed by the court because they are considered to be gratuities. Private carriers, unlike public agencies, can settle or compromise a contested claim in case of "problem" claimants, a mechanism which permits them to deal efficiently and conveniently with troublesome cases.

Similar trends in legislation regarding rehabilitation seem to have evolved in recent decades in some eighteen countries studied by the United Nations.[55] While some countries like Germany had rehabilitation programs for special disability groups long before World War II, it was only after the war that all these countries enacted legislation which viewed rehabilitation as an integral process aiming at developing the physical, educational, social, psychological, and vocational potentialities of the disabled person. Although the range of categories of disabled entitled to rehabilitation services varies considerably and tends to be larger the higher the level of social and economic development in a country, the emphasis placed upon vocational rehabilitation seems to be universal. Not all countries restrict rehabilitation services to only those who have working potential, but rehabilitation efforts are concentrated mostly upon returning the disabled to gainful employment. And while some countries, like Switzerland, have done away with differentiation based upon the cause of the disability under the Federal Disability Insurance Act (passed January 1960), benefits are still provided only when the disability causes a diminution of the earning capacity (or of the capacity for work in the case of the housewives).[56]

Such an "economic" definition of disability presents definite shortcomings, although Switzerland's system is thought to be a step ahead of other European rehabilitation systems. There seems to be a universal consensus that a general governmental disability insurance program for all the disabled regardless of type or cause of disability (such as that in England and Switzerland) is a more advanced system of rehabilitation than segmentalized rehabilitation schemes such as that provided by workmen's compensation—provided, of course, that such a general disability insurance program is extended equally to all the disabled regardless of their work potential and "placeability."[57] Some writers indicate that this disproportionate preoccupation with the return of the disabled to gainful employment (often without great concern about the quality of the work or the level of pay) is an undesirable leftover from the puritanical Victorian era when only the "deserving" poor and disabled were helped—deserving meaning only those who were willing to accept any type of work, under any conditions, and at any level of pay.[58]

Poland has pioneered in the vocational rehabilitation of the disabled through the establishment of cooperatives managed and operated by the disabled for those so severely handicapped that they cannot work in the open competitive employment market. This solution seems to be much more satisfactory than compulsory systems (in terms of quota or of types of jobs reserved for the disabled) and may be especially promising for developing countries and the rural disabled. This solution also presents some interesting features because the disabled can work and act under a principle of self-determination without being socially segregated and isolated. Old people, widows of men who died in active service, and up to 25 percent of "healthy" individuals of any category and age group can also be members of the Invalids' Cooperatives, thus ensuring the social integration of the handicapped.[59]

In Finland, a country with an advanced social security system, rehabilitation (medical and vocational) is included as an integral part of many insurance and pension schemes and is also provided by the government to many categories of disabled. Thus, persons incurring automobile or work accidents or occupational diseases in need of rehabilitation services are eligible for such services under the auspices of the relevant plans. Under some plans, provisions are made for the rehabilitants to receive a reasonable income during rehabilitation and vocational training so that financial problems will not interfere with the successful outcome of rehabilitation. For example, those disabled at work receive, regardless of the actual degree of disability, 60 percent of their former earnings, if single, and 80-90 percent, if married. Recent recommendations of Finnish rehabilitation and insurance experts include the extension of free vocational rehabilitation services to all disabled regardless of age, degree of disability, and level of education, and of full insurance benefits throughout the entire rehabilitation program. Two distinctive features of the Finnish rehabilitation program are: (a) The direction and content of the recent rehabilitation movement (since 1938) has been predominantly influenced by the needs of the disabled rather than the projected plans and growth of social agencies; and (b) there has been a tendency to integrate the different facets of rehabilitation into existing social structures and institutions rather than proliferating the number of specialized agencies. For example, medical rehabilitation has often been relegated to hospitals, where such services can be offered at an early stage and become incorporated into the entire plan of medical treatment.[60]

In the 1960s an increased interest in rehabilitation, and especially in vocational rehabilitation of the disabled, marks several of the Western European countries and in particular those belonging to the European Common Market. Large-scale efforts are being made to assess the overall social problems created by disability, to find solutions, to suggest legislation and to evaluate existing programs. For example, in December 1967 there was a monumental report on the general condition of the handicapped in France by Bloch-Lainé, followed by seven other more specific reports dealing with the financial, administrative, statistical, employment, and social aspects of the disabled's problems.[61] These quite sophisticated reports pointing out the inadequacies of present legislation and operating societal mechanisms for the social reintegration of the physically and socially disabled and suggesting a variety of possible solutions will probably bring about a number of legislative and administrative reforms and innovations in France.

Another example is provided by a detailed study of the reemployment of old and handicapped workers in Germany, France, Belgium, and Holland undertaken in 1966 under the auspices of the European Coal and Steel Community. A wealth of data on societal mechanisms and on recent legislation passed in these countries that facilitates the reemployment primarily of handicapped workers are presented and evaluated. For example, legislation passed in 1963 in Germany and Belgium according to which employers could be paid a part of the disabled worker's salary (up to 50 percent) for a length of time ranging between 26 and 52 weeks did not prove to be successful. The reason given is that the actual job performance of the disabled worker acts as a much stronger incentive in the employer's decision to keep or fire him than financial incentives. The four countries also enacted legislation to provide financial remuneration for unemployed disabled workers who must move in order to find suitable employment or to finance public works for the employment of unskilled, old, and disabled workers who are not willing to move where jobs are available in order to improve these workers' chances of securing gainful employment. The study also indicates that protective quota legislations for the employment of the disabled has resulted more in the retainment of those workers already working for the company who become disabled rather than in the employment of new workers who are disabled.[62] Finally, the Danish Institute of Social Research conducted a major study of disability dealing with the statistical picture of disability: the employment, transportation, housing, and psychological problems of the disabled in Denmark.[63]

In most countries, the financing of rehabilitation programs is partially governmental and partially private and voluntary.[64] There is, however, a tendency for governments to assume increased financial responsibility. According to the U.N. survey previously cited, Poland and England represent the two countries with the greatest governmental financial responsibility for rehabilitation. In the U.S.S.R. and Yugoslavia, state agencies are responsible for rehabilitation programs; only in Argentina are rehabilitation services exclusively financed by voluntary nongovernmental organizations.

It is evident, therefore, that at present society responds to disability and its consequences with at least some kind of rehabilitation effort. Although there is considerable variation in the scope and nature of rehabilitation programs and their financing, by now most countries have some system to cover at least partially the medical care and financial needs of severely disabled persons and their families, at least for some categories of disabled (especially war veterans, industrial workers, the blind, and the deaf). The more developed the country and its welfare system, the more rehabilitation benefits are extended to more of the disabled and the greater the emphasis upon vocational rehabilitation. Developing countries with high rates of unemployment cannot ordinarily assimilate disabled workers except under federally subsidized workshops. And while through successful and appropriate vocational rehabilitation programs the disabled have been helped to become reintegrated (or integrated) into the occupational world, as we shall see in later chapters, such programs have not always been effective. Often those who are being helped are those who would find employment even without the aid of rehabilitation services because of the level of skills they possess. Or the disabled are helped to find routine and sometimes degrading jobs that diminish their morale instead of enhancing it. At other times the kinds of job opportunities open to the disabled are such (for example, sheltered workshops or industries for the disabled) that they further contribute to their social segregation and isolation.

But most countries have failed to include a comprehensive system of societal reintegration of the disabled in their rehabilitation programs. Some countries have started to acknowledge the existence of prohibiting architectural barriers which interfere with the disabled's societal integration, but very few are tackling the problem with effective solutions. Unfortunately, the easier solution sometimes appears to be construction of buildings accessible to the disabled but concentrated in one neighborhood—a form of ghetto. And even less has been done to break down the psychological barriers that prevent the societal integration of the disabled. It seems, then, that no society has been successful in organizing a rehabilitation system conducive to the effective societal integration of the disabled in all social spheres.

Rehabilitation Under Disability Programs in the United States and Canada

As we have already seen, there are several disability programs in the United States—federal, state, and private—which make some provision for rehabilitation services to be offered to beneficiaries. The extent of such services, the eligibility requirements, and the administrative machinery differ widely from program to program and under the same program from state to state. Because of the great variability of conditions under which rehabilitation is offered, it is quite possible that the rehabilitation process follows different paths and, consequently, the outcome varies considerably. Other benefits offered by the same or different programs, such as compensation or maintenance income, may be competing with or facilitating the rehabilitation of the beneficiaries. Administrative procedures may also facilitate or inhibit early and comprehensive rehabilitation. Variations are even greater if we compare the disability programs of different countries. We shall now see how the presence of benefits competitive to rehabilitation, the variety of bureaucratic regulations and procedures, and conflicting professional interests affect the disabled's chances for and the quality of rehabilitation under different programs.

There are a number of hypotheses about which conditions are conducive to the rehabilitation of the beneficiaries of disability programs and which ones inhibit adequate rehabilitation, but there have been no systematic comparative studies of rehabilitation under the different disability programs in the United States and abroad. Most of the available studies concentrate on the chances and the quality of rehabilitation under workmen's compensation programs in the United States, and only fragmentary comparative data exist concerning rehabilitation under other disability programs. We shall therefore first examine in detail rehabilitation under the workmen's compensation plan and then whatever other data are available about other programs. According to 1960 data, 23 state and federal laws include provisions for at least some aspects of rehabilitation, and four states (Ohio, Oregon, Rhode Island, and Washington) operate rehabilitation facilities as part of their workmen's compensation administration. But even today more than half the states make no provision in their compensation laws for rehabilitation.[65]

Besides the fact that rehabilitation provisions under workmen's compensation are neither universal nor uniform, they are all reported to fail to effectively rehabilitate the disabled workers covered. And the same degree of failure is reported when physical or vocational rehabilitation are used as criteria for the determination of successful rehabilitation. The criticisms voiced against workmen's compensation programs state specifically that not only are the disabled workers not encouraged to receive a high quality of medical care and rehabilitation, but that, in addition, the nature of the legislative basis of the program and most of its administrative procedures seriously interfere with and hinder rehabilitation. The following factors inhibiting rehabilitation are usually discussed in the literature:

1. Because the usual amount of income maintenance granted to

a worker during rehabilitation is inadequate to meet the needs of his family, he is often obliged to forego vocational rehabilitation altogether or to withdraw from rehabilitation before the program is completed. The normal temporary disability benefits from workmen's compensation are low, and either the worker is made ineligible for additional maintenance by the vocational rehabilitation service or his family needs are such that the maximum $100 a month allowed by the vocational rehabilitation service is grossly inadequate.[66] In some cases, when injured workers find that they cannot live on the weekly payments or when such payments (or payments for medical care) are not regularly forthcoming or are cut off by the insurance company in order to force them to go back to work, the serious lack of funds pressures them into accepting a lump sum settlement. This money, usually a small sum, is generally used to pay accumulated debts and to meet living expenses rather than to support the injured worker's physical or vocational rehabilitation.[67] Other alternatives open to the disabled worker are to accept welfare in order to be able to continue with the rehabilitation or to get a job (any job, even if it pays very little or is unsuited to his physical condition), thus increasing the probability of his suffering additional injury, aggravating his condition, or getting fired. Since the last choice means that both rehabilitation and compensation have been seriously compromised, this solution is not very popular, especially among semi- and unskilled workers. Thus, when rehabilitation is foregone, all efforts tend to concentrate on compensation rather than return to gainful employment—at least until the case is settled.

2. Workmen's compensation awards are made not on the basis of physical injury, but on the basis of the disability produced by an injury at work. The fact that it is the disability rather than the injury that is compensable does not motivate the worker to recover from his injury as fully as possible and as soon as possible. On the contrary, it often makes him attempt to accentuate his disability in order to obtain a larger compensation for his injury. On this basis, rehabilitation becomes a threat to potential compensation, while conservation of the disability (at least until the compensation case is heard and adjudicated) constitutes a promise to recover for the injury what "is due to them." As Larson has specified, there are two ingredients in the legal definition of disability: One is the medical aspect of

disability, and the second is a de facto inability to earn wages. While the first aspect of the legal definition often deters injured workers from receiving adequate medical care and physical rehabilitation, the second element usually contributes to their unwillingness to undergo vocational rehabilitation or to return to gainful employment before their case is closed.[68]

The unwillingness to work despite opportunity or ability is reinforced by the worker's not always unfounded fear that he might soon be dismissed because of true or alleged disability-connected absenteeism or low level of performance or that he might suffer another injury. Faced with the difficulties and uncertainties involved in finding and holding a job when disabled and with a legal definition of disability that will deprive them of any recovery for their injury, some injured workers have almost no motivation to work. Highly skilled persons, whether white collar or blue collar workers, however, who usually have much more to gain from working than from being idle, seldom become involved in litigation and usually successfully complete vocational rehabilitation programs whenever they need such services. The only exceptions are some older skilled workers who see the possibility of a lump sum settlement for their disability claim as an opportunity to realize their lifelong dream of establishing a small shop of their own.[69] But a considerable number of compensation claimants are older semi- or unskilled workers with low work morale, poor identification with their job, and frequently rather serious occupational maladjustments.[70] These workers when disabled may be tempted to grasp at the social semilegitimation offered by disability to withdraw from the unsuccessful performance of the working role and live on the low but steady compensation check, a sum of money not much lower than their usual seasonal wages or low average wages due to frequent periods of unemployment.[71]

Because of their social characteristics (age, race, level of education), this category of disabled people realistically have very little chance to be reemployed even after they have been more or less physically rehabilitated; and if they are able to find a job, it will usually be even more marginal in terms of financial reward, security, and interest than the jobs available to them before the disability. On the other hand, vocational training that could hold out a promise of upgrading their skills and making them more employable, as we shall see later in this book, is frequently not available to them; and when it is, the rate of success is low because it usually has all the shortcomings of formal education. But, in general, rehabilitation services are most often denied this group of disabled, who are usually labeled "unmotivated," "uncooperative," and "interested only in compensation."[72] Therefore, it seems that the workmen's compensation program particularly fails to rehabilitate the great bulk of semi- and unskilled workers for whom the compensation payments understandably represent a solution preferable to complete physical recovery and a return to work.

3. The legal or semilegal procedures involved in workmen's compensation that emphasize cash benefits seriously obstruct effective medical care and consequently the successful rehabilitation of injured workers. Regardless of how the consulting physicians are chosen (whether by the employer or the employee), they often do not offer objective medical opinions and disability evaluations because they may become involved in nonmedical issues and take sides with the employer or the employee. Accordingly, they tend to either minimize or maximize the existing degree of disability. This is especially true because, whether the physicians were hired by the employer or by the employee (who is often guided by his lawyer), the selection is often made not so much on the basis of medical competence but rather on the basis of the physician's willingness to "cooperate" and testify adeptly in court.[73]

What is probably more crucial for his long-term rehabilitation is the fact that many times the injured worker does not receive adequate or effective medical care.[74] Some physicians refuse to treat compensation patients altogether, and some surgeons are reluctant or refuse to operate on injured workers before their cases are settled and closed.[75] This reluctance has often been attributed to the fact that compensation patients usually delay seeking treatment for a considerable time and do not respond as satisfactorily to surgical intervention as do private patients.[76] But there is some evidence that the payment of medical bills plays also a crucial role. For example, a California survey of doctors showed that more than one-third of the doctors rarely or never accept compensation cases mainly because the fees are inadequate, there is too much paper work required, or they prefer to treat private patients only.[77] But the doctors who treated compensation cases mentioned as problems (in order of importance): inadequacy of fees, choice of physicians (should be free), forms and amount of paper work, annoyances caused by the insurance carrier or the employer and the "system," and abuses by other physicians. These trends were not equally distributed among all medical specialties. Psychiatrists more than any other specialty predominantly reported that they never treat compensation cases, and all types of surgeons (regardless of the degree to which they treat compensation cases) complained about the inadequacy of fees, followed by opthalmologists, internists, and heart specialists.

Another study of contested cases in New York has thrown some light on the quality of medical care received by all controverted cases but especially those who are finally judged to be incompensable. In controverted cases, a claimant has no right to receive medical care until the question of liability has been settled; he must pay for whatever care he receives unless the employer or carrier is willing to assume costs "without prejudice." Therefore, in these cases physicians as well as claimants are usually reluctant to go beyond conservative treatment (only in one-third of the cases was some type of surgery reported) and very rarely is rehabilitation undertaken.[78]

The emphasis on a financial settlement has another negative influence upon the worker's chances for good medical care and successful rehabilitation because of the hiring of a lawyer who has a vested interest not only in winning the case but also in settling for a large sum of money. He is therefore mostly interested in lump sum settlements and in preserving and accentuating his client's degree of disability. He usually advises the worker which physician to consult (if the choice is up to the employee), and he advises him against rehabilitation and return to gainful employment. The lawyer, then, sometimes becomes the person the worker feels he can trust most since he is unquestionably "on his side" and can even be depended on for some financial aid; in some cases, he may represent the most powerful obstacle to rehabilitation. This especially applies in the case of older, unskilled workers who have little to lose by never returning to work. (See Chapter 7 for a detailed discussion of the role of the lawyer.)

4. The provision of the compensation law permitting the employer to reopen a previously closed case for reevaluation and re-

rating because the disabled person seems to have improved makes the worker even more suspicious of rehabilitation and its aims, since he is most often referred to a rehabilitation facility by the workmen's compensation commission. If he is legally obliged to accept rehabilitation, he will go along but may remain uncooperative until he is discharged if he is afraid that his physical improvement will jeopardize his compensation in any way. It is, of course, quite possible that some disabled manage to improve their physical status during rehabilitation but systematically refuse to admit any such improvement and keep on complaining of symptoms and pains.[79]

5. A variety of administrative, legislative, and informal mechanisms are often responsible, directly or indirectly, for a significant delay in the worker's being referred to and receiving rehabilitation services. For example, very few controverted cases are referred for rehabilitation, and some rehabilitation centers refuse services to those primarily preoccupied with compensation until their case is closed.[80] Also, in some cases the insurance carriers do not want the claimant to be contacted by the vocational rehabilitation agency because they are afraid the claimant may be informed and initiate action against the carrier.[81] Early referral for rehabilitation is neither guaranteed nor facilitated by workmen's compensation programs, and since medical care is not supervised by the programs, the disabled worker may in some cases be doomed to stay disabled regardless of how motivated he is to overcome his disability.[82]

Now that we have examined the criticisms voiced against the American workmen's compensation programs, let us see how other programs fare in terms of the extent to which rehabilitation is facilitated or inhibited. The most applauded foreign workmen's compensation program is that of Ontario, Canada, mainly because it is reported to be the most conducive to rehabilitation. The main reason for this seems to be the fact that the amount of compensation is determined by the degree of physical injury and permanent physical disability regardless of future earnings. Thus, workers are more willing to be rehabilitated and return to work since the amount of pension to be received will not be influenced by either activity. However, the Ontario program has a number of other distinctive administrative differences: the workmen's compensation agency administers an exclusive state fund, supervises all medical care, and provides vocational rehabilitation and placement services to the covered workers. In addition, the adjudication of compensation claims is in the hands of the Workmen's Compensation Board and not the law courts, and appeals can be made only to an organization within the board.[83]

No systematic studies exist about the rehabilitation success (physical and vocational) of the disabled workers covered, nor are there controlled, comparative studies of rehabilitation success under the Ontario and other programs differing in some criteria. It is therefore difficult to state with certainty that the Ontario workmen's compensation program is the best. Even if rehabilitation success among the same populations of disabled workers would prove to be higher in Ontario than in any American state, we would still need carefully planned, controlled comparative studies to help us understand which particular feature of the Ontario legislation is conducive to which aspect of rehabilitation and for which populations of disabled workers.[84]

A European study evaluating the effects of compensation legislation on the vocational rehabilitation of the disabled throws some light on the relationship between the legal basis for a disability pension and the disabled worker's chances to return to work. In those countries in which the disabled do not lose their compensation payments for work-connected disabilities when employed, the slightly and moderately disabled are quite motivated to work, since they can then enjoy both a low compensation check and a high salary level. In the case of non-work-connected disability, when (as in France and Belgium) the social security invalidity pension cannot be combined with a salary, it becomes a real obstacle to the reemployment of seriously disabled workers.[85]

The sporadic data that exist comparing the response of compensation cases to medical care and rehabilitation with that of private cases are by no means conclusive or "solid." One of the reasons for the questionable quality of the findings is the fact that other factors, such as occupation, education, social class, and age, were not taken into consideration during the analysis. One study, for example, reports that compensation patients with low back injuries do not respond as satisfactorily to surgery as private patients do, and another reports that fewer compensation than private patients with low back pain were rated as improved at the time of discharge.[86] The patients,

however, were considered unimproved if they still complained of
pain and did not return to work—regardless of their degree of physical improvement. In terms of our discussion concerning compensation legislation, we can assume that if objective physical improvement was used as the criterion in these studies and the quality of medical care was the same, most probably there would be no significant
difference between the two groups of patients. The only real difference may have been the fact that the compensation patients did not
want to admit any improvement and go back to work because they
did not wish to affect the amount of compensation they would receive. Furthermore, the social class composition of private patients
is probably very different from that of the compensation patients, and
social class differentials may well account for differentials in the
quality of the medical care received as well as in the response to medical care and rehabilitation.

Because of the severe disability of the people covered by the
Old Age, Survivors, and Disability Insurance (OASDI) program,
only 1 percent qualify for vocational rehabilitation services and even
these cases are mostly concentrated in the group below fifty years
of age. There are no data concerning rehabilitation success and no
studies evaluating the degree of vocational rehabilitation achieved
after the 1960 legislation permitting the continuation of benefits during a trial work year. Such legislation is assumed to encourage a
return to work because the disabled are then not afraid to try to
work, since they know they will not lose their pension if they do not
hold their jobs.[87] We cannot be sure of the value of such legislation,
however, until controlled comparative studies are carried out.

A variety of other programs provide rehabilitation services; for
example, the Liberty Mutual Insurance Company, some unions (the
Amalgamated Clothing Workers of America), veterans' programs,
state vocational rehabilitation programs, and so forth. Again, no
definite conclusions can be drawn about the quality of rehabilitation
offered under different disability programs since there are no systematic and controlled comparative studies of outcome that could
indicate the legislation, the types of provisions, and the administrative
structures most conducive for rehabilitation success, both physical
and vocational.

Adequacy of Existing Rehabilitation Programs

Regardless of the quality and effectiveness of the rehabilitation services offered under the different disability programs, a different kind of question must be raised: How adequate are the present available rehabilitation facilities in terms of the present and predicted number of disabled? And if these facilities do not suffice for all the disabled, who are left out?

Let us first examine the current disability picture in the United States. The simple question, however, of how many disabled there are cannot be answered easily or accurately. The answer varies considerably from study to study and depends upon the definitions and the methodology used, the former often influenced by the value orientation of the investigator. Usually the performance of the major role of the individual (according to age and sex) is considered the crucial arca of concern. So the U.S. National Health Interview Survey (July 1, 1957–June 30, 1961) shows that 2.2 percent (or 3,776,000 persons) of the civilian population (exclusive of persons residing in institutions) are unable to carry on their major activity, and 5.5 percent (or 9,574,000 persons) are limited in amount or kind of major activity.[88] More specifically, 7.3 percent of all persons 17 and over are limited in their ability to work.[89] If limitations in other activities such as participation in social, civic, recreational, or sport activities are to be included, then 10.4 percent of the population is in some way disabled. The proportion of chronic disability increases with age and becomes considerable after age 45; 13.6 percent of those at ages 45–54, 22.6 percent of those at 55–64, and 37.2 of those over 65 have a chronic limitation.[90] However, a 1966 Social Security survey of disabled adults has shown that disability is much more prevalent than the quoted statistics indicate.[91] According to those figures, 17.2 percent of the noninstitutionalized population 18–64 years old (or 17.8 million persons) were found to have been disabled longer than 6 months. Of these disabled, 6 million (or 4.7 percent of the male population and 7 percent of the female population) were severely disabled in that they could not work altogether or work regularly; 5 million (or 4.9 and 4.8 percent of the male and female population, respectively) had to work part-time or to change the type

of work, and the remaining 6.6 million (or 7.6 and 5.4 of the male
and female population, respectively) had limitations on the kind or
amount of work they could perform. The extent of disability varies,
of course, with age, sex, and race. Thus only 9.9 percent of white
men are disabled between the ages of 18–44, compared with 34.6
percent between ages 55–64. The figures for nonwhite men in the
same age groups are 11.9 and 51.0 percent, respectively.

These survey statistics do not cover the prevalence of "sociopsychological" chronic limitation which may result from a disability
or the so-called psychic losses, such as feelings of inadequacy, in-
security, inferiority, and rejection. The presence of such a limitation
would not be reflected in the statistics quoted because it may not
limit the disabled person's ability to perform activities, even though it
affects his emotional well-being and the nature of his interpersonal
relations and interferes with the successful performance of such
familial roles as father, mother, husband, wife. The degree of chronic
limitation the presence of a disability may represent for the happy
and well-integrated family life of the disabled person as well as for
the nondisabled family members is completely ignored. These sur-
veys suffer from two further limitations resulting from the omission
of (a) those who adjust to their chronic condition by accepting a
less productive employment or by changing their major activity to
housekeeping (in the case of previously working wives); and (b)
the omission of mental retardation and alcoholism from the checklist
of chronic conditions.[92]

Furthermore, the same factors that are responsible for the rise
in numbers of disabled people in the last few decades will most probably be operating in the future. These are:

1. Medical, surgical, and pharmaceutical progress which has
helped control most acute illnesses and infections and has permitted
the maintenance of the chronically ill and the survival of the seriously
ill or injured who usually died in earlier times. The statistics on death
rates from specific diseases show that there has been a dramatic
decline in deaths from infectious diseases (typhoid fever, dysentery,
tuberculosis, syphilis, etc.). In contrast, little progress has been made
in the control of chronic diseases, as evidenced in the death rates
from cancer, diabetes, heart disease, and ulcers, which are quite high
and have increased considerably since 1900.[93] The treatment of

chronic diseases (even when nonfatal) is far below a satisfactory level, expensive, and with an uncertain prognosis. No effective prevention or early diagnosis is usually possible. However, some types of infirmities are better controlled at present so that the afflicted individuals are maintained in life and can function at least in some social roles. For example, while of 400 American paraplegic veterans of World War I only 2 were alive twenty years later (the others having died from decubitus ulcer or other complications), more than 80 percent of the 2,500 paraplegic veterans of World War II were alive and working or attending school in 1958.[94] The fact, however, that fewer tuberculars and paraplegics die now means that many more must learn to live and to work with a more or less arrested pathological condition which imposes some definite chronic restrictions on their activities.

2. The extended and ever-increasing use of the automobile, which is still the most dangerous and crippling means of transportation, as evidenced by the ever-increasing number of accidents. From 1962 to 1967 the number of drivers rose from 90.5 to 102 million, and 126 million drivers are forecast by 1975.[95] But what is even more crucial is the rising number of crippling but nonfatal automobile accidents; thanks to surgical progress, more of such victims survive but with a chronic disability. While recent studies indicate that the use of the safety belt decreases to a considerable extent the number of fatalities in automobile accidents, they do not report estimates of the degree of disability that is incurred by the surviving drivers and passengers.[96] It may be that further safety measures will help reduce fatalities but multiply disabling injuries.

3. The life expectancy of most people around the world (especially the Western world) has been constantly increasing in our century, a trend that leads to an ever-larger number of surviving older people (65 and over) who are much more susceptible to chronic diseases.[97] Thus, while one-sixth of the population under age 15 in the United States and two-fifths of the people 15–44 years of age suffer from one or more chronic conditions, the proportion increases to three-fifths at ages 45–64 and to slightly over the three-fourths at ages 65 and over.[98] Similarly, the degree of limitation in major activity rises rapidly with age; while one-fourth of the men and one-fifth of the women with a chronic condition are thus limited at ages 45–64,

nearly three-fifths and two-fifths, respectively, are similarly limited at ages 65 and over. These facts, in combination with the tremendously rapid increase of elders in comparison to the rest of the population, seriously multiply the problem of chronic disabilities.[99] Furthermore, it is known that acute conditions cause a greater amount of individual disabilities at ages 65 and over than in any other age group and probably also aggravate existing chronic conditions.[100]

In conclusion, it seems that medical and public health progress have not diminished in any way the spread of chronic diseases; on the contrary, they have contributed to their accentuation by helping people live longer. Medical, surgical, and pharmaceutical progress have also contributed to the increase in chronic disabilities by saving the lives of the seriously ill or injured. This apparent paradox is due to the fact that medical and public health efforts have failed to prevent or cure chronic diseases and most other disabling conditions.

Some writers, such as Conley, find that all of the conditions discussed above do not necessarily lead to a continuous rise in the prevalence of chronic conditions. His argument is based on a U.S. Department of Commerce forecast that there will be a slight decline in the percentage of population 45 and over and on the fact that since many diseases causing disabilities have already been eliminated, in the future the disabling effects of chronic conditions might also be eliminated through prevention or cure.[101] It is possible that the prevalence of disabling chronic conditions may not continue to multiply rapidly in the future, but the prospects are not good. Despite the fact that epidemiological studies indicate what social and sociopsychological factors are associated with the occurrence of chronic conditions, it is quite problematic—and often impossible—for public health or any other agency to influence these in any concerted, coordinated way. Such changes require a good understanding of human values and of the techniques effective in altering them.[102]

This is the disability picture in the United States; now let us see how well quantitatively rehabilitation has met the social problems created by disability. Recent figures indicate that the impact of rehabilitation programs is too small and too selective. In 1966, it is reported that 200,000 disabled were rehabilitated under formal vocational rehabilitation services.[103] This number of rehabilitated persons represents slightly more than 1 percent of the total disabled and less than the annually added number of disabled. Of course, an additional number of disabled (the number of which is not known) are being rehabilitated through other rehabilitation agencies, but most probably their total number is much smaller than 200,000. Outside the 90 state vocational rehabilitation agencies, some one-disability facilities, and some well-known hospital insurance, union- or company-operated rehabilitation facilities, it is difficult to assess whether or not some so-called rehabilitation units of hospitals, companies, and agencies can be truly classified as such.[104] Sometimes the rehabilitation services offered in the latter settings are so elementary and inadequate that the label "rehabilitation unit" is a misnomer.

Statistics available for 1965 also indicate that about 10 percent of the cases served by federal vocational rehabilitation programs were closed before or after a rehabilitation plan was initiated.[105] And a national study of state vocational rehabilitation agencies has shown that those who are not accepted for services need these services equally with or even more than those accepted and are predominantly old (over 50), severely disabled, or judged to be "inadequately motivated."[106] This latter category, as we shall see in the following chapters in greater detail, consists mainly of disabled persons of low socioeconomic status with a low level of educational achievement and occupational skills.[107] Thus, despite the recent proliferation of rehabilitation facilities, very few of the disabled have been helped. There is some evidence that available rehabilitation facilities are not always used to capacity and that many disabled are never told by their private physicians about the different types of rehabilitation services partially because many of the physicians are not themselves aware of the possibilities.[108]

Furthermore, those who are not accepted for rehabilitation (despite their needing such services) or those whose status remains unimproved by rehabilitation services are not always financially helped through some kind of assistance program. Actually, more than half the severely disabled received no income from public income-maintenance programs during 1965 or any other kind of disability-related benefit; and three-fourths of them were women.[109] Thus, three-fifths of the severely disabled women but only two-fifths of the severely disabled men do not receive any type of public assistance. Most of these women are married; one-fourth of them, however, are single, divorced, or widowed, so it may be misleading to always assume that there is a man who can support the disabled woman.[110]

On the basis of the available statistics, we could conclude that American society has a long way to go before it can meet in a systematic and comprehensive manner the social problems created by disability. At present neither rehabilitation services nor public assistance programs reach all those who need physical and/or vocational rehabilitation or income assistance because of incurred disability. And whatever short-range predictions have been made about future medical or population trends do not suggest that the causes of disability will be soon eradicated or that fewer people will be needing rehabilitation services or income assistance.

After having examined the types of societal response to the social problem of disability not only in the United States but also historically and cross-culturally, we turn now to the study of the actual experiences of the disabled. Throughout the following chapters we shall look at different aspects of their lives and experiences at different stages of their disability career. Because there are no data from other countries about all topics treated in this book, in some cases we shall base our discussion only upon American studies. Data from other countries will be incorporated in the discussion of several topics on which studies conducted in Canada, Australia, and Europe are available.

NOTES

1. Much of the material throughout this section of the chapter is based on two previously published articles: Constantina Safilios-Rothschild, "Social Prejudice Against the Sick and the Disabled," in *Industrial Society and Rehabilitation—Problems and Solutions, Proceedings of the Tenth World Congress, International Society for Rehabilitation of the Disabled* (Heidelberg, 1967), pp. 33–34; and Constantina Safilios-Rothschild, "Prejudice Against the Disabled and Some Means to Combat It," *International Rehabilitation Review*, 19, 4 (October 1968), 8–10, 24. Unless there is a specific reason to

refer the reader to the original article, there will be no indication each time a sentence or paragraph is quoted.

2. For an excellent discussion of the confinement houses in
Europe, of the mentality that led to them, and of the beliefs
concerning mental illness, see Michel Foucault, *Madness and
Civilization* (New York: Pantheon, 1965).

3. Henry E. Sigerist, *Civilization and Disease* (Ithaca, N.Y.:
Cornell University Press, 1945), pp. 68–70.

4. *Ibid.*; see also Robert Strauss, "Social Change and the Rehabilitation Concept," in Marvin B. Sussman (ed.), *Sociology
and Rehabilitation* (Washington, D.C.: American Sociological
Association, 1966), p. 3.

5. Sigerist, *op. cit.*, pp. 68–70.

6. Talcott Parsons, *The Social System* (New York: Free Press,
1951), pp. 428–33.

7. Beatrice A. Wright, "Spread in Adjustment to Disability,"
Bulletin of the Menninger Clinic, 28 (July 1964), 198–208.

8. Constantina Safilios-Rothschild, "Deviance and Mental Illness
in the Greek Family," *Family Process*, 7, 1 (March 1968),
100–17; G. Alivisatos and G. Lyketsos, "A Preliminary Report of Research Concerning the Attitudes of the Families of
Hospitalized Mental Patients," *International Journal of Social
Psychiatry*, 10, 1 (1964); and John Cumming and Elaine
Cumming, *Closed Ranks* (Cambridge, Mass: Harvard University Press, 1957).

9. Strauss, *op. cit.*, pp. 3, 7.

10. For an interesting and detailed discussion on the historical
trends and the actual status of the blind in society as well as
the societal responses to their problems, see Jacobus tenBroek
and Floyd W. Matson, *Hope Deferred: Public Welfare and
the Blind* (Berkeley and Los Angeles: University of California
Press, 1959).

11. "Relations with Employers, Job Induction and Follow-up,"
in *Manual on Selective Placement of the Disabled* (Geneva:
International Labour Office, October 1965), chap. IX.

12. David S. Abbey, "Attitude Formation and Change" (paper
presented at the CARC Tenth Annual Conference on Mental
Retardation, Quebec, September 19–22, 1967).

13. Jerome Siller and Abram Chipman, "Perceptions of Physical
Disability by the Non-disabled" (paper presented at the
American Psychological Association Meetings, Los Angeles,
September 1964).

14. Fred Davis, "Deviance Disavowal: The Management of
Strained Interaction by the Visibly Handicapped," *Social
Problems*, 9, 2 (Fall 1961), 120–32; Robert Kleck, "Emotional
Arousal in Interactions with Stigmatized Persons," *Psycholog-*

ical Reports, 19 (1966), 1226; Robert Kleck, Hiroshi Ono, and Arbert H. Hastorf, "The Effects of Physical Deviance and Face-to-Face Interaction," *Human Relations*, 19, 4 (1966), 425–36; also Erving Goffman, *Stigma: Notes on the Management of Spoiled Identity* (Englewood Cliffs, N.J.: Prentice-Hall, 1963); and J. Edwin Thomas, "Problems of Disability From the Perspective of Role Theory," *Journal of Health and Human Behavior*, 7, 1 (Spring 1966), 2–14.

15. See the original article, Safilios-Rothschild, "Prejudice Against the Disabled and Some Means to Combat It," *op. cit.*, pp. 10, 24.

16. Whenever the voice of the disabled has been heard, it has demanded that they be integrated into normal society. A good example is the collection of autobiographical notes in Paul Hunt (ed.), *Stigma: The Experience of Disability* (London: Chapman, 1966).

17. "Current Trends in National Rehabilitation Legislation, A Summary of a United Nations Survey," *International Rehabilitation Review*, 18, 4 (October 1967), 9–10.

18. For some reason, seamen but not soldiers were in most countries one of the earliest or the earliest working groups to be covered by some form of rehabilitation legislation or by workmen's compensation. (It may be that a deep-seated fear of the sea and its hazards had a greater emotional appeal to legislators.)

19. Neil J. Smelser, *Social Change in the Industrial Revolution* (Chicago: The University of Chicago Press, 1959), pp. 274–81.

20. Smelser's entire book (see Note 19) is a theoretically exciting analysis of the social changes which took place before and after the advent of the Industrial Revolution in England. The discussion of these issues here is based on his book.

21. George Rosen, "The Evolution of Social Medicine," in Howard E. Freeman, Sol Levine, and Leo G. Reeder (eds.), *Handbook of Medical Sociology* (Englewood Cliffs, N.J.: Prentice-Hall, 1963), pp. 20–21.

22. Strauss, *op. cit.*, pp. 7–8.

23. Boaz Siegel, "History of the Enactment of the Workmen's Compensation Law in the State of Michigan" (unpublished master's thesis, Wayne State University, 1940), pp. 1–4; also Frank Lang, *Workmen's Compensation Insurance* (Homewood, Ill.: Irwin, 1947), pp. 4–6.

24. Crystal Eastman, in Paul U. Kellogg (ed.), *Work Accidents and the Law—The Pittsburgh Survey* (New York: Charities Publication Committee, 1910), p. 170.

25. Siegel, *op. cit.*, pp. 3–9. Siegel's entire thesis is a fair historical

discussion of legislation related to workmen's compensation and its shortcomings, as well as of the social conditions out of which different legislation arose. See also Lang, *op. cit.*, pp. 5–6. A much more sophisticated discussion from a legal and a sociological point of view is provided by Lawrence M. Friedman and Jack Ladinsky, "Social Change and the Law of Industrial Accidents," *Columbia Law Review*, 67, 1 (January 1967), 50–82.

26. Siegel, *op. cit.*, p. 12.
27. *Ibid.*, pp. 21, 25–26.
28. Magaret S. Gordon, "Industrial Injuries Insurance in Europe and the British Commonwealth Before World War II," in Earl F. Cheit and Margaret S. Gordon (eds.), *Occupational Disability and Public Policy* (New York: Wiley, 1963). Gordon's entire chapter (pp. 191–220), as well as the following chapter on "Industrial Injuries Insurance in Europe and the British Commonwealth Since World War II" (pp. 221–53), are good sources of information about the history of European legislation on workmen's compensation.
29. Strauss, *op. cit.*, pp. 8–11.
30. Henry H. Kessler, *Low Back Pain in Industry* (New York: Commerce and Industry Association, 1953), p. 13; and Siegel, *op. cit.*, p. 31.
31. Herman Miles Somers and Anne Ramsay Somers, *Workmen's Compensation* (New York: Wiley, 1954), p. 8.
32. Siegel, *op. cit.*, pp. 29–31.
33. *Ibid.*, p. 32.
34. Strauss, *op. cit.*, p. 8.
35. Lang, *op. cit.*, pp. 7–8.
36. Arthur Larson, "Compensation Reform in the United States," in Cheit and Gordon, *op. cit.*, p. 11.
37. Strauss, *op. cit.*, pp. 14–15.
38. Ronald W. Conley, *The Economics of Vocational Rehabilitation* (Baltimore, Md.: Johns Hopkins Press, 1967), p. 40.
39. Larson, *op. cit.*, p. 11.
40. Somers and Somers, *op. cit.*, p. 26.
41. Monroe Berkowitz, *Workmen's Compensation: The New Jersey Experience* (New Brunswick, N.J.: Rutgers University Press, 1960), pp. 5–6.
42. Somers and Somers, *op. cit.*, pp. 26–27.
43. Constantina Safilios-Rothschild, "The Reactions to Disability in Rehabilitation" (unpublished Ph.D. dissertation, Ohio State University, 1963), Kessler, *op. cit.*, pp. 13–14.
44. W. Scott Allen, *Rehabilitation: A Community Challenge* (New York: Wiley, 1958), p. 4.
45. Talcott Parsons and Renee Fox, "Illness, Therapy, and the

46 DISABILITY AND REHABILITATION

Modern Urban American Family," in E. Gartly Jaco (ed.), *Patients, Physicians and Illness* (New York: Free Press, 1958). Absence of a core family member because of hospitalization will also be disrupting, but probably less so than having to care for him (her) at home; also through removal from familial well-being and dependency, motivation for a speedy recovery will tend to be greater; and finally, it is assumed that the quality of care received will be more effective, systematic, and consistent.

46. Strauss, *op. cit.*, p. 20.
47. There is, of course, a shortage of manpower in several skilled, professional, and semiprofessional occupations, but most of these jobs could not be filled by the usual clientele of rehabilitation services because the level of training required would not ordinarily be obtainable by this population for a variety of reasons (see Chapter 5).
48. "Special Education and Rehabilitation," *Hearings Before the Sub-committee on Education of the Committee on Education and Labor,* U.S. House of Representatives, 87th Congress, 1st Session, August 1961, p. 97.
49. Julius S. Cohen, Robert J. Gregory, and John W. Pelosi, *Vocational Rehabilitation and the Socially Disabled* (Syracuse, N.Y.: Syracuse University Press, 1966), pp. 7–8, 29–31.
50. For a detailed description of the disability programs in the United States, see Leo Price, "Disability Programs in the United States," *Journal of Occupational Medicine,* 7 (July 1965), 341–47. Most of the basic description has been taken from this article.
51. Bernard Popick, "The Social Security Disability Program," *Post Graduate Medicine,* 40, 2 (August 1966), A89–A92.
52. Arne Fougner, "For Auto Accident Victims—A New Kind of Insurance," *The Reader's Digest,* May 1961; *Rehabilitation Center Program,* a leaflet of the Liberty Mutual Insurance Company, Boston.
53. Price, *op. cit.*, pp. 341–47.
54. Leo Price, "Scope and Size of Some Disability Programs," *Journal of Occupational Medicine,* 7 (July 1965), 286–90.
55. United Nations, Department of Economic and Social Affairs, *Study on Legislative and Administrative Aspects of Rehabilitation of the Disabled in Selected Countries* (New York: United Nations, 1964), pp. 159–60. Most of the discussion about legislation and the administration of rehabilitation programs in other countries has come from this publication.
56. Albert Granacher, *Rehabilitation in Switzerland* (Berne: Federal Office for Social Insurance, 1961).
57. Friedman and Ladinsky, *op. cit.*, pp. 79-81.

58. TenBroek and Matson, *op. cit.*, pp. 261–63. They are saying that the present-day sheltered workshops may be the equivalents of the seventeenth- and eighteenth-century workhouses for the poor.

59. Tomasz Lidke, "Rehabilitation of the Disabled in Poland"; Aleksander Futro and Kazimierz Rysiewicz, "The Role and Tasks of Cooperatives for the Disabled in Poland"; Miroslav Gersdorf, "Legal and Organizational Aspects of Cooperatives for the Disabled in Poland"; and "Final Conclusions," in *Report to Participating Governments on the I.L.O. Interregional Seminar on Vocational Rehabilitation* (held in Warsaw, May 16–June 4, 1966; Geneva: International Labour Office, 1966), pp. 7–19, 110–20, 121–30, 214. See also Aleksander Futro, *Invalids' Cooperatives in Poland* (Warsaw: Publishing House of the Central Agricultural Union of Cooperatives, 1964).

60. Aulikki Kananoja, *Rehabilitation in Finland* (Helsinki: The Finnish Committee of the International Society for Rehabilitation of the Disabled, 1966), pp. 8–23; Viekko Niemi, "Rehabilitation as a Form of Workmen's Compensation," *Insurance in Finland*, 1 (1964), 12; and Viekko Niemi, "A Plan for the Development and Reorganization of Rehabilitation in Finland," *Rehabilitation in Finland, op cit.*, pp. 24–25.

61. M. François Bloch-Lainé, *Etude du problème général de l'inadaptation des personnes handicapées* (report presented to the Prime Minister, Paris, December 1967).

62. *Problèmes du reemploi des travailleurs agés ou handicapes* (Luxemburg: Communauté Européenne du Charbon et de l'Acier, December 1966), pp. 44–48, 93–105.

63. Bent Rold Andersen, *Fysik Handicappede I Danmark* (Copenhagen: Teknisk Forlag, 1964), vols. I–V.

64. *Study on Legislative and Administrative Aspects of Rehabilitation of the Disabled in Selected Countries, op. cit.*

65. U.S. Department of Labor, Division of Labor Standards, *State Workmen's Compensation Laws: A Comparison of Major Provisions With Recommended Standards*, Bulletin 212, revised (Washington, D.C., December 1961), pp. 11–12. According to another source, 25 states, the federal laws, and all Canadian provinces have specific rehabilitation provisions. In addition to these, all states have accepted the provisions of the Federal Rehabilitation Act, which provides federal funds for retaining disabled workers. See *Analysis of Workmen's Compensation Law* (Washington, D.C.: Chamber of Commerce of the United States, 1966), p. 12.

66. Z. L. Gulledge, "Summary Statement: Vocational Rehabilitation of Industrially Injured Covered by California Workmen's

Compensation Laws," in A. J. Jaffe (ed.), *Research Conference on Workmen's Compensation and Vocational Rehabilitation* (New York: Bureau of Applied Social Research, Columbia University, 1961), p. 117.
67. James N. Morgan, Marvin Snider, and Marion G. Sobol, *Lump Sum Redemption Settlements and Rehabilitation* (Ann Arbor, Mich.: Survey Research Center, Institute for Social Research, 1959), pp. 13–14, 27, 64–81, especially p. 77.
68. Arthur Larson, *The Law of Workmen's Compensation* (Albany, N.Y.: Matthew Bender, 1952), vol. II, p. 2. Z. L. Gulledge, *The Rehabilitation of Industrially Injured Workers Covered by Workmen's Compensation Laws* (Sacramento, Calif.: Department of Education, Vocational Rehabilitation Service, 1961). Some people (disabled and nondisabled) feel strongly that physical loss can never be adequately compensated for by money and that society has a definite debt to the injured person. See J. S. Keifer, M. W. Zucker, J. J. Regan, and M. Z. Eubank, *Studies in Workmen's Compensation* (New York: Commerce and Industry Association of New York, 1954), p. 70.
69. Safilios-Rothschild, "The Reaction to Disability in Rehabilitation," *op. cit.*, p. 10. See also Ely Chinoy, *Automobile Workers and the American Dream* (New York: Random House, 1955), p. 8; Morse and Weiss, "The Function and Meaning of Work on the Job," in Sigmund Nosow and William H. Form (eds.), *Man, Work, and Society* (New York: Basic Books, 1962), pp. 193 and 197. But of course very few skilled workers ever succeed in establishing a repair shop even when they have obtained a lump sum settlement: The lump sum is seldom over $3,000 (in Michigan, for example, only 33% settle for more than $3,000), and after the lawyer's fees and accumulated debts are paid, there is not enough capital left to open a small shop; their families may object to their plans; and skilled workers do not usually know enough about running a small business. The overall rate of success of small businesses is generally low. According to a survey study of workers who received lump sum settlements in Michigan, only 6% used the money to start their own businesses. See Morgan *et al., op. cit.*, p. 13.
70. See Safilios-Rothschild, "The Reaction to Disability in Rehabilitation," *op. cit.*; and Noel Lawrence Moyer, "Occupational Variables and the Role of the Sick," (unpublished Ph.D. dissertation, Ohio State University, 1963).
71. In the author's study of back-impaired rehabilitants, it was found to be the semiskilled and unskilled workers who most often had low morale and did not return to work. See Safilios-

Rothschild, "The Reaction to Disability in Rehabilitation," *op. cit.*

72. The term "compensionitis" is sometimes used by rehabilitation personnel to refer to those disabled who seem to be more preoccupied with the settlement of their compensation case than with improving their abilities. Some rehabilitation centers refuse to admit such people for services till their case has been settled, and by the time it is settled it is often too late for them to become rehabilitated, from a psychological and physiological point of view.

73. Earl F. Cheit, *Injury and Recovery in the Course of Employment* (New York: Wiley, 1961), pp. 8, 49–54. See also Alex P. Aitken, "Rehabilitation in Workmen's Compensation," in *International Association of the Industrial Accidents Boards and Commissions Proceedings* (Washington, D.C., 1952), p. 2. It also seems that workmen's compensation medicine is less acceptable than independent private practice or academic medicine, and it is therefore possible that it tends to attract a greater percentage of "marginal" doctors. Probably this lesser acceptance is due to the fact that some physicians treating injured workers under workmen's compensation "have been shown to have been guilty of such abuses as overtreatment, kickbacks, poor service, and willingness to testify to anything for a fee." See Leon Lewis, "Medical Care Under Workmen's Compensation," in Cheit and Gordon, *op. cit.*, p. 154.

74. For example, it was found that compensation patients (who already because of class-linked experiences tend to mistrust doctors) often receive inadequate therapy for a prolonged period of time (for example, heat therapy as the only kind of physical therapy), so that they develop even stronger prejudices and extreme resentment against doctors, hospitals, physical therapy, and treatment in general. See E. M. Krusen and Dorothy E. Ford, "Compensation Factors in Low Back Injuries." *The Journal of the American Medical Association,* 166, 10 (March 8, 1958), 1131.

75. Louis S. Reed, *Medical Care Under the New York Workmen's Compensation Program* (Ithaca, N.Y.: Cornell University, Institute of Hospital Administration, 1960), pp. 103–13.

76. Krusen and Ford, *op. cit.,* p. 1131. R. K. Diveley, R. H. Kiene, and P. W. Meyer, "Low Back Pain," *The Journal of the American Medical Association,* 160, 9 (March 3, 1956), 731.

77. *The California Workmen's Compensation System: Attitudes and Experiences of a Cross-section of California Physicians* (San Francisco: California Medical Association, July 1964).

78. *Controverted Cases—New York State Workmen's Compensa-*

tion (Washington, D.C.: U.S. Department of Health, Education and Welfare, Vocational Rehabilitation Administration, 1964).

79. Gulledge, "Summary Statement: Vocational Rehabilitation of Industrially Injured Covered by California Workmen's Compensation Laws," *op. cit.*, p. 118.

80. *Controverted Cases—New York State Workmen's Compensation, op. cit.*, pp. 58–61.

81. Gulledge, "Summary Statement: Vocational Rehabilitation of Industrially Injured Covered by California Workmen's Compensation Laws," *op. cit.*, pp. 116–17.

82. Although the optimum time of referral for rehabilitation is not necessarily an early referral but one carried out as soon as the first stage of mourning has passed, it seems that compensation claimants are usually referred or accepted for rehabilitation well beyond the optimum time. It has been argued that an early referral (2–3 months after the injury), even when it does not lead to acceptance for rehabilitation services, plays an important role because it informs the disabled worker of the rehabilitation alternative.

83. Samuel B. Horowitz, "Selections From: Rehabilitation of Injured Workers—Its Legal and Administrative Problems," in Jaffe, *op. cit.*, pp. 136–37; Gulledge, "Summary Statement: Vocational Rehabilitation of Industrially Injured Covered by California Workmen's Compensation Laws," *op. cit.*, p. 123. See Also "Vocational Rehabilitation Plays a Major Role in the Ontario Compensation Plan" [draft] (Toronto: The Workmen's Compensation Board, 1968); and John Lauer, "Modern Rehabilitation As Seen by an Industrial Physician," *Industrial Medicine and Surgery,* 30, 1 (January 1961), 12.

84. It is interesting to note that in the Research Conference on Workmen's Compensation and Vocational Rehabilitation in 1960 the need for comparative studies of rehabilitation under different types of workmen's compensation legislation (including that of Ontario) was emphasized. Despite this, no such comparative study has been carried out. See "Some Areas for Basic Research," in Jaffe, *op. cit.*, pp. 27–40.

85. *Problèmes du reemploi des travailleurs agés ou handicapés, op. cit.*, pp. 31–33.

86. Diveley *et al., op. cit.*, p. 731; Krusen and Ford, *op. cit.*, p. 1129.

87. Arthur Hakenen, "Social Security Disability Benefits and Rehabilitation," *Journal of Michigan State Medical Society,* 61 (May 1962), 606–7.

88. U.S. Public Health Service, *Health Statistics From the U.S. National Health Survey,* series B, no. 36 (October 1962), p.

22; also no. 31 (January 1962), p. 11; and no. 11 (July 1959), p. 11. See also Theodore D. Woolsey, "Classification of Population in Terms of Disability" (paper presented at the United Nations World Population Conference, Belgrade, August 30–September 10, 1965).

89. U.S. Department of Health, Education and Welfare, National Center for Health Statistics, *Selected Health Characteristics by Occupation,* series 10, no. 21 (Washington, D.C.: July 1961–June 1963), p. 1.

90. Woolsey, *op. cit.*

91. Lawrence D. Haber, *Prevalence of Disability Among Noninstitutionalized Adults Under Age 65: 1966 Survey of Disabled Adults,* Research and Statistics Note 4 (Washington, D.C.: U.S. Department of Health, Education and Welfare, Social Security Administration, Office of Research and Statistics, February 20, 1968).

92. Conley mentions marital instability as a possible result in some cases and impaired care and training of children. Conley, *op. cit.,* pp. 5–7, 15–16.

93. Saxon Graham, "Social Factors in Relation to the Chronic Illnesses." in Freeman, Levine, and Reeder, *op. cit.,* pp. 68–70.

94. H. Robert Blank, "The Challenge of Rehabilitation," *Israel Medical Journal,* 20, 5–6 (1961), 127.

95. Metropolitan Life Insurance Company, *Statistical Bulletin,* 48 (November 1967), 3.

96. Donald F. Heuelke and Paul W. Gikas, "Causes of Deaths in Automobile Accidents," *The Journal of the American Medical Association,* 203, 13 (March 25, 1968), 1100–7.

97. Metropolitan Life Insurance Company, "International Trends in Survival After Age 65," *Statistical Bulletin,* 46 (January 1965), 8–10.

98. Metropolitan Life Insurance Company, "The Prevalence of Chronic Conditions," *Statistical Bulletin,* 44 (September 1963), 3–5.

99. In 1965, there were 18.2 million persons in the United States at ages 65 and over, a gain of 1.6 million over 1960 and of 5.9 million over 1950; by 1975, the number is expected to exceed 21 million and by 1985, 25 million. See Metropolitan Life Insurance Company, "The Population of Elders," *Statistical Bulletin,* 46 (November 1965), 1.

100. The acute conditions account for an average of about 10 days of restricted activity annually instead of 7½ days at ages 45–64. See Metropolitan Life Insurance Company, "Health Characteristics of the Older Population," *Statistical Bulletin,* 46 (October 1965), 10.

101. Conley, *op. cit.,* pp. 25–26.

102. Edward S. Rogers, "Public Health Asks of Sociology," *Science,* 159, 3814 (February 2, 1968), 506–8.
103. Lawrence D. Haber, "Demographic Correlates of Disability" (paper presented at the meetings of the Population Association of America, Boston, April 1968). In all previous years, the annual number of rehabilitated individuals was much lower; see Conley, *op. cit.,* pp. 53–55.
104. A study undertaken by Martin Dishart in 1964 reports that there were 90 state vocational rehabilitation agencies. Since that time it is quite possible that many more such facilities have become available. See Martin Dishart, *A National Study of 84,699 Applicants for Services From State Vocational Rehabilitation Agencies in the United States* (Washington, D.C.: National Rehabilitation Association, October 1964).
105. U.S. Bureau of the Census, *Statistical Abstract of the United States: 1966* (Washington, D.C., 1966), p. 301.
106. Dishart, *op. cit.* Similarly, in the case of the blind, it has been found that only children and young, educated, trainable, and employable adults are being served by the multiple agencies for the blind. Even in the case of children, multiply-handicapped ones are not often accepted. Robert A. Scott, *The Making of Blind Men: A Study of Adult Socialization* (New York: Russell Sage Foundation, 1969), pp. 69–70.
107. For an interesting review of the characteristics of those who do not receive the benefits of rehabilitation services, see Conley, *op. cit.,* pp. 100–19 and 8–9.
108. Written communication by Theodor Litman from his commentary to the first draft of this chapter. See also R. Castro De la Mata, G. Gingras, and E. D. Wittkower, "Impact of Sudden, Severe Disablement of the Father Upon the Family," *The Canadian Medical Association Journal,* 82 (May 14, 1960), 1015–20.
109. Haber, "Demographic Correlates of Disability," *op. cit.*
110. Lawrence D. Haber, "Disability, Work, and Income Maintenance: Prevalence of Disability, 1966" Report 2 (Washington, D.C.: Social Security Administration, Office of Research and Statistics, May 1968), pp. 6–7.

CHAPTER 2

The Career of the Disabled

From the moment that the first symptoms (or an accident) are experienced to the eventual stage at which no further effort is made to alter the extent of residual disability, disabled persons follow different types of "careers." By "career" we mean what Roth has defined as ". . . a series of related and definable stages or phases of a given sphere of activity that a person goes through on the way to a more or less definite and recognizable end-point or goal. . . ."[1] The notion of a career also implies the existence of some kind of normative data about how others in similar positions have or are behaving with which to compare one's passage from one phase to another. In the presence of injuries, of physical or mental symptoms, the goal of those bearing the symptoms is preferably to get rid of the symptoms—or if some permanent disability is unavoidable, to learn how best to live with it. Depending upon their social and sociopsychological characteristics as well as their previous experience with illness and medical care, the disabled will tend to recognize, define, and cope with symptoms differentially; will enter into different types of patient-doctor relationships, thereby receiving a different quality of medical care; and finally, will tend to define themselves as either temporarily or permanently vocationally handicapped. In this chapter we will examine all the steps through which a person usually proceeds from relative health to disability, partial or total, temporary or permanent. The factors affecting the first stages involving the assumption of the "sick" role, the initial patient-doctor relationship, and the quality of medical care received will be elaborated at greater length. In the remaining chapters we shall discuss the career of the disabled in more detail, proceeding from the time they are faced with the possibility of some degree of permanent disability; that is, from the time they become probable candidates for the "disabled" role.

From Health to Illness

Except for the congenitally disabled, most people go through some type of transition which leads them from a state of relative health to an awareness of "abnormal" symptoms and eventually, to the assumption of the sick role.[2] In the case of most disabling illnesses, the beginning is slow and insidious, and cultural, social, and sociopsychological factors are crucial in determining the nature of the process from health to illness. In the case of most accidents, however, the involved individuals are forced into the sick role abruptly and without choice.

The first conceptual difficulty encountered in this analytical discussion is the ambiguity of the definition of health. When is a person healthy? And is a person ever completely healthy? If health is defined as the absence of illness, how is illness to be defined: in terms of the presence of clinical (or subclinical) symptoms or in terms of the presence of "disabling" symptoms which interfere with the individual's functioning? Medical authorities by and large favor the former, while most lay people may in fact apply the latter. On the other hand, the use of a comprehensive definition of health, such as the one proposed by the World Health Organization: "a state of complete physical, mental, and social well-being," is impractical.[3] Even if accurate and operational indexes could be established to measure this ideal and comprehensive state of health, very few people would be judged healthy.

Another basic problem encountered in the definition of health or illness revolves around the question of whether it should be based on medical criteria only, lay individual criteria only, or a combination of both. Physicians tend to rely predominantly upon a *clinical* definition of illness based upon the presence of identifiable pathological symptoms of a specified disease entity or of a nonclearly delineated pathological condition. Strictly speaking, only those who are seen by a physician and are diagnosed as having pathological symptomatology can therefore be clearly labeled as sick. However, doctors will date an illness as having begun prior to consultation, perhaps at the time when friends and relatives of the afflicted were making their own diagnoses and suggesting home remedies. Furthermore, they would define as illness conditions treated and cured by home remedies only as well as those given professional medical attention.

Definitional problems that represent either overdefinitions or underdefinitions of illness arise from this approach. There is evidence that physicians, when unsure if a patient is really sick or if his complaints are unimportant and within the "normal" range, tend to define him as sick and check him thoroughly until the state of sickness is either validated or discarded.[4] There is, then, a tendency for the physician to overdefine illness in order to safeguard his position in case his client is actually sick. On the other hand, there is also some contrary evidence of a serious underdefinition of illness when the physician does not attach any particular significance to the patient's complaints and, in the absence of gross pathology, dismisses them altogether without checking further.[5] No systematic study has yet been made of the nature of the cases in which the physician, instead of overdefining, is inclined to underdefine illness. Is it when patients are "chronic complainers" about minor, unimportant symptoms that he tends to also place more serious, nonspecific symptoms within the range of normality? Or is it when an illness is in a very early stage and the patients' vague, nonspecific complaints or symptoms are not clearly indicative of a particular disease entity? A related definitional problem is the following: Can those who suffer from an undiagnosed disease—at an early stage, before any serious physiological changes have come about which could affect behavior, alter fatigue level, degree of activity, or emotional states—be considered ill during these early stages? Even if a physician examined them at that point, he would most probably not find any definite pathological indications. Probably only when the pathological malfunctioning starts affecting the stamina, emotional and physical well-being, or the playing of social roles can an individual be considered ill whether he is conscious of his illness or not, because now his condition is clinically diagnosable.[6]

Scheff has also pointed out that medical diagnoses may be more or less influenced by stereotypes and well-known conceptual "packages" about standard or prevalent diseases. Of course, the greater the reliance upon such diagnostic stereotypes, the less the probable accuracy of the diagnosis. Such stereotypes may be used by some physicians in certain settings or in the case of some categories of patients (lower class patients) more often than in others not only as guiding hypotheses for further investigation, but also as the final result of the diagnostic procedure.[7]

A physician decides that one is sick by recognizing the presence of clearly identifiable pathological symptoms of disease entities and by making specific tests to determine that some bodily functions are below or above the normative range (for example, that one's tension is too high or too low). The range within which physiological functioning is considered to be normal is established on both a statistical and an "ideal" basis.[8] When the physiological functioning of most people does not fall within a more or less well-defined range, they exhibit disabling symptoms. It is true, however, that some individuals may be able to function adequately and without disturbance even when outside this normative range, a fact that sometimes may complicate the diagnostic process. Also, in some developing societies certain symptoms or types of physiological malfunctioning may be so widespread that the ailing persons themselves may not define their condition as abnormal.[9] But a physician who compares their state of being and level of functioning with an "ideal"; that is, a state that could be enjoyed under different conditions of nourishment, housing, and medical care (and is being enjoyed by people in countries with a higher standard of living), would diagnose them as sick despite the prevalence of the condition. For example, in rural Guatemala practically the entire population is malnourished; as correlates, the people are small in size, infant mortality is high, intestinal parasites are endemic, disease resistance is low, and the life span short.[10] But the fact that intestinal parasites are endemic does not make this condition nonpathological.

In the case of mental health, however, the model of adequate mental functioning is not well developed, and there is considerable variability in the definition of "normal" functioning under different living conditions. When some symptoms of mental malfunctioning are found to be prevalent, one could raise the question of whether or not the concept of mental health should be so redefined as to include these symptoms within the "normal" range. For example, when the Midtown study in Manhattan showed that 81.5 percent of the noninstitutionalized population was not "normal" with respect to several mental symptoms, one could question whether or not the presence of certain symptoms clinically considered as deviant and abnormal is a sufficient condition for labeling those individuals as "abnormal" or "mentally ill." One could further speculate that for people living in a certain type of society (at a certain level of industrialization, with cultural values concerning a high level of achievement, and so forth), the presence of these symptoms up to a certain level of frequency and intensity is "normal" and even necessary for successful functioning.[11]

While physicians may vary in their degree of reliance on an absolute "ideal" of functioning (or rather on one relative to the patient's life conditions and idiosyncrasies) as well as in their tendency to underdefine or overdefine illness, the patient usually comes to the physician with an altogether different conceptualization. The patient's view of health and illness is influenced, and by and large determined, by cultural and subcultural, social, sociopsychological, and psychological factors. There are definite cultural uniformities in the definitions of health and illness, in the attitudes toward medical care, physicians, and hospitalization, as well as toward the sick and the disabled, that distinguish those belonging to one culture or cultural area from those belonging to another. Despite these cultural uniformities, however, a variety of social factors of which social class is the most prominent may produce a great degree of variability within one cultural group. And this variability, as we shall see, may be so great that those belonging to one social class in one culture have more in common with those of the same social class in another culture (or cultural area) than they have in common with the other classes in their own culture. Furthermore, additional variability with respect to the definition of illness and illness behavior may be produced among people belonging to the same social class and culture by their differing sociopsychological and psychological characteristics that specify the mode in which they will define the situation. Thus, it is possible that some middle class Americans in some particular types of interpersonal relations and roles may define and handle illness in the same way as some lower class Americans do and not at all similarly to other middle class Americans. Finally, the type of illness—that is, the rapidity and acuteness of onset, the nature of the symptoms, and the degree of their ambiguity—further influences the definitions and behaviors of the ailing persons. We shall now examine in some detail both the uniformities and the variabilities in definitions of illness and illness behavior produced by cultural, social, sociopsychological, and psychological factors as well as by the illness.

At the most general level, health and illness may be conceptualized in terms of collective types of perception and labeling of pathological conditions and modes of reacting to them prevalent in a particular culture or subculture. The process of perceiving, defining, and reacting to symptoms is largely influenced by the values prevailing in a cultural milieu, especially those values concerning health, illness, the sick role, required levels of role and task performance, and cultural attitudes toward physicians and medical care. For example, the Anglo-Saxon values concerning health—which may be representative of the values prevailing in highly industrialized societies —appear to be rational because they are based upon a "mechanistic approach to the body and its functions culminating in the view that the body is a machine to be well taken care of, periodically checked, and taken to an expert to 'fix' any defect that may appear."[12] Such cultural values tend to encourage both an early definition of a very wide range of symptoms as pathological and the seeking of expert medical care without such emotional complications as denial or fear about the illness. Also the overall preoccupation of Americans with deviance, to the extent that any (even minor) deviation from the "normal" must be corrected, is conducive to early detection of symptoms and medical care. But it seems that social class plays an important role, since among Americans, the higher the socioeconomic status, the greater the preoccupation with any type of deviance, including illness; the lower the socioeconomic status, the greater the probability that the "deviant" will experience a "deviant" status while he is treated for his deviance. Therefore, lower class patients experience much more social isolation and "primary-group disvaluation of the patient-role" while they are being hospitalized than do middle class patients.[13]

In contrast, most developing countries are characterized by a nonscientific orientation toward health and illness and a distrust of doctors and medical care. These attitudes are responsible for a considerable degree of symptom toleration, for considerable delays in seeking medical care, for lack of confidence in medical advice and recommendations, and therefore for a hesitancy or even a complete refusal to follow recommendations, especially if they involve hospitalization and/or surgery.[14] The opinion of family members and trusted friends is at least as equally respected as medical opinion and, indeed, often challenges the latter. Of course, the "folk" type of social structure and mentality prevalent in developing countries may also be found among some groups and subcultures living in highly industrialized societies. Suchman found, for example, that in the United States people belonging to closely-knit, ethnocentric, traditional communities in which friendship and family ties were the strongest tended to have a nonscientific orientation toward health, to distrust impersonal medical care, to have poor factual knowledge about illnesses, and to depend upon their own group in case of illness.[15] Also, there is evidence indicating that the American lower class holds values toward health and medical care as well as attitudes toward physicians very similar to those held by the majority of people in traditional, developing countries.[16]

Probably the most important factor in determining what range of symptoms will be more quickly experienced and consequently treated is the social role(s) particularly emphasized in each culture. Physical or emotional symptoms interfering with the effective performance of this social role (or roles) soon draw the attention of the afflicted individual or his significant others, and some kind of corrective action is taken. Parsons' definition, according to which "Health may be defined as the state of optimum *capacity* of an individual for the effective performance of the roles and tasks for which he has been socialized," seems to be cross-culturally valid.[17] Thus in Spain, where the roles of father, husband, and protector of the family are the emphasized male roles and that of mother and housewife the female, symptoms diminishing men's strength, virility, and ability to protect the honor and interests of the family or affecting women's fertility or ability to take care of their children and husband would be definitely defined as illness.[18] Otherwise, suffering resulting from symptoms which do not interfere with the ideal social roles would simply be tolerated as an annoyance or as a cross to bear. Similarly, a cultural definition of adequate functioning in basic roles —such as the one held by the Spanish-speaking villagers of New Mexico and Colorado, based upon a high level of physical activity, a well-fleshed body, a "healthy" appearance, and the absence of pain —results in the tolerance of all kinds of upper respiratory infections, tuberculosis, and other "internal" diseases when they do not relate to their health criteria.[19]

Among Anglo-Saxons (and probably some other highly industrialized cultural groups), interference with adequate functioning in basic roles is also the primary criterion for defining a symptom or condition as illness and seeking medical care for it. The criteria for defining what constitutes "adequate functioning," however, may be more exigent than in developing countries. And in the case of men, for whom the occupational role is the most important, medical care is usually sought for symptoms or conditions interfering with effective functioning in vocational activities.[20]

The degree of social stigma attached to an illness within a culture greatly affects also an individual's (or his significant others') willingness to adopt the sick role. For example, because in Greece tuberculosis and mental illness carry a social stigma for the afflicted individual and his family that cannot be removed regardless of the outcome of treatment, afflicted persons are strongly motivated to deny and hide their symptoms as long as possible. When the symptoms can no longer be denied, the individual or his family may finally accept his condition but still keep it, as well as the required treatment, a secret.[21] Finally, whether or not falling sick carries a connotation of moral weakness seems to influence the afflicted individual's tendency to accept the fact that he is ill and to then seek medical care.[22] In the United States, whenever the individual is not held responsible for his state and his affliction is considered beyond his control, a considerable number of ailing individuals may tend to accept their state of illness more easily. However, even for the United States it is debatable to what extent "falling sick" may be considered to lie totally out of one's control, since the importance of social, sociopsychological, and psychological factors in aggravating symptoms, rendering them more noticeable and bothersome, and bringing about the "need" for medical care is being given more and more attention. In some cultures, such as those of rural Greece and Bali, where there is a belief that people must battle with symptoms and not "give in" to them because then, and only then, will they fall ill or die, a relatively larger number of people will try to function despite pain, discomfort, and other more or less incapacitating symptoms.[23]

Of course, such generalizations at the cultural level may be misleading, since they refer to model behavior and in reality there is at least as much variation in the illness and help-seeking behavior of Greeks and of Americans as there is between the two. And the modes of variation within each cultural group will be determined by the combined effect of a number of social and sociopsychological factors which in the presence of clinically diagnosable symptoms may influence the afflicted individuals to either define or not define themselves as sick and to seek or not seek medical care accordingly. As Maclachlan says: "It may seem too much to assert that a man 'is as sick as he feels,' but there is considerable evidence to support such a statement."[24] It is the person's definition of his symptoms rather than the sheer presence and nature of them that really determines at which point on the health-illness continuum he will consider himself to be sick as well as whether or not he will seek medical care.

This subjective evaluation and definition of the symptoms that determine the course of action deemed appropriate has been called by Mechanic and Volkart "illness behavior."[25] A variety of factors

may influence illness behavior, such as: (1) The individual's status
in the society, that is, "the differentiated type of role and corresponding task structure, e.g., sex or age"; level of education; marital status;
religion; income level; number and age of dependents; and occupational and social status.[26] (2) His values concerning health (how
important health is in the value hierarchy); inclination to adopt the
sick role; value placed on self-reliance (or negatively stated, the
strength or dependency needs); membership in "cosmopolitan" or
"parochial" social structures; nature of cultural values regarding
health and degree of adherence to them, plus the belief that most
illnesses will go away by themselves or, conversely, only through the
administration of special care (not necessarily medical).[27] (3) The
types of "lay" definitions and "lay referral" systems available to him.
(4) The types of life crises, griefs, and stresses the individual is
undergoing in his family life, his work or both. All these social and
sociopsychological factors, together with a person's psychological
state, life stresses, and past experience with illness, may combine in
a variety of ways to account for the high degree of variability in illness and help-seeking behavior among individuals. We shall now discuss in detail some of the factors about which there is considerable
research documentation.

Assuming that he believes in the purposefulness and efficacy
of medical care, it could be hypothesized that whether or not an
individual assumes the sick role with all its rights and obligations
will depend on a balance between the perceived sanctions for his
well-being (that is, the perceived danger to health involved in the
neglect of observable symptoms as well as their possible interference
with the effective performance of basic social roles) and the perceived severity of sanctions that accompany falling ill (in terms of
expense, loss of income, loss of time, the relinquishing of binding
responsibilities, and actual interference in role performance generated
by illness, and so forth). The accuracy of a person's perception of
the degree of danger involved in symptoms depends to a great extent
on his degree of factual knowledge about illness,[28] but also upon his
personal acquaintance with the symptoms either through a previous
illness of his own or the illness of a loved one. Although we know
some of the factors that influence the level of anxiety about a particular illness—such as the level of perceived incidence of a disease, the

perceived susceptibility to the disease, the level of education and income—we do not know the effect of the level of anxiety about a particular disease upon illness behavior with respect to symptoms related to this disease.[29] Probably a moderate level of anxiety about a disease may motivate an individual to seek medical care more quickly. A very high level of anxiety may generate paralyzing fear and a medical diagnosis may be avoided because of its potential threatening content.

Individuals with demanding occupational, educational, or family responsibilities may be inclined to "define away" symptoms unless they perceive serious danger as a consequence of neglect or unless these symptoms interfere seriously with normal role functioning. For example, a mother of several small children and a wife of a busy (and often absent) upwardly mobile husband who shoulders the entire family responsibility, or a highly skilled professional, or a top executive whose decisions affect the functioning of entire plants may be reluctant to assume the sick role, especially the dependent patient role. They may admit that they are ill but continue their role performance as best as they can, because there is (or they think there is) nobody who could replace them. Of course, in the case of upper middle class men, it is possible that physicians themselves are reluctant to impose vocational inactivity and the dependent patient role (especially hospitalization) because they deem their patient's social function too important to be in any way curtailed or interfered with. When hospitalization is necessary, it is as brief as possible.[30]

Significant others are also important for the individual's illness behavior because they are usually the "lay" diagnosticians to whom symptoms or feelings are first described. Freidson's research on the "lay referral systems" has shown that the usual process followed by those who perceive the presence of abnormal symptoms is to resort to self-diagnosis and simultaneously to consult with significant others within or outside the household.[31] Then, if the condition is bearable and the "lay" people consulted do not favor consultation with a doctor, the ailing individual may or may not apply self-treatment and postpone seeing a doctor unless his condition worsens. However, the degree of severity and visibility of the symptoms again may determine whether or not the physician will be consulted directly and without the intermediate stage of the lay referral system.[32] It has also been found that lower class persons tend to rely much more heavily upon lay consultants than do middle and upper middle class persons.[33] The latter tend to rely upon themselves for the initial diagnosis and the determination of when to consult a physician.

Recent research has shown that when a spouse is used as lay consultant, women and men were equally often legitimately granted the sick role,[34] but the younger their age and the less frequent the occurrence of "abnormal" symptoms, the greater the tendency to legitimize their being sick with all the accorded rights and obligations.[35] In reality, of course, there are several types of significant others (spouse, children, co-workers, employers, friends, and relatives) who may not agree among themselves whether or not the consulting "other" is sick or what treatment or course of action is appropriate. A recent study dealing with two significant others— wives and co-workers—concluded that the husband's tendency to avoid responsibility was greater when both his wife and his co-workers defined his symptoms as "sickness," thus legitimizing the temporary relinquishing of role performance in the occupational, social, and familial spheres.[36] In the case of conflicting definitions of symptoms on the part of the wife and co-workers, the degree of the husband's dependency determined which of the two sets of significant others was the most influential. Dependent husbands tended to be more influenced by their wives' definition and dominant husbands by their co-workers' definition. Furthermore, other studies have indicated that the nature of the relationship between significant family members significantly influences their definition of symptoms as an illness requiring medical care or hospitalization.[37]

There are also some indications that people tend to pay more attention to already existing and largely unattended physical complaints (and it is rather questionable if one is ever symptom-free), defining them as symptoms requiring medical diagnosis and treatment when they experience either grief or a depressive reaction due to the actual or symbolic "loss of a valued object, be it a loved one, a cherished possession, a job, status, home country, an ideal, a part of the body, etc."[38] In such instances the individual may experience feelings of hopelessness, meaninglessness or helplessness and lose interest in living. He may even wish in a sense to die; however, he does not take the drastic step of suicide but instead finds refuge in illness, a mild kind of "suicide substitute." In many clinical and survey studies it has been found that some kind of "crisis," whether defined as an incapacity to cope with changing environmental stresses, as domestic conflict, as disruption of social participation patterns, or as an unresolved conflict, precedes the onset of various diseases.[39] This series of events has sometimes been explained causally; that is, the "crisis" or unresolved conflict causing the disease by decreasing physical resistance or by altering the body's physiology. However, such a causal explanation may not always hold true, since depressive symptoms (as well as a variety of other psychiatric symptoms) can be found almost as frequently among people not attending doctors as among those attending them.[40] And just the opposite direction of causality may sometimes hold true; that is, decreased physical stamina due to pathological symptomatology could create or precipitate a life crisis.

Probably emotional factors (such as depressive reactions or grief from an actual or symbolic loss) or crises draw the individual's attention to physical symptoms which are already present, and by rendering them more "visible" make the demand for diagnosis and treatment imperative. While it is quite difficult to ascertain which has come first—the crisis and stress or the physical symptoms—it seems that the presence of emotional factors alone or the presence of physical symptoms alone may not always be sufficient to send a person to a doctor. The compound effect, however, of emotional factors and physical symptoms very often leads the afflicted individual to the physician's office.[41] This interpretation probably helps to explain why at any given time there are almost as many persons not consulting doctors who present the same range of physical symptoms as do those who consult doctors, and why people suddenly decide to see a doctor for symptoms they may have been having for quite some time.[42]

Up to now we have examined a variety of factors relating to the individual's cultural and social origins, personality organization, and type of interpersonal relations, as well as life experiences and stresses that influence perception of symptoms and consequent behavior. We can now turn to examine the role of the nature of experienced symptoms in the way in which they will be explained and acted upon by different types of people. There are some indications that the nature of the symptoms may bring about similar types of illness definition and illness behavior among ailing persons with a variety of cultural, social, sociopsychological or psychological backgrounds. For example, it has been found that when the symptoms are severe, continuous and incapacitating, indicating a serious illness, there is usually considerable uniformity in recognition of the illness and in seeking medical care.[43] When the symptoms are of long duration, regardless of degree of severity or ambiguousness, a similar uniformity of behavior can be observed.[44] Thus, the presence of threatening, severe, and incapacitating symptoms of recent origin tend to diminish considerably differences in illness behavior between lower class and middle class people, between young and old, educated and uneducated, between those living in highly industrialized societies and those living in folk societies.[45]

Most of the variability in illness behavior, then, can be accounted for by the common, nonserious, familiar, and predictable-outcome illnesses where the individual can take a certain amount of risk without having necessarily to pay a severe health penalty. And this variability is determined by the different combinations of cultural, social, sociopsychological, and psychological factors found in different individuals. Each of these factors affect the individual's illness behavior with a differential intensity and often in a different direction. In order to be able to predict illness behavior, therefore, a complicated predictive index will have to be constructed. Keeping in mind that individuals within the proposed typological categories will exhibit a great amount of behavioral variability, we can proceed to delineate some rough overall typologies of illness careers.

1. There are those who, either immediately or soon after the appearance of abnormal but not severe and incapacitating symptoms (excluding routine and temporary annoyances), define them as potential illness and consult a physician for diagnosis and care. These individuals have confidence in the physician's diagnosis and prescribed treatment and faithfully follow his directions. While this illness behavior is considered to be the most "rational" alternative within the American culture, its absolute rationality can be questioned, since at least some people "appear to regain their health most of the time whether or not adequate therapeutic techniques are utilized." More middle and upper middle than lower class Americans have been reported to follow this type of "career"; they are usually quick to

obtain adequate explanation about diagnosis, treatment, and prognosis.[46]

2. There are those who consult a physician only after self-determined or lay-determined treatment has failed to ameliorate their condition and their "lay consultants" finally refer them to a physician or after their condition has become severe and visible. While they are delaying seeking medical care, they may either do nothing special to alleviate the condition and expect the illness to go away by itself or use such home remedies as rest, special diet, entertainment, alcoholic beverages, massages, etc., while continuing to function as best they can in all their roles. On the other hand, they may selectively and temporarily omit or curtail certain activities or tasks they feel are not essential or even definitely detrimental to their actual state of health. Since this relinquishing of tasks and activities is not legitimized by a physician, the degree of acceptance and support this decision receives from the significant others may well vary from family to family, from social class to social class, and from culture to culture, depending upon whether or not medical legitimation of the ill state is necessary. By and large in the American culture (and probably in most other highly industrialized countries as well), only medical diagnosis legitimizes the sick state of the individual as well as his temporary exemption from normal social roles, especially the vocational role, if this is deemed essential to recovery. In many developing countries—for example, Greece—a sick person may be exempted without medical legitimation from the performance of tasks required in some roles (including the vocational) while he continues to enjoy the rights and privileges accorded some of his roles, especially his family roles (for example, he may make important decisions or run the entire life of the family from his bed). Medical legitimation is not necessary because those claiming "sick" status in the Greek culture are not bound by the obligation to seek competent medical help. This is probably due to a mistrust of physicians and a devaluation of the effectiveness of medical care in the Greek culture. In America, lower class more often than middle class persons have been reported to follow the same type of illness career, tending to "check" the physician's diagnosis or prescribed treatment with their lay referral system and discarding diagnosis, treatment, or both if their significant others disapprove or suggest a "better" doctor.[47]

3. Those who, despite their awareness of abnormal symptoms,

which they may or may not define as illness, are unwilling to assume
the sick role and forfeit their social roles. Mostly these individuals
are those who cannot "afford" to fall sick or who cannot take the
time. They may, however, treat their symptoms either through self-
prescribed patent medicines or by medical prescriptions obtained by
calling their private physicians. They may "give in" to their illness
only when it becomes so severe that it drastically interferes with the
performance of the very social roles which they deem to be crucial
in their lives. Upper middle class men with strong career attachments
and their wives (when they have young children) may well follow
this type of illness career. A subcategory of this type may be those
who do not assume the sick role because they have no faith in physicians or medical care. Some lower class or working class Americans
have been reported to fall in this subcategory.

From Illness to Disability

Theoretically at least, once the individual has assumed the sick
role, he should: (a) be exempted from social responsibility (after his
sick state has been legitimized, preferably by a physician); (b) not
be expected to take care of himself; (c) want to get well; and (d)
seek medical advice and cooperate with medical experts.[48] This theoretical conceptualization represents the physicians' point of view—
that is, how they would like people to behave when they "fall sick."[49]
Each point may be challenged as to whether or not and to what
extent it represents the optimal behavioral alternative for all individuals. Research has shown that regardless of whether or not these
behavioral alternatives are best for them, not all persons suffering
from "abnormal" symptoms and considered "sick" by themselves as
well as by others are necessarily bound by all the rights and obligations attached to the sick role. Some may relinquish social responsibilities even without medical legitimation because significant others
nurture their dependency. Others may delay seeking medical care or
diagnostic tests, or following the required treatment, either out of
fear (as in the case of those who think they may have cancer) or out
of disbelief in the effectiveness of medical care. And others may not
always cooperate fully with medical experts without questioning or

challenging medical opinion, an attitude which necessarily results in slower recovery or poor prognosis.

Gordon's validation study of the Parsonian model showed that only when prognosis is believed to be serious and uncertain do the reported role expectations come close to those described by Parsons.[50] When, on the contrary, prognosis for an illness is known and non-serious, the afflicted individual can legitimately assume only the "impaired" role for which expectations tend to support normal behavior in terms of activities and involvement and to discourage seeking medical care. It was also found that the more the prognosis was unknown, serious, and uncertain, the more the person was exempted from social responsibilities and the care of self and the more he was treated as dependent by medical experts and his significant others. Gordon also found that low-income and low-education groups significantly more often than high-income and high-education groups defined the disabled (deaf and amputees) as sick rather than "impaired" and therefore fostered dependency in them.[51] Most probably, of course, a variety of other social, sociopsychological, and psychological factors besides those examined by Gordon (social class, education, and occupation) would further differentiate the "sick role" and the variations of its meaning to different people. It seems, then, that the basic inadequacies of the Parsonian theoretical postulates of the sick role are: (a) the assumption that everyone regardless of type of illness, sociopsychological characteristics, and values about health will behave in a similar manner; and (b) the fact that they represent the physicians' point of view.

With the one exception we have already mentioned (unwillingness to totally cut oneself off from social responsibilities), the degree to which a patient's behavior resembles the physician's expectations of the ideal sick role is a significant factor in determining the type of medical care he will receive and the degree to which he may recover. However, the way in which three of these role obligations are individually defined seems to be the most important for the outcome of the illness: (1) the wish to get well, (2) nondelay in seeking medical care, and (3) willingness to follow essential medical directions and regimen.

Another factor which by and large determines the extent to which the patient's behavior coincides with the physician's expectations and is crucial in predicting the type of medical care he will receive is his social class. Despite the fact that physicians are expected to be "affectively neutral" and use "universalistic" criteria in offering their services—that is, share their attention and efforts equally among patients regardless of whether or not they like them and their sociopsychological characteristics—there is ample evidence that they are greatly affected by the patient's characteristics, especially social class.[52] Treatment is clearly stratified according to social class both at the doctor's office and at a clinic or hospital. The higher the patient's social class, the better treatment he receives, the greater the experience and reputation of the physician (intern versus faculty member), the more time the physician spends with the patient, and the harder he tries to return him to health.

The reasons for the differential medical care may be attributable to a number of factors, such as (a) the "human" and "natural" attraction physicians feel for people similar to themselves in terms of socioeconomic background; (b) the greater prestige given by patients in the upper echelon of the social scale to their physician in exchange for his services; and (c) the greater ease with which patients of similar or higher social position than their physician ask questions and require discussion of the illness process and treatment procedures, their knowledge of what "good" medical care is, and their insistence on receiving nothing but the best care. Of course, not all doctors are expected to show the same degree of discrimination toward patients of low socioeconomic status.[53] Recent research findings indicate that members of occupational groups energetically striving for professional status are negatively oriented toward lower class or poor people.[54] It may also be possible that within a high- or low-striving occupational group, those members who are more conscious of and involved in this striving for professional status tend to discriminate most against the lower class clients. Thus physicians, nurses or other health personnel who are most upwardly mobile and ambitious tend also to concentrate their efforts exclusively on middle and upper middle class patients. Only such patients may symbolically mark their "having made it" since they no longer "mess around" with undesirable lower class patients.

Because of these occasionally dramatic differentials in treatment and medical care, even persons with exactly the same type of initial physical or mental affliction may be left with varying residual effects that are sometimes unwarranted on the basis of their initial condition. This is not to imply that physicians through conscious and intended malpractice are responsible for a considerable extent of disability in lower class patients. But by their indifference, their unwillingness to spend time with these patients, their custom of placing the treatment of lower class patients in the hands of the least experienced physicians and giving them last priority, they may be contributing to some extent to the greater prevalence of disability among lower class patients.

Regardless of the extent of medically diagnosable disability, however, what is of more crucial importance is the degree of disability that an individual is willing to admit, that is, the degree to which he is willing to define himself as "disabled." The process by which one arrives at defining oneself as physically disabled bears a considerable degree of similarity to the labeling process involved in the self-definitions of deviance and mental illness. Both processes lead to the social "stigmatization" of the individual; the afflicted individual is therefore motivated to try anything in order to avoid these labels. The differences among the labels of deviance (the presence of abnormal symptoms), sickness (in mental symptoms corresponding to the label of nerves, shaken nervous system), and disability (or mental illness) lie in the degrees of severity and permanency implied by each. Thus, the label of deviance, regardless of the degree of permanency implied, connotes a low degree of severity in the existing condition. The label of sickness, although it may imply severity, also implies a temporary condition which can, through some kind of intervention (usually medical), be made to disappear. It is only the label of disability that carries the connotation of permanency and irreversibility regardless of the degree of severity of the condition. Because of this distinctive connotation, an individual is much less willing to accept it as a label. And some disabled, as we shall see in the next chapter, never accept it even when they have to sacrifice reality in order to avoid the negative effects of its stigma. They may reject the disability label either by playing down their disability and claiming that they are completely "normal" (only troubled by human aches and pains) or by never relinquishing the label of illness and therefore the hope of returning to normal health through further medical (or semimedical) intervention.

Again, the afflicted individual's significant others play an important role in influencing him to either accept or reject the labels. Sometimes, however, they may define him in a way that he himself is never willing to accept. Our earlier discussion dealt with the influence that significant others can play in the recognition of abnormal symptoms and the assumption of the sick role. In the case of the disability label, available research in mental illness has shown that the nature of the husband-wife relationship prior to the onset of the disabling symptoms is crucial in determining whether the nonafflicted spouse will accept the stigmatized label of permanent disability or resist the negative label even at the expense of reality.[55] Spouses highly satisfied with their marriage before the onset of an illness refuse the label of mental illness, to them a permanent and irreversible label, even after psychiatric diagnosis and lengthy hospitalization. But spouses who were dissatisfied with their marriage prior to the onset of the illness are eager to accept the permanent and seriously stigmatizing label of mental illness and the psychiatric diagnosis. These spouses seem to welcome a serious and irreversible disability, probably because it reinforces the already-present desire to dissociate themselves from the stigmatized spouse. This dissociation may come about either as a complete break of the marital relation by means of divorce, or through a process of alienation by which the mentally ill spouse is denied the chance of rehabilitation and reintegration within his family and within society.[56]

Although similar studies of married disabled persons are not available, similarities and dissimilarities to the patterns described above can be theoretically posited. Some of the dissimilarities which may influence the process are: First, the disabled person may or may not accept the disability label and his spouse may or may not accept that label. Thus four typological categories are possible, depending on whether both spouses accept or refuse the disability label or whether one of them accepts it while the other refuses to do so. We know very little about the dynamic process that takes place in each of these typological categories when the disabled is urged by "significant" persons, such as co-workers, treating physicians, employers, friends, lawyers, and insurance people, to accept or refuse the disability label, and the same holds true for the implications of each typological category for the disabled person's chance of eventual rehabilitation.[57] Second, in the case of physical disability, we may find that sometimes the acceptance of the disability label (regardless of the degree of severity of the condition) may be motivated by a wish of the non-disabled spouse to take on some of the afflicted's roles. This acceptance of the disability label may not necessarily lead to the disintegration of the marital relationship if the disabled spouse is willing to relinquish these roles. Thus, it has sometimes been found that the wives of disabled workers who had always wished to work (and were trained to do so, for example, nurses) tend to encourage their husband's dependency and foster his inability to work in order to have the opportunity of assuming the vocational-breadwinner role and that middle-aged disabled husbands tend to accept this role rearrangement.[58]

If the research findings concerning the mentally ill could be extended to the physically disabled, it could be expected that eager acceptance on the part of the significant others of the disabled status may result in the poor social rehabilitation of the physically disabled and resistance to the disability label may be functional for the outcome of their social rehabilitation. We do not know to what extent this is true. There is some evidence that the physically disabled may become socially rehabilitated more easily when they are well motivated, expected to succeed, and emotionally supported to do so.[59] However, since a certain amount of physical restriction and incapacity is often unsurmountable, the disabled person may at some point feel quite discouraged and frustrated because no matter how hard he tries, there are some things that he cannot do or, worse, that some physical limitations remain no matter how many operations or treatments he receives. Specific studies of the definitional process of physical disability are greatly needed so that we can gain insights into the types of family dynamics that encourage or discourage rehabilitation.[60]

From Disability to Rehabilitation: The Disabled Role

From the time that the illness or condition is expected to leave residuals and not go away altogether, medical personnel assign the individual the "disabled" role whether or not he himself wishes to assume it. The way physicians and rehabilitation people conceptualize the disabled role is of course based upon how they would wish the disabled to behave. Since an empirical validation of the role is not available, we do not know to what extent it reflects actual behavior or the range of variability of actual behavior with different combinations of social, sociopsychological, and psychological factors.

Since residuals are usually a result of serious illnesses or accidents, the afflicted have enjoyed a more or less long period of dependency fostered by medical personnel as well as by their significant others. This is due to the seriousness of their condition as well as to the uncertainty of prognosis. However, once prognosis can be made with a greater degree of certainty and the seriousness of the condition diminishes, physicians usually expect the patient to make a relatively rapid shift from a state of almost total dependence to a state of relative independence and self-reliance. The patient thus experiences a considerable amount of stress because of a drastic discontinuity in what seems to be expected of him.

Examination of medical and sociological literature indicates that physicians as well as rehabilitation personnel would like the disabled individual to behave as follows:

1. When the disabled individual is told by medical authorities that the degree of his physical disability cannot be further diminished (or completely eliminated), *he should accept his disability and start learning how to "live with it."*[61] This expectation becomes effective after the disabled has fulfilled his responsibilities as a sick person, that is, after he has availed himself of expert medical care, has cooperated with medical experts, and has been motivated to get well. One basic difficulty with the enactment of this role expectation is the disabled's unwillingness to accept the fact that medical science can do no more for him. It is accepted with difficulty not only because psychologically the disabled individual cannot accept the fact that he will remain disabled, but also because the different physicians who have been consulted may not entirely agree on the prognosis or can give no specific and certain prognosis because of the nature of the disability. The smallest ambiguity or ambivalence on the part of any of the treating physicians encourages the disabled's everpresent desire to cease being disabled altogether. Anybody who offers the promise of diminishing the pain or the degree of disability will therefore be consulted in order that the painful acceptance of permanent disability can be postponed indefinitely. The disabled continues going from

physician to physician, to osteopaths, chiropractors or even quacks who are willing to promise unrealistic, miraculous results.[62] Because the uncertainty of the prognosis is thus prolonged, the individual is probably sometimes able to get away with an extension of dependency and exemption from at least some social responsibilities.

There is, of course, an equal danger that the disabled person will give up the required medical treatment and restorative modalities too soon and attempt to resume his normal social roles under the burden of unnecessary physical restrictions and undue pain. Because of such unfavorable conditions, he may suffer a recurrence of his illness or another accident or simply such pain and discomfort that he often has to be absent from work or perform at an unsatisfactory level. Or he may have to compromise his performance of social and emotional roles to such an extent that he loses his job or injures his marital relationship and becomes totally discouraged. This expectation raises the serious question of what constitutes the optimum length of medical care to assure the sick person of adequate treatment without developing "invalidism" or making him cling to false hopes. As some researchers have remarked, however, because the determination of this optimum cannot be made accurately by medical technology on the basis of the nature of the illness, it is instead often "bargained" among physicians, administrators, and patients on the basis of many criteria irrelevant to the illness and the effectiveness of necessary treatment.[63]

2. Once the disabled person has accepted the permanency of his disability, he is supposed (in contrast to what is expected of the "sick") to *"pull himself together" and start carrying on his normal social roles by utilizing to the utmost his capacities and abilities within the restrictions set by the physical impairment.* Since it is believed that the extent to which physical impairment becomes a vocational and/or social handicap largely depends on his own will, he is therefore under obligation to make every possible effort to minimize the degree of handicapping, especially in the vocational area. In some cases, of course, the limitations imposed by the physical disability are such (in nature or intensity) that the afflicted individual has to be, in essence, thoroughly resocialized by learning new vocational and/or social and emotional skills in order to adequately perform his social roles. When the performance of the vocational role is interfered with by the physical limitations present, the disabled person not only has

access to, but is under an obligation to avail himself of, vocational rehabilitation services.[64] If, however, the physical impairment does not dictate any necessary change in the vocational role, the disabled person must not use the vocational rehabilitation services in order to bring about a change from an undesirable occupation. Here, of course, there is again a difficulty: Who should pass judgment as to whether or not the physical disability necessitates a change in the usual vocation? Should the individual be entitled to define his needs or must his definition of "need" be overruled by an expert who knows better what they are since allegedly he can make an objective judgment?[65]

3. Up to the time the degree of permanent disability is not stabilized, the disabled, as with all the sick, is expected to be motivated to "get well." *Once, however, the disability is stabilized and no further improvement can be expected, the disabled's motivation must be geared toward effective utilization of remaining abilities in order to resume as many of the "normal" social roles as possible.* Often the disabled person has to be trained how to use his remaining abilities effectively or must have his ability implemented through the addition or use of artificial parts or devices. In such cases, he must usually avail himself of rehabilitation services and be willing to cooperate with the rehabilitation team in finding solutions for his problems. The rehabilitation team will not perform miracles; the disabled must become an active member of the team and work toward mutually agreed goals. Rehabilitation, in essence, can teach him how to use his abilities more successfully and how to control his physical condition and/or prevent its aggravation, as well as help him find ways of coping with his life and responsibilities. But it is always assumed that disabled people, regardless of their nature and level of disability, are interested and willing to master their environment and go on struggling with life and meeting its requirements. All those who do not fit this assumption are considered to be not interested in helping themselves and are dismissed from rehabilitation programs.

But in order for a disabled person to be able to use his remaining abilities, he must know what they are. This presupposes that physicians (and other medical personnel) are able and willing to tell him clearly and specifically the exact extent of his abilities and disabilities— namely, the activities in which he can comfortably indulge, those activities he should never participate in, and the precautions he should

take in performing certain activities or movements. Such a clear deline-
ation of the extent of ability is seldom, if ever, given to the disabled
person at the time he is told that no further physical improvement
can be expected through medical treatment. The reasons are two-
fold: (1) Physicians are not always able to assess so accurately the
extent of the disability and the range of activities that the individual
can still perform.[66] (2) Physicians do not want to take the time to
explain to patients their physical condition in detail, especially if
they are uneducated, lower class patients. Physicians usually give
vague, ambiguous evaluations to the disabled and rationalize their
behavior by saying that their patients would not be able to understand
more elaborate statements and that specific information about their
condition could often harm them rather than benefit them.[67] Thus, the
disabled are left on their own to figure out how disabled they are
and how much exactly they can still do with only some unclear, brief,
and often misunderstood information received from their physician.
In this way their fears and fantasies about their condition can easily
take over and their emotions and needs can color their physical
status. And by repeatedly unsuccessful trial and error efforts to
perform different types of activities and roles, the disabled may finally
become frustrated, discouraged, lose motivation, and embrace the
dependent status.[68]

   4. *The disabled person with a stabilized degree of physical
impairment is not legitimately exempted from the performance of
his social roles, tasks, and activities—especially when he is am-
bulatory.*[69] Even the severely disabled are supposed to manage to take
care of themselves with the aid of specially designed devices and to
find ways of working and earning an income. In the area of social
activities and social interaction, even the ideal societal expectations are
not very clear. On the one hand, while self-reliance, independence,
and autonomy are highly valued and emphasized, disabled persons
seem to undergo societal pressures directing them toward assuming
a helpless, handicapped role, at least when they interact socially with
the nondisabled. Probably, this "negative" pressure exists because the
total assumption of the handicapped role facilitates interaction for the
nondisabled who can then, usually on the basis of stereotypic impressions, rather easily assess the limits and restrictions which the
disability imposes upon the mode of interaction. Because of a norma-

tive ambiguity concerning their expected behavior in social contacts with the nondisabled, there is evidence that the disabled go toward either of two extremes: "normalization" or excessive handicapping.[70]

5. When the disability is compensable through workmen's compensation or some other type of insurance program, an additional set of societal expectations—an extension of the role expectations discussed above—are applied to this category of disabled persons: *First, he is expected to focus upon physical recovery and return to gainful employment rather than live on compensation.* As a result, he must never get involved in litigation. Emphasis upon compensation is socially disapproved because the amount of compensation is maximum only when the amount of permanent disability is maximum. The disabled who is interested in maximizing the compensation he is to receive is not motivated to minimize his disability (that is, to get as well as is medically possible) and thus fails to fulfill one of the basic expectations of the sick role. He is not subsequently willing to "make the most" out of his remaining abilities or to "pull himself together" and go on performing his social roles as well as possible. Of course, this pattern of behavior may persist only up to the time that the case is settled; after that time, the disabled may become a "model" actor. *Second, he is supposed to seek the best available medical care to aid him in regaining the maximum functioning that is realistically recoverable instead of seeking out physicians who will emphasize the disability and testify in court to raise the amount of compensation. Moreover, he is expected to avail himself of rehabilitation, if such services are indicated, and to cooperate with every rehabilitative effort aimed at returning him to gainful employment and to a satisfactory level of performance in the other social roles.*

From Rehabilitation to What?

Not all who assume the disabled role necessarily assume the rehabilitant role, either by choice or because they are not permitted to assume it. Those who never become rehabilitants fall into two major categories: First, those with a slight or moderate disability and the cultural, social, sociopsychological, and personality attributes that permit them to fulfill the "ideal" sociocultural expectations. They are able to accept their disability to the extent that is necessary and to use their remaining abilities in order to resume their vocational as well as other social roles as soon as they are medically improved. They usually seek competent medical care and respond well to it; and while they are disabled, they become only minimally handicapped. Second, those who are old, severely disabled, unskilled and poorly educated (and often black) and are therefore very poor vocational rehabilitation risks, since they are most often unplaceable. Because they have little chance of appearing in "success statistics" and because they are often not interested in returning to work, they are usually rejected from rehabilitation programs as "unmotivated" either immediately or after a short diagnostic period. This category of people is practically doomed to remain burdened by severe disabilities (which could probably be decreased and controlled), since they usually receive poor medical care during the acute phases of their condition and are rarely given a chance later to benefit from physical rehabilitation. Here, of course, the question could be raised as to whether or not this category of disabled "needs" rehabilitation and help except in the minds of physicians and social workers. While it may be true that they themselves may not necessarily think they "need" rehabilitation, it must be remembered that recognition of a need requires a certain level of knowledge and awareness of alternatives. There may be considerable debate about whether or not they "need" vocational rehabilitation, but there can be little doubt they would benefit from it.

There is also considerable controversy over what constitutes the *optimum timing* for rehabilitation after the onset of the illness, but a considerable degree of agreement in rehabilitation personnel's conceptualization of the rehabilitant role.[71] Here again there are no systematic studies empirically validating the rehabilitant role, so we cannot describe the spectrum of variation in rehabilitant behavior when an individual does assume this role. Therefore, we shall have to limit ourselves to rehabilitation personnel's expectations of how these roles should be fulfilled. Of course, there may be variation within each occupational category of rehabilitation personnel (for example, between physicians and occupational therapists, or between physicians and social workers) in their conceptualization of the disabled or the rehabilitant role; furthermore, there may be variation among physiatrists, vocational counselors, or social workers in their expectations of how the disabled should act. But we do not possess information even about this type of variability. With these limitations in mind, we may consider the "ideal" role expectations of a rehabilitant.

1. He must be actively involved in his rehabilitation and in essence be an agent of change rather than a passive object in the hands of the rehabilitation team. He must not only comply with suggestions or cooperate with the team members' efforts, but also innovate and improvise new ways to circumvent his physical restrictions.[72] The degree to which this ideal is enacted varies largely from rehabilitation setting to rehabilitation setting and according to the sociopsychological background of the disabled person. Middle and upper middle class disabled people may conform more closely to this role expectation because they have been accustomed to excercise a certain degree of mastery over their lives. Working and lower class disabled people, on the contrary, socialized to comply and follow orders and not to be self-reliant, particularly those whose prevalent mode of behavior has been passive compliance, may have difficulties fulfilling this expectation. When these people arrive at a rehabilitation center, they may perceive it as a hospital where passive compliance is required and rewarded. And despite the fact that the difference between the rehabilitation setting and a hospital has usually been briefly explained as well as the new set of expectations, they may also be rewarded for passive compliance, especially by the custodial personnel with whom they may better identify and relate. Thus, because of often short and inadequate explanations as well as contradictory messages, they may fail to become "socialized" into the acceptable rehabilitant role.

There is, however, some evidence suggesting that the desirable rehabilitant role (in the eyes of rehabilitation workers) is a compliant one, with total acceptance of the rehabilitators' definitions of the disability as well as their formulations of rehabilitation goals. Therefore, any innovation or improvisation on the part of the rehabilitant must be in line with the set rehabilitation program if it is to be acceptable and rewarded. Because of this observed "dependency" orientation, sometimes creative, well-educated disabled persons withdraw from a rehabilitation agency.[73]

2. Because in assuming the rehabilitant role a disabled person is

temporarily institutionalized, during his stay at the rehabilitation center *he is temporarily and conditionally exempted from the performance of his normal social roles and activities.* This exemption is granted on the condition that he will concentrate all his efforts on again being able to perform competently and as soon as possible his normal social roles, especially the vocational. There is, however, evidence indicating that the disabled who manage to keep up all their contacts with significant others and employers and who have not in fact entirely relinquished any of their social roles while being rehabilitated have a better chance for a successful rehabilitation outcome.[74]

Some sociologists have been questioning the content of the rehabilitant role because an individual assumes that role within a particular setting—some type of rehabilitation facility, usually a rehabilitation center. As a consequence, a certain number of tasks and duties that result from the internal rules and regulations of the particular rehabilitation facility may or may not coincide with the "ideal" rehabilitation requirements or each rehabilitant's personal needs and goals. Because of these possible incongruencies, a disabled person may be rehabilitating himself as much as he wishes and in the areas that he wishes, but fail to rehabilitate himself according to the judgment and the criteria of the rehabilitation team. Some members of the team may also be urging the rehabilitants to achieve and improve in those areas more "functional" for the institution than the individual, since they lead to less trouble for the custodial personnel.[75] And some types of behavior may be discouraged or negatively sanctioned not so much because they are not helpful for the final rehabilitation outcome, but because they tend to disrupt institutional routines and interfere with "smooth" functioning.[76] These observations raise a number of other questions: When a disabled person is "successfully rehabilitated," what is he prepared for? Is he more or less fitted to become reintegrated into society than those who are partially rehabilitated, only subjectively rehabilitated or who have been refused rehabilitation services? What does it mean when a disabled person has failed to become rehabilitated or has been refused rehabilitation? We shall examine these questions in detail in Chapters 6 and 7. Next, we turn to a close study of the sociology and social psychology of disability and rehabilitation.

NOTES

1. Julius A. Roth, *Timetables* (Indianapolis: Bobbs-Merrill, 1963), p. xviii and throughout the book.
2. It is questionable whether or not anyone is perfectly healthy from a clinical point of view. One may be, however, healthy to the extent that he functions adequately in all his roles without difficulty or impediment and without experiencing any type of incapacitating pain.
3. Saxon Graham, "Sociological Aspects of Health and Illness," in Howard E. Freeman, Sol Levine, and Leo G. Reeder (eds.), *Handbook of Modern Sociology* (Chicago: Rand McNally, 1964), p. 312. The concept of "optimum" physical, emotional, or social functioning is quite elusive, even in the case of optimum physical functioning, by far the most tangible and measurable one. There can be a variety of optimum physical functionings for different ages, environmental conditions, "natural" biological cycles, "normal" variations, and finally types and content of activities that may be used as criteria, so that the concept is not a useful ideal construct.
4. Thomas J. Scheff, *Being Mentally Ill: A Sociological Theory* (Chicago: Aldine, 1966), pp. 105–27.
5. Raymond S. Duff and August B. Hollingshead, *Sickness and Society* (New York: Harper & Row, 1968). In some of the case studies presented in this book, the first complaints connected with a serious illness were "underdefined" and neglected by the first doctor consulted; see especially pp. 109, 311, 314–15.
6. Some people have pointed out that if illness were measured objectively on the basis of signs or conditions that can be labeled "clinical entities," the majority of the population might be ill. See Irving Kenneth Zola, "Some Effects of Assumptions Underlying Sociomedical Investigations," in Gerald Gordon (ed.), *Proceedings of the Conference on Medical Sociology and Disease Control* (New York: National Tuberculosis Association, 1966), pp. 9–17. And if all those whose incipient symptoms could not be diagnosed were added, probably everyone would be a medical case (as the Sterling County studies have concluded)—and the concepts of health and illness would become meaningless.
7. Scheff, *op. cit.*, pp. 178–87.

8. For a more detailed discussion of the doctor's views of disease and the patient, see David Mechanic, *Medical Sociology* (New York: Free Press, 1968), pp. 90–114. Mechanic points out that neither the "ideal" nor the statistical norms of "perfect" health are so clearly defined that all doctors can make consistent and uniform judgments. On the contrary, there is a considerable degree of variability from doctor to doctor and from case to case.

9. John Maclachlan, "Cultural Factors in Health and Disease," in E. Gartly Jaco (ed.), *Patients, Physicians and Illness* (New York: Free Press, 1958), pp. 94–96; Irving Kenneth Zola, "Culture and Symptoms—An Analysis of Patients Presenting Symptoms," *American Sociological Review,* 31, 5 (October 1966), 615–18.

10. The discussion of the Guatemala example is taken from a written communication to the author by Dr. David Kallen, scientific administrator at NICHHD, included in his comments to the first draft of this chapter.

11. The breakdown of this percentage is as follows: 36.3% had a mild symptom formation; 21.8%, a moderate symptom formation; and 23.4% were mentally impaired. Despite considerable methodological controversy over these findings, they probably give a fairly accurate and valid picture. See Leo Srole, Thomas S. Langner, Stanley T. Michael, Marvin K. Opler, and Thomas A. C. Rennie, *Mental Health in the Metropolis* (New York: McGraw-Hill, 1962), vol. I, pp. 138–45.

12. Irving K. Zola, "Socio-cultural Factors in the Seeking of Medical Care: A Progress Report," *Transcultural Psychiatric Research,* no. 14 (April 1963), 64–65.

13. Richard J. Ossenberg, "The Experience of Deviance in the Patient Role: A Study of Class Differences," *Journal of Health and Human Behavior,* 3, 4 (Winter 1962), 277–82.

14. Greece is a typical example of such cultural values prevailing among all social strata except perhaps the upper middle and upper class. See Constantina Safilios-Rothschild, "Sociopsychological Aspects of Psychiatric Practice in Greece," *Transcultural Psychiatric Research,* 4 (October 1967), 177–78; and Constantina Safilios-Rothschild, "Deviance and Mental Illness in the Greek Family," *Family Process,* 7, 1 (March 1968), 110–12.

15. Edward A. Suchman, "Social Patterns of Illness and Medical Care," *Journal of Health and Human Behavior,* 6 (Spring 1965), 7.

16. Lee Rainwater, "The Lower Class: Health, Illness and Medical Institutions" (background paper prepared for a study of medical facilities planning conducted by Anselm L. Strauss for the

Institute of Policy Studies, March 1965); also Duff and Hollingshead, *op. cit.*; and Eliot Freidson, *Patients' Views of
Medical Practice* (New York: Russell Sage Foundation, 1961).
17. Talcott Parsons, "Definitions of Health and Illness in the Light
of American Values and Social Structure," in Jaco, *op. cit.*, p.
176.
18. Michael Kenny, "Social Values and Health in Spain: Some
Preliminary Considerations," *Human Organization*, 21 (Winter
1962–1963), 280–84.
19. Sam Schulman and Anne M. Smith, "The Concept of 'Health'
Among Spanish-speaking Villagers of New Mexico and Colorado," *Journal of Health and Human Behavior*, 4 (Winter
1963), 228–32.
20. Barbara Baumann, "Diversities in Conceptions of Health and
Physical Fitness," *Journal of Health and Human Behavior*,
2, 1 (Spring 1961), 40–46; and Dorian Apple, "How Laymen
Define Illness," *Journal of Health and Human Behavior*, 1,
3 (Fall 1960), 219–25. In both these studies all respondents
were middle class; and in the latter one, symptoms had to be
of recent origin. See also Zola, "Socio-cultural Factors in the
Seeking of Medical Care," *op. cit.*; and Irving Kenneth Zola,
"Illness Behavior of the Working Class: Implications and
Recommendations," in Arthur B. Shostak and William Gomberg
(eds.), *Blue Collar World* (Englewood Cliffs, N.J.: Prentice-
Hall, 1964), pp. 354–55. Zola found that interference with
specific vocational activities is the reason for seeking medical
care in the case of Americans of Anglo-Saxon origin, but not
for those of Irish or Italian origin. Educational and social class
similarities, however, blurred ethnic distinctions. Thus, in the
latter study he shows that middle class Irish, Italian, and Anglo-
Saxon men came to see a physician because of an "interference
with vocation or a vocational activity" and because of "the
nature and quality of the symptoms," while working class men
of all ethnic groups came because of an "interpersonal crisis,"
"social interference," or "the presence of sanctioning."
21. Safilios-Rothschild "Deviance and Mental Illness in the Greek
Family," *op. cit.*
22. The scientific explanation of illness based on the "germ" theory
aided in shifting the responsibility for falling sick from the
individual to neutral external factors. However, the recognition
of the importance of sociopsychological factors for all illnesses
and the theoretical conceptualization of illness as deviant behavior (and possibly an unconscious or semiconscious escape
from normal responsibilities) has partially shifted the responsibility for having become ill back on the ailing individual.
Presently, patients, especially those in categories such as factory

workers or college students, may be suspected by the examining doctor as well as by employers, professors, etc., of being potential malingerers.

23. Jane Belo, "The Balinese Temper," in Douglas G. Haring (ed.), *Personal Milieu and Cultural Milieu* (Syracuse, N.Y.: Syracuse University Press, 1956), pp. 160–61.

24. Maclachlan, *op. cit.*, p. 96.

25. David Mechanic and Edmund H. Volkart, "Stress, Illness Behavior, and the Sick Role," *American Sociological Review,* 26, 1 (February 1961), 51–58.

26. On social status, see Parsons, *op. cit.*; and Edward A. Suchman, "Stages of Illness and Medical Care," *Journal of Health and Human Behavior,* 6, 3 (Fall 1965), 114–28. On level of education, a beautiful example of the "definition of symptoms" is provided by pregnant women who, depending on their sociopsychological characteristics (such as education, aspiration for mobility, and sick role expectations), assume or do not assume the sick role. See William R. Rosengreen, "The Sick Role During Pregnancy: A Note on Research in Progress," *Journal of Health and Human Behavior,* 3, 3 (Fall 1962), 213–18. Another study indicates that education is more important than social class in determining an individual's level of health knowledge, and the latter influences illness behavior. See Julian Samora, Lyle Saunders, and Richard F. Larson, "Knowledge About Specific Diseases in Four Selected Samples," *Journal of Health and Human Behavior,* 3, 3 (Fall 1962), 176–85. Also, Kutner found a negative relationship between level of education and delay in seeking medical care, especially in the case of cancer symptoms. See Bernard Kutner and Gerald Gordon, "Seeking Care for Cancer," *Journal of Health and Human Behavior,* 2, 3 (Fall 1961), 176–77. On religion, see David Mechanic, "Religion, Religiosity and Illness Behavior," *Human Organization,* 22, 3 (Fall 1963), 202–8. Mechanic found that Jewish populations show a greater tendency to seek medical care than Protestant and Catholic populations, particularly among middle class people. Income level has sometimes been included in the computation of the socioeconomic status index, and in these cases we do not know to what extent the relationships to illness behavior are due to the income level or the level of educational accomplishment or the type of occupation. See Suchman, "Stages of Illness and Medical Care," *op. cit.* One study at least has, however, shown that delay in seeking medical care is significantly and variably affected by income level. See Kutner and Gordon, *op. cit.* On occupational and social status, Kutner found a negative relationship between socioeconomic status and length of delay in seeking medical

care for cancer symptoms but not other symptoms; see Kutner and Gordon, *op. cit.*, pp. 175–76. Suchman, on the other hand, found that persons of lower socioeconomic status report a slightly higher rate of incapacitation than those in higher status levels but that there are no differences in the degree of severity and concern attributed to these symptoms and in their being interpreted as illness. However, their lay referral system tended to interpret symptoms as serious illness more often in high status than in low status persons. See Suchman, "Stages of Illness and Medical Care," *op. cit.*, pp. 119–20.

27. On inclination to adopt the sick role, see Mechanic and Volkart, *op. cit.*, pp. 51–58. Mechanic and Volkart define "inclination to adopt the sick role" as "a more or less learned pattern of behavior influenced by situational contingencies, [indicating] the probability with which individuals will react to a given set of symptoms." Therefore, those more inclined to adopt the sick role would tend to define a wider spectrum of symptoms as illness and to seek medical care quickly. On self-reliance, see Derek L. Philips, "Self-reliance and the Inclination to Adopt the Sick Role," *Social Forces*, 43, 4 (May 1965), 555–63; and Mechanic and Volkart, *op. cit.,* p. 55. On kind of social structure, see Suchman, "Social Patterns of Illness and Medical Care," *op. cit.*, pp. 7–14. On cultural values, see John A. Ross, "Social Class and Medical Care," *Journal of Health and Human Behavior*, 3, 1 (Spring 1962), 35–40. It has been also found that belief in the efficacy of medical care is positively related to income and education; see John P. Kirscht *et al.*, "A National Study of Health Beliefs," *Journal of Health and Human Behavior*, 7, 4 (Winter 1966), 253.

28. Kutner found that when the level of general medical knowledge is high, people are less concerned about noncancer symptoms than about cancer symptoms and vice versa. And in the case of cancer symptoms, the least delay of treatment was found among those who had the highest degree of cancer information. In Kutner and Gordon, *op. cit.*, pp. 177–78.

29. Gene N. Levine, "Anxiety About Illness: Psychological and Social Bases," *Journal of Health and Human Behavior*, 3, 1 (Spring 1962), 30–34.

30. Suchman, "Stages of Illness and Medical Care," *op. cit.*, pp. 122–25. See an analogy in Field's data: Mark Field, *Doctor and Patient in Soviet Russia* (Cambridge, Mass.: Harvard University Press, 1957).

31. Freidson, *op. cit.*, especially pp. 142–51.

32. Petroni found that visibility and urgency of a condition automatically legitimized the sick role and the significant others' acceptance of the ill state without any doubts. See Frank A.

Petroni, "The Influence of Age, Sex and Chronicity in Perceived Legitimacy to the Sick Role" (paper presented at the Midwest Sociological Association meetings, Omaha, April 1968).

33. Freidson, *op. cit.*, pp. 150–51.
34. Another study lumping lay consultants together has shown that while women tend to discuss their symptoms with others more than men, their symptoms are less often interpreted by their lay consultants as indicative of a serious illness. See Suchman, "Stages of Illness and Medical Care," *op. cit.*, p. 120.
35. Frank A. Petroni, "Significant Others and Illness Behavior: A Much-neglected Sick Role Contingency" (paper presented at the Southwestern Sociological Association meetings, Dallas, April 12, 1968).
36. Gerald D. Bell and Derek L. Philips, "Playing the Sick Role and Avoidance of Responsibility" (paper read at the Sixth World Congress of Sociology, Evian, France, September 4–10, 1966).
37. The author found that only when the mentally disturbed symptoms of a spouse were directed against the marital relationship or the "normal" spouse did the latter define the condition as requiring medical care and hospitalization. See Safilios-Rothschild, "Deviance and Mental Illness in the Greek Family," *op. cit.*; also in Bursten's study, wives suggested hospitalization for their husbands—who had long had untreated physical symptoms—when their marital relationship was thrown into serious disequilibrium. See Ben Bursten, "Family Dynamics, the Sick Role, and Medical Hospital Admissions," *Family Process*, 4, 2 (September 1965), 206–15.
38. J. D. Stoeckle and G. E. Davidson, "Bodily Complaints and Other Symptoms of Depressive Reaction," *The Journal of the American Medical Association*, 180, 2 (April 14, 1962), 134–36. See also George L. Engel, "Is Grief a Disease?" *Psychosomatic Medicine*, 23, 1 (January–February 1961), 18–19.
39. Arthur H. Schmale, Jr., "Relationship of Separation and Depression to Disease," *Psychosomatic Medicine*, 20, 4 (July–August 1958), 269–71; E. Lindemann, "The Meaning of Crisis in Individual and Family Living," *Teachers' College Record*, 57, 5 (February 1956), 310–15; and J. D. Stoeckle and G. E. Davidson, "The Use of 'Crisis' as an Orientation for the Study of Patients in a Medical Clinic," *Journal of Medical Education*, 37, 6 (June 1962), 604.
40. Norman G. Hawkins, Robert Davies, and Thomas H. Holmes, "Evidence of Psychosocial Factors in the Development of Pulmonary Tuberculosis," *American Review of Tuberculosis and Pulmonary Diseases*, 75, 5 (May 1957), 768–80.

41. Irving Kenneth Zola, "Sociocultural Factors in the Seeking of Medical Aid" (unpublished Ph.D. dissertation, Harvard University, 1962). Mechanic also writes that the finding showing that those who are ill have experienced stress cannot suffice for "an assertion of causality." See David Mechanic and Edmund H. Volkart, "Illness Behavior and Medical Diagnosis," *Journal of Health and Human Behavior*, 1, 2 (Summer 1960), 93–94.

42. The question still remains, of course, of why the emotional factors described led to physical rather than psychiatric illness. It may be that the presence of definite physical symptoms or other serious emotional difficulties (or an individual's personality organization, ego strength, etc.) will determine if and in what direction additional, complicating socioemotional stress will affect health. See Schmale, *op. cit.*, p. 271. Also it may be due to the lack of social acceptance of mental disorders in a society or in particular cultural groups. Emotional symptoms such as depression, anxiety, and feelings of inadequacy are often unacceptable because they connote weakness and because they imply an "internal" failing of the individual. Thus, a mentally disturbed individual may try to present his disorder in a more socially acceptable way, as a physical illness. See Safilios-Rothschild, "Deviance and Mental Illness in the Greek Family," *op. cit*; R. C. Behan *et al.*, "Disability Without Disease or Accident," *Archives of Environmental Health*, 12 (May 1966), 655–59; A. H. Hirschfeld and R. C. Behan, "The Accident Process: III. Disability: Acceptable and Unacceptable," *The Journal of the American Medical Association*, 197 (July 11, 1966), 85–89; and Barbara L. Blackwell, "Upper Middle Class Adult Expectations About Entering the Sick Role for Physical and Psychiatric Dysfunctions," *Journal of Health and Human Behavior*, 8, 2 (June 1967), 83–95.

43. Zola includes an excellent review of studies presenting relevant evidence in Irving Kenneth Zola, "Culture and Symptoms—an Analysis of Patients Presenting Symptoms," *American Sociological Review*, 31, 5 (October 1966), 615–17.

44. Mechanic found that only in the case of common, relatively familiar, predictable and probably nondangerous illnesses was illness behavior related to the afflicted person's tendency to adopt the sick role. See Mechanic and Volkart, "Illness Behavior and Medical Diagnosis," *op. cit.* Also, Suchman, "Stages of Illness and Medical Care," *op. cit.*, pp. 118–19.

45. Apple, *op. cit.*, pp. 224–25.

46. There is evidence that even in folk societies in which Western-style physicians are not yet quite accepted, they are usually consulted in the case of nonchronic, severe, incapacitating illnesses. See Harold A. Gould, "The Implications of Techno-

logical Change for Folk and Scientific Medicine," *American Anthropologist*, 59, 3 (1957), 507–16; and Charles John Erasmus, "Changing Folk Beliefs and the Relativity of Empirical Knowledge," *Southwestern Journal of Anthropology*, 8, 4 (1952), 411–28. See also Lionel S. Lewis, "Rational Behavior and the Treatment of Illness," *Journal of Health and Human Behavior*, 4 (Winter 1963), 239.

47. Freidson, *op. cit.*, pp. 140–51, 180–81.
48. *Ibid.*, pp. 140–42, 145–46; and Duff and Hollingshead, *op. cit.*
49. Talcott Parsons, *The Social System* (New York: Free Press, 1951), pp. 433–34.
50. Freidson, *op. cit.*, pp. 189–91.
51. Gerald Gordon, *Role Theory and Illness: A Sociological Perspective* (New Haven, Conn.: Yale University Press, 1966), pp. 99–101.
52. Parsons, *The Social System, op. cit.*, pp. 434–35.
53. Duff and Hollingshead, *op. cit.*, entire book, but especially pp. 217–47 (see, in particular, tables 30 and 32, pp. 234 and 236).
54. James Leo Walsh and Ray H. Elling, "Professionalism and the Poor—Structural Effects and Professional Behavior," *Journal of Health and Human Behavior*, 9, 1 (March 1968), 16–28.
55. John Clausen, "The Marital Relationship Antecedent to Hospitalization of a Spouse for Mental Illness" (paper presented at the Fourth World Congress of Sociology, Stresa, 1959); Charlotte Green Schwartz, "Perspectives on Deviance—Wives' Definitions of Their Husbands' Mental Illness," *Psychiatry*, 20, 3 (August 1957), 275–91; and Safilios-Rothschild, "Deviance and Mental Illness in the Greek Family," *op. cit.*
56. Safilios-Rothschild, "Deviance and Mental Illness in the Greek Family," *op. cit.*
57. A study by New *et al.*, has presented some data concerning the degree of agreement between a patient's evaluation of the degree of dependence he exhibits in the activities of daily living (ADL) compared with his spouse's, children's, and friends' evaluations, as well as that of the rehabilitation personnel. While their study does not deal specifically with the dynamic process taking place in each agreement-disagreement typology and its effects upon the rehabilitation of the disabled person, some implications could be hypothesized on the basis of their data. See Peter Kong-Ming New *et al.*, "The Support Structure of Heart and Stroke Patients: A Study of the Role of Significant Others in Patient Rehabilitation," *Social Science and Medicine*, 2, 2 (June 1968), 185–200.
58. Safilios-Rothschild, "The Reaction to Disability in Rehabilitation, *op. cit.*
59. For studies relating the effect of marital status or of some

aspect of the family system on definitions of disability and re-habilitation outcome, see discussion and notes in Chapter 7.

60. Medical as well as sociopsychological literature points out the importance of the "acceptance of the disability." For the former, see M. Grayson, "The Concept of 'Acceptance' in Physical Disability," *Military Surgeon*, 107 (September 1950), 221–26; D. A. Thom, C. F. Von Salzen, and A. Fromme, "Psychological Aspects of the Paraplegic Patient," *Medical Clinics of North America*, 30 (1946), 473–80; and Harry Prosen, "Physical Disability and Motivation," *Canadian Medical Association Journal,* 92 (June 12, 1965), 1264. For sociopsychological literature, see Theodor J. Litman, "Self-conception and Physical Rehabilitation," in Arnold M. Rose (ed.), *Human Behavior and Social Processes* (Boston: Houghton Mifflin, 1964), pp. 556–58; Edwin J. Thomas, "Problems of Disability From the Perspective of Role Theory," *Journal of Health and Human Behavior,* 7, 1 (Spring 1966), 5; and T. Dembo, G. Ladieu-Leviton, and B. A. Wright, "Acceptance of Loss Amputations," in J. F. Garrett (ed.), *Psychological Aspects of Physical Disability* (Washington, D.C.: Office of Vocational Rehabilitation, n.d.), Rehabilitation Service Series, no. 210, pp. 80–96.

61. Of course, sometimes quacks may in fact attend to and facilitate an often-neglected part of the rehabilitation process: the emotional rehabilitation. Sometimes a patient "cured" by the "miraculous" treatment of a quack is willing to accept his disability and go on living within the restrictions of his condition by using what ability remains. The element of faith or magic involved in a quack's treatment may sometimes help bring about psychological acceptance of the disability.

62. Herbert S. Rabinowitz and Spiro B. Mitsos, "Rehabilitation as Planned Social Change: A Conceptual Framework," *Journal of Health and Human Behavior,* 5, 1 (Spring 1964), 5–9.

63. Julius Roth, "The Treatment of Tuberculosis as a Bargaining Process," in Rose, *op. cit.,* pp. 575–88.

64. Walsh and Elling, *op. cit.*

65. The question of what is a "need" and who should define it was raised by Dr. Julius A. Roth, professor of sociology at the University of California, Davis, in his written commentary on the first draft of the book.

66. In Chapters 6 and 7 we shall see in detail the physicians' difficulties in making accurate evaluations of the extent of the disability present and of the potential of a particular disabled person, as well as some of the reasons for these inaccuracies.

67. Rainwater, *op. cit.*; Duff and Hollingshead, *op. cit.,* especially pp. 124–50, 283; and James K. Skipper, Jr., "Communication

ate:

and the Hospitalized Patient," in James K. Skipper, Jr., and Robert Leonard (eds.), *Social Interaction and Patient Care* (Philadelphia: Lippincott, 1965), pp. 61–82. The latter two studies mention that uneducated, lower class patients hesitate and are afraid to ask questions from doctors and that this attitude on their part increased further the communication gap between them and their treating physicians.

68. John R. Barry and Michael R. Malinovsky, *Client Motivation for Rehabilitation: A Review*, Rehabilitation Research Monograph Series, no. 1 (University of Florida, February 1965).

69. Gene G. Kassebaum and Barbara O. Baumann, "Dimensions of the Sick Role in Chronic Illness," *Journal of Health and Human Behavior*, 6, 1 (Spring 1965), 18–19.

70. Thomas, *op. cit.*, pp. 9–13; and Lawrence E. Schlesinger, "Disruptions in the Personal-Social System Resulting From Traumatic Disability," *Journal of Health and Human Behavior*, 6, 2 (Summer 1965), 95–98.

71. Research concerning the factors related to rehabilitation success suggests that "there probably is an optimum time for beginning rehabilitation. It should begin neither too soon nor too long after the injury." See Barry and Malinovsky, *op. cit.* Some writers have been lamenting the fact that five or seven years elapse between the onset of the disability and the beginning of rehabilitation. See Robert D. Wright, "Rehabilitation's Wave in the Future," *Archives of Physical Medicine and Rehabilitation* (August 1962), p. 395; and Jacobus tenBroek and Floyd W. Matson, *Hope Deferred: Public Welfare and the Blind* (Berkeley and Los Angeles: University of California Press, 1959), p. 176. However, some research has shown that one to two years should go by before rehabilitation is undertaken for optimum results. See Saad Z. Nagi *et al.*, "Back Disorders and Rehabilitation Achievement," *Journal of Chronic Diseases*, 18 (February 1965), 181–97, especially 188.

72. Szasz and Hollander, *op. cit.*, p. 585; and Eddy, *op. cit.*, p. 69.

73. Robert A. Scott, *The Making of Blind Men: A Study of Adult Socialization* (New York: Russell Sage Foundation, 1969), pp. 72–80, 108–10; and Fred A. Novak, *A Program for Serving the More Severely Disabled Individuals in Nebraska* (Lincoln, Neb.: Division of Rehabilitation Service, April 1965).

74. Rabinowitz and Mitsos, *op. cit.*, pp. 11–12.

75. There is often an actual dilemma between the therapeutic goals which ought to be primarily pursued and the custodial goals which ensure the efficient and smooth functioning of the intitution. The irrelevancy of the rehabilitation goals is also indicated by the fact that often "success" may be nothing more than the attainment of goals chosen by the rehabilitant rather

than those set by the institution. This, however, tends to be more accentuated the more the rehabilitation facility is operated as a total institution and to be less true the more permeated it is by a permissive philosophy. See Julius A. Roth and Elizabeth M. Eddy, *Rehabilitation for the Unwanted* (New York: Atherton, 1967), pp. 78–80, 142, 170–71.

76. Actually Roth and Eddy report that sometimes a rehabilitant has to become rebellious and "dysfunctional" to the institutional peace if he wants to get things done so that his rehabilitation may progress. *Ibid.*, p. 142.

CHAPTER 3

The Sociology
and Social Psychology
of Disability

In this chapter we shall examine those aspects
of the disabled's career which are relevant to
its final stages; that is, beginning when he is
faced with the possibility (or certainty) of some
degree of permanent disability. The likelihood
of remaining permanently disabled (even to a
small degree) precipitates more or less serious
reactions and demands more or less basic
psychological readjustments on the part of the
disabled, the nature of which depend partly
upon the type and degree of the disability and
partly upon the way the disabled define it.
Therefore, in order to understand the disabled's
career patterns and the type of reorganization
they often must bring about in their self-con-

cept, we must take into consideration two important typologies: a disability typology and a typology of the disabled's profiles.

At the social level, the presence of a disability, partially because of the limitations it imposes upon the disabled's range of activities and behavior, but mainly because of the nondisabled's reaction to the disability, renders the disabled "deviant." Such a societal labeling, attributed to the disabled regardless of whether they define themselves as disabled or "deviant," considerably influences interactions between the disabled and the nondisabled and the latter's chances for societal integration. Furthermore, whether or not the disabled and his significant others accept the disability and the "deviance" label further modifies the mode of his relating to the nondisabled as well as his interest in and capacity to integrate into the "normal" society. And finally, we shall examine the degree of prejudice directed toward all disabled as well as the types of disabilities which are more or less stigmatized in their variation from culture to culture, from subculture to subculture, from social class to social class, from type of family to type of family, and from individual to individual depending upon cultural values, beliefs, stereotypes, and upon social structures and requirements.

For the sake of conceptual clarity, the different social aspects of disability will be grouped and treated under three major headings: disability at the personality level, at the social system level, and at the culture level. In each of these sections we will analyze disability with a different central point of reference, although as we shall see, the analysis at these three levels is interrelated and a considerable number of conceptual junctions can be found.

The Disability at the Personality Level

In order to examine disability at this level, we must first point out the direct impact that a disability has upon one's body image. With the exception of congenital disabilities or those experienced in early childhood which oblige the afflicted individual to incorporate the disability into the formation of his body image, all other disabilities require changes in the already-established body image. Such changes may be overt and dramatic, as in the case of amputations or disfigurements, or more or less subtle and gradual, as in the case of organic chronic diseases.

Body image includes a conception of appearance to others; a conception of physical stamina, capacities, and endurance; a conception of degree of attractiveness and therefore differential emotions attached to preferred or admired bodily assets or characteristics; and a conception of what constitutes a state of physical "normality" or "well-being."[1] Disability may affect one or more of these body conceptions simultaneously and thus oblige the disabled person to reconsider his past body image because his earlier conceptions no longer coincide with his present sensations and experiences. For example, a chronic disease may decrease physical endurance appreciably, so that an individual cannot work many hours at a time and requires long hours of rest, whereas he was formerly able to work long hours without feeling fatigued. Paraplegia may seriously impair mobility; a leg amputation, although it may not significantly impair a young woman's mobility, may seriously upset her body image because her once shapely legs were greatly admired and therefore quite central to her self-concept as an attractive woman.

Available evidence indicates that there is a considerable degree of resistance to altering one's body image, especially when the necessary alterations are negative, disagreeable, and devaluative to one's self-esteem.[2] An interesting exception is provided by positive and desirable changes. Examples of such changes may be individuals undergoing corrective plastic surgery for birth defects or undesirable facial characteristics (too big or too small a nose) or those who changed from a handicapped to a nonhandicapped position (cured cardiac cases and cases of arrested tuberculosis). However, we do not have much understanding of the dynamics involved in incorporating desirable changes into the body image. What we do know is that persons with facial disfigurements who had adequately incorporated their disability in their self-concept were satisfied with improvement achieved through plastic surgery.[3] The opposite holds true for those who had never accepted their disability and had not incorporated it into their self-concept, since they were hoping for a total cure as the outcome of surgery. This finding suggests that probably desirable changes can be rather easily incorporated into the body image and self-concept if the person eagerly discards the previously held negative self-images. Also, amputated individuals experience a "real" and not an imagined "phantom limb" because of an almost physiological tendency and need to keep the body image and bodily sensations intact even after significant changes have come about.[4]

The degree of resistance to incorporating bodily changes into the body image and later into the self-concept will depend to some extent upon the practical consequences of the experienced change but mainly upon the symbolic meaning the physical change comes to have for the disabled person. There is, of course, a normal stage of mourning over the experienced loss, a period of a situational reaction. After this initial stage, however, the disabled person may view his disability as a misfortune that has reduced him to being a "half-person," or he may come to accept it as a part of living. In such cultures as the American, in which the body beautiful is highly valued and people are not prepared to accept psychological suffering as a part of living, it is difficult to accept physical disability, to change one's values and body image accordingly, and to live with the disability.[5] Whenever a person's appearance is changed as a result of disability, the mode of interpersonal relations will also be greatly influenced. These marked changes in the interaction process will finally affect the individual's self-perception, although the extent and depth of such an effect will depend greatly upon his willingness to perceive these changes and interpret them as significant.

It seems that the more an individual has a chance to hide his disability or the more the resulting limitations are diffused and mal-defined, the more he tends to avoid integrating the necessary changes into his body image and self-concept. Also, the more readily and specifically he can evaluate his abilities and disabilities, the more he may be willing to "accept" his disability and bring about the necessary changes (unless the assessed disabilities are too severe or too threatening). Thus, it has been found that an amputation was incorporated into the disabled's self-concept more adequately and with less general damage than an all-pervasive illness such as tuberculosis.[6] This is probably due to the greater ease with which the individual can evaluate and to a considerable degree control the limitations resulting from amputation. In the case of tuberculosis as well as of similar disabilities, the uncertainty of prognosis and of the extent of limitations may keep the individual in a state of anxiety, since he may be continuously fluctuating between extreme optimism and extreme pessimism about his condition. Accordingly, he may hope that he will get well completely, he may try to hide his disability and refrain from incorporating his illness into his self-concept, or he may despair about the eventual outcome and bring about more drastic changes in his self-concept than are realistically warranted.

Among those disabled who have always placed great value on bodily integrity, strength, and attractive appearance and who therefore tend to view a physical disability as a misfortune and a disaster, the most probable reaction to an incurred disability may be the denial of its existence. Such individuals desperately attempt to remain "normal" and nondisabled; and in order to prove their "normality" try to keep the predisability patterns and activities of their lives as unchanged as possible. Depsite the fact that these persons are often admired in activistic and optimistic cultures such as the American, they never "come to terms" with their disability. Because some aspects at least of their lives and interactions with others are necessarily changed, they will never be "adjusted," contented men.[7] They will always be met with more or less significant frustrations because they will never take into consideration their inescapable physical limitations and disability-determined restrictions. While it is true that a certain degree of physical handicapping may be overcome through sheer will power (for example, by working while in pain), the disability and its resulting limitations cannot be entirely avoided by "making-believe" that they do not exist. If a worker cannot lift an object over a certain weight and tries to go beyond this limit in his effort to appear normal, he may only further injure his back and increase the degree of his physical disability.

It is possible, however, that the mechanism of denial may enable these disabled to become rehabilitated up to a certain point, since they are extremely motivated to "get well" and return to their former job and mode of life. Their motivation, however, tends to be misplaced, since it drives them toward complete normalcy. And at the point at which it becomes obvious that no matter how hard they try, some limitations remain, they can lose interest altogether in the rehabilitation which forces them to face undesirable realities.[8] If their physical limitations permit them to resume their former jobs and to live more or less the lives they led before their disability, supported in their efforts by congruent actions on the part of their significant others, they may be fairly well "adjusted" to their disability. If, however, their disability does not permit them to function in their previous jobs (or they are denied those jobs because of it), or they no longer are sexually potent, or their significant others' definition of them has changed so that they are now clearly considered disabled and deviant, they may go from doctor to doctor and treatment to treatment in the vain hope of complete recovery.[9] They may finally become quite alienated and disturbed and go on refusing to be anything less than "normal" and to learn how to live with their disabilities.[10]

Some disabled persons who greatly value their physique and their strength are able to accept the fact that something has changed in their appearance or in their bodily sensations and physical capacities without being plunged into helplessness and despair. They can still feel that they are "worthwhile" persons who can go on living a meaningful and full life by capitalizing upon their unchanged capacities, physical and nonphysical. They are able to change their values concerning the body whole and the body beautiful as well as health in general by enlarging them so as to encompass their present state of health as acceptable, although not ideal.[11] Finally, a third type of disabled seem to be able to bring about the "necessary" changes in body image all too easily and painlessly and even eagerly accept physical limitations and restrictions that could be overcome. This category of disabled usually makes no attempt to minimize the degree of disability and to utilize the remaining physical capacities to the maximum.

At this point it must be said that the distinction among the three prevalent modes of reacting to physical disability and incorporating such disability into the body image cannot always be made clearly or accurately. It is not always easy to determine the extent to which a physical handicap may be overcome by sheer motivation and will. Thus, some disabled persons may be encouraged to deny their disability when they are urged by different therapists to use their abilities and not to concentrate on their ills and pains; others may interpret the therapists' advice to "accept" the fact that they are disabled as meaning they can now take on the disabled status and capitalize upon it without having to make any further effort to perform tasks and roles to the extent of their remaining capacities. It seems, then, that the therapists' emphasis upon either the need to use the remaining resources or the need to accept the physical disability may be easily misinterpreted according to the disabled person's needs and predisability personality. This is more probable if the medical staff does not take the time to clarify not only the extent of the disability and its resulting restrictions, but also the capacities and abilities remaining. Acceptance of the disability in the context of this book will refer to a relatively *optimal condition* in which the disabled person brings about such changes in his body image (and possibly his self-concept) as are absolutely necessary so that reality is not sacrificed. There is general consensus in the medical as well as in the sociological literature that this "realistic" type of acceptance is the reaction most conducive to successful rehabilitation and societal reintegration (See Chapter 6 for detailed discussion and references). There is some evidence, however, that at least some of the disabled who have "rejected" their disability, according to the criteria used by rehabilitation agencies, are successfully rehabilitated vocationally and socially, and without the help of any agency.[12] Also there is some evidence that physicians and other rehabilitation team members hold their own norms as to what constitutes a "normal" reaction. Any deviance from this norm is disapproved of, even when the deviance is "positive." Thus, if the disabled person can accept his disability and adjust well to it, he may be met with disbelief and mistrust by the very people who encourage him to do exactly what he did.[13]

In order to explain this differential degree of incorporation of change brought about by the presence of physical disability, the phenomenon must be examined in a wider perspective, namely, that of self-concept. A person's body image—including physical appearance, bodily sensations, beliefs and emotions about the body—makes up part of his self-concept. The importance of body image within the self-concept will vary mainly according to the nature and intensity of values and emotions invested in it.[14] The "centrality" of physical appearance and physical strength in an individual's self-concept; that is, "the degree to which they determine the person's self-esteem," varies from person to person.[15] In the case of a very attractive woman who primarily thinks of herself as a beautiful woman or of an unskilled worker employed in heavy labor who primarily sees himself as a physically tough and strong man, body image is of crucial importance to self-concept. In contrast, a plain-looking college professor who primarily sees himself as an intellectual has most probably received psychological rewards, satisfaction, and pride from his intellectual accomplishments rather than from his strength or beauty. Therefore, his body image may not be imbued with very intense emotions. For this reason, physical changes which do not seriously interfere with his mobility or his ability to perform his professional tasks may be inconvenient but not shattering or threatening, since they tend to be peripheral to his self-concept.

Generally, when the body image does not have a prominent and central position in a disabled's self-concept, the degree of unavoidable physical disability as well as the necessary changes that must be brought about in body image and self-concept can be assessed quite realistically. The nature and degree of the physical disability, however, also seem to play an important role. Thus, when the nature and degree of physical disability are such that survival is threatened or mobility seriously interfered with, even the disabled who did not primarily value their body image may show great resistance to incorporating such changes into their self-concept.

When the body image has always occupied central importance in the disabled's self-concept, impeding changes due to the incurred physical disability will be greatly resisted because such changes would mean self-devaluation.[16] These disabled will refuse to accept the possibility that they may now be something less than "normal" (less than what they used to be) and will strive continuously to eliminate all disability residuals by resorting to scientific, parascientific, and "magical" treatments. When they finally are forced to face the fact that they are disabled, they may "make-believe" that their disability does not exist and reject it completely, at the expense of reality, attempting to live their predisability life as if nothing had happened.[17] The devaluating change in the body image is avoided at any price because it would also mean a drastic change in self-concept, a threatening and self-diminishing change that cannot be tolerated.

Whether or not the individual's "core" self-concept can ever change radically has been somewhat of a controversy within the symbolic interaction school of social psychologists. The prevailing notion, however, seems to be that presented by such social psychologists as Shibutani and Strauss. They propose that the self-concept once fixed tends to be self-sustaining and persistent through a continuous process of selective perception by which inconsistencies or undesirable changes are discarded, explained away, or go by unnoticed.[18] The individual usually needs to feel that his core identity persists despite everyday changes, and the effect of persistence of identity is realized only to the extent that the individual is willing and interested in maintaining a feeling of "sameness" and consistency about who he is and how he behaves.

We shall now attempt to explain the disabled's basic modes of reacting to disability by applying the above theory of continuity in the core self-concept. When the afflicted part of the part image or the values and emotions attached to it are not central to the disabled's self-concept, acceptance of the disability is relatively easy because, unless it is a serious condition, the required changes can be more or less localized in some self-images (which are always more flexible) without the individual feeling that his core identity has basically changed. The disabled is thus permitted (because of the peripheral importance of the afflicted part of the body image) to think that he is basically the same person, but because of his physical disability must make some changes and adjustments in order to successfully cope with it.

When, however, the afflicted part of the body image as well as the values and emotions attached to it are central to the disabled's self-concept, the physical disability is usually rejected because its acceptance would require such a major change in self-concept that he would have to experience a serious discontinuity in his identity—a discontinuity that may lead to a negative, devalued identity depriving him of self-esteem and self-acceptance. Because of the great threat it represents to the disabled's identity, the impending change is therefore discarded at the price of reality.

Finally, Shibutani's and Strauss' theoretical frameworks explain why the third category of disabled persons not only are able to tolerate a discontinuity in their identity, but seem to welcome and even embrace it when "objectively" (medically) it is not necessary to do so. Such persons are motivated to perceive and capitalize upon a discontinuity in their identity. They claim that their disability has brought about "shattering" changes, while exactly the same type and degree of disability may well have been "rejected" or "accepted" by other disabled. Usually, they seem to be motivated by a negative predisability self-concept, reinforced by social and/or occupational maladjustments and failures, to perceive and overemphasize their physical disability and the resulting "necessarily drastic" changes.

An individual may have a negative predisability self-concept regardless of whether or not any part of the body image and the values and emotions attached to it have played a central role in its organization. Furthermore, it is known that if a person is sufficiently motivated, any part of the body image that becomes afflicted can be invested with the appropriate emotional meaning and significance. Thus, the disabled person and his "significant others" can be convinced that its loss or incapacity is important enough to bring about a major discontinuity in the disabled's indentity. The disabled, by unconsciously or semiconsciously (but only rarely completely consciously, as in the case of the true malingerer) wishing to bring about a change in his disagreeable and often intolerable negative self-concept, finds the physical disability the "perfect alibi." By now conceiving of himself as disabled, he no longer blames himself for his failures, but instead blames the disability. The discontinuity in identity from "normal," "healthy" to "disabled" is desirable, because it makes it possible for the individual to reconcile himself with negative, unacceptable life experiences, or socially undesirable needs (such as intense dependency) or wishes (to stop working before retirement age and have his wife be the breadwinner).[19]

Disabled persons who react in this way are often referred to in the literature as those who derive "secondary gains" from their disability.[20] Data from case studies indicate that this reaction is rather frequent among those over 45 years of age, especially if they are unskilled or semiskilled workers with histories suggesting some kind of occupational maladjustment.[21] Because the presence of the disability and its resulting changes serve a definite purpose in the personality organization of these persons, they may consciously or unconsciously decide that their identity has to be discontinued regardless of the severity of the disability. They may even resist further medical treatment or other rehabilitation services if they fear that such treatment or services could bring about changes that would seriously challenge their newly adopted disabled identity.

Up to now we have been conceptualizing about disability as an entity, since all disabilities have common features and often similar consequences for the lives of afflicted persons regardless of specific medical differences. However, some characteristics of the disability may vary significantly, and this variation may have significant effects on the degree to which the disabled can incorporate it into their body image and self-concept.

TABLE 1.
Disability Typology

Age at Onset	Nature of Onset	Prognosis	Visibility & Stigma	Area & Degree of Impairment	Nature of Functional Limitation	Financial Reward
Birth, child-hood	Sudden (accident, discovery of disease)	Stable (no further medical care or diet required)	Visible, stigmatized (facial)	ADL none slight moderate severe	Clear-cut General-ized, diffuse	Compensable Noncompensable
Adolescence, early adulthood	Insidious (slow progression of symptoms)	Stable if controlled (medical care, diet, exercise)	Visible, nonstigmatized (amputation, paralysis)	Social none slight moderate severe		
Adulthood						
Later years (after age 45)		Degenerative (but slow progress)	Non-visible, stigmatized (TB)	Vocational none slight moderate severe		
		Terminal (imminent death)	Non-visible, non-stigmatized (heart disease)			

Table 1 presents some possible variations in disability according to seven criteria: (1) age at onset of disability, (2) nature of onset, (3) prognosis, (4) visibility of disability and degree of stigma, (5) area and degree of impairment, (6) nature of functional limitation, and (7) financial reward. For example, amputation of one leg or arm can occur at any age; usually has a sudden onset (but not necessarily the illness that led to it, for example, diabetes) and a stable course; is visible but not significantly stigmatized; has varying areas and degrees of impairment depending on the individual's definition of his amputation; has more or less clearcut limitations; and can be compensable (result of an accident) or noncompensable (result of a

TABLE 2.
Typology of Disabled's Characteristics

Sex	Age	Education	Occupation	Income	Social Class
M	Child (1–13)	Elementary	Professional, high admin.	Very Low ($0–3,000)	Lower
F					Working
	Adolescent (14–19)	Some high school	Lesser professional, admin.	Low ($3,000–6,000)	Lower middle
	Adult (20–40)	Some high school & vocational training	sional, admin.	Average ($6,000–10,000)	Middle
	Middle-aged (41–60)	High school graduate	Semiprofessional, low admin.	Above Average ($10,000–15,000)	Upper middle
	Old (60 +)	High school & business school	Business (large & medium)	High ($15,000–50,000)	Upper
		College graduate	Business (small)	Very High ($50,000–over)	
			Sales & clerical		
			Skilled worker		
			Semi- & unskilled worker		

* Equil. = equilibrated; Disequil. = disequilibrated.
† Left, S = satisfactory, U = unsatisfactory; right, S = stable, U = unstable.

nonoccupational illness). On the other hand, heart disease occurs mostly among adults, especially middle-aged ones; is often sudden; usually stable if controlled; nonvisible and nonstigmatized; has areas and degrees of impairment dependent largely upon the disabled's definition of his disability; has generalized and diffuse limitations; and

Status Profile Type & Stability*	Marital Status	Significant Others' Relation to Disabled†	Significant Others' Acceptance of Disability	Disabled's Predisability Self-concept	
				Positive	Negative
Equil. high	Single	S, S	Accepted	Bodily integrity, strength and/or attractiveness central	Attributes other than bodily integrity, strength and/or attractiveness central
	Married	U, S	Denied		
Equil. med.		S, U			
	Widowed		Eager accept-		
		U, U	ance,		
Equil. low	Divorced, separated		secondary gains		
Disequil., high positions stable					
Disequil., high positions unstable					

is debatably compensable even when it occurs at work. These two examples suffice to show the utility of grouping disabilities with the same time and nature of onset, the same prognosis and course, the same degree of visibility and stigma, the same nature of functional limitations, and the same potential for compensation in order to be able to proceed with productive comparative analyses and draw valid theoretical conclusions and generalizations. The fifth criterion, "area and degree of impairment," has been omitted from the suggested grouping because it varies more according to the disabled's definition of the disability than according to the nature and severity of the disability itself. Thus, having controlled all other characteristics, we could study more clearly the role played by the disabled's profile of social and sociopsychological characteristics. Table 2 presents a typology of the disabled's characteristics which, although tentative and incomplete, could be used to derive working hypotheses.

By combining the profile of the disability with the disabled's sociopsychological profile, we should be able to determine the type and degree of impact that the disability has had upon the disabled's personality as well as his reaction and mode of adaptation. Some existing studies about types of disabilities illustrate how well information referring to both typologies can predict the disabled's reaction. A series of studies refers more to the disability typology than to the characteristics typology. For example, one study showed that diabetics (a stable if controlled chronic illness, nonvisible and nonstigmatized and usually without any or with only slight functional limitations) more than other chronically ill tend to deny the sick role and emphasize autonomy and individual responsibility for their physical condition.[22] This may suggest that they can accept the few functional limitations resulting from their condition and the necessary treatment and precautions they must ordinarily take without over- or under-accepting their illness. Probably, then, they can also incorporate only the necessary changes into their body image and self-concept without feeling threatened or devalued.

Other studies have shown that partial loss of hearing or sight provokes more depression in the afflicted persons than does total loss.[23] Does this mean that those who have suffered a partial loss tend to deny their affliction and hope for a recovery? Since they deny their affliction, they do not change their body image or self-concept in any way and thus have the same range of self-expectations (as well as expectations from others) as before. Everyday reality must be challenging to their make-believe world and therefore plunge them into depression.

The impact of the severity of disability is also well illustrated by the extreme situation of patients facing potential or imminent death. When survival is so drastically threatened and the changes that the person is forced to accept and incorporate into his self-concept so upsetting and shattering, we could question whether or not the same patterns can be observed as in the case of other disabilities. The kind of changes that imminent death requires in self-concept cannot be accommodated within the existing framework without a major re-organization, unless the individual has been able to gradually change his self-concept during the slow degenerative progression of a chronic illness. The research available, however, indicates that the same basic alternatives are open to those facing terminal illnesses: to deny or to accept the imminence of death.[24] The alternative, of course, of "secondary gains" to be derived from an unwarranted acceptance of the condition is not present among patients who are really dying. It can, however, exist among some chronically ill who may exploit their condition by wielding their potential death as a means of manipulating people and situations. In Greece, this type of exploitation is well known and prevalent among middle-aged women who can thus dominate the life of an entire family.

There are no data about the characteristics of those who can accept their imminent death, those who are not well informed (and never demand clear-cut information), and those who deny the possibility of their dying even after they receive definite cues indicating clearly that this is a fact.[25] Probably the same characteristics that help people accept their disabilities also help them accept their coming death, but in this case the person must have the facilitating characteristics and qualities to a very high degree.

One interesting reaction of some of the people who have accepted the fact that they are dying is their willingness to participate in experimental projects with new and uncertain drugs and treatments.[26] Obviously, their motivation is the hope that a new treatment or medicine will work a miracle. In this sense their reaction is not radically different from that of those who seek treatment by quacks, except that their need for a "magic" cure is turned to a socially acceptable outlet, the research physician. But what does this reaction mean in terms of degree of incorporation of the fact of death into the self-concept? Most probably those persons who still hope to find some way to cling to life have not accepted death beyond the level of "fictional acceptance." Their trying different medicines and experimental methods is thus nothing but a socially approved form of denial of death, eagerly encouraged by hospital personnel.

A few studies have examined the effect of some social and sociopsychological characteristics of the disabled upon the nature of his disability with or without attempting to relate this type of definition to some characteristics of the disability. A study of handicapped adolescents showed that severely disabled females had a more negative self-concept and were less self-accepting than mildly disabled females. The same relationship did not hold true for males. It was also found that girls with obvious or severe disabilities had a much more unfavorable self-concept and accepted themselves much less than did boys afflicted with similar disabilities.[27] Thus, it seems that sex is quite an important factor in determining the differential impact upon the self-concept, at least in the case of adolescents.

Although the disabled's age seems to be related to successful rehabilitation (see Chapter 6), there is inconclusive and contradictory evidence as to whether or not the age of onset plays an important role in the degree of impact upon the disabled's self-concept and reaction to it.[28] On the one hand, it is true that those afflicted with a congenital disability do not have to incorporate changes into their body image and self-concept, since they can tailor their self-concept according to their disabled status. However, this does not preclude their developing very negative feelings about their body image and self-concept as they internalize the majority values about physical integrity, competence, and beauty. Or they may deny their disability, attempt to build their self-concept as if they were "normal," and try whenever they can to pass as "normal." Thus, it is possible that despite the fact that some differences exist among disabled who incurred their disability at different stages of their lives, the basic dynamics are similar.

Finally, if we look at such characteristics as education, occupation, income, social class, and status profiles, we could hypothesize that the more "resources" a person has at his disposal, the less threatened he may be by the functional limitations imposed by a disability, unless the nature or severity of the disability is such that he can no longer have access to or use any of his valued resources. One evidence of this is the fact that highly educated and skilled persons or quite wealthy persons seldom appear in rehabilitation centers not only because they usually have access to needed services on a private basis, but also because they can "adjust" to their disability in a satisfactory manner without special aid. That, of course, does not mean that they all accept their disability.[29] Some may deny it because their high status position is threatened by the social stigma of the disability or because their status profile is unequilibrated and unstable and could be pulled to its lowest level by compromises necessitated by the functional limitations of the disability.[30]

Much more research is needed in the area of sociopsychological characteristics that are significantly related to acceptance, denial, or use of the disability for secondary gains. Only then will we be able to predict the type of reaction to disability of a given category of individuals or even hopefully the reaction of a particular disabled individual as well as formulate a complete theory concerning the impact of disability upon the disabled's self-concept.

The Disability at the Social System Level

In this section we shall consider the disabled as a segment of society, the place the disabled hold in society, and the relationship vis-à-vis the disabled and the "healthy" majority of the nondisabled. The disabled will then be studied as a "minority" group adapting to the larger society as well as the individual disabled adapting to his significant others, friends, colleagues, and acquaintances. In addition, we shall look at the group and individual adaptation of the nondisabled to both the collectivity of the disabled and to individuals. Thus our analysis will be macro- and microsocietal in order to provide a fairly complete picture of the disability at this level of conceptualization.

There is some controversy as to whether or not the disabled can be conceptualized as a "minority" group and as to what constitutes the differences between the collectivity of disabled people and other minority groups.[31] We shall separately examine those features that the collectivity of the disabled share with other minority groups as well as those in which they differ; then we shall evaluate the consequences of these differences for the validity of conceptualizing the disabled as a minority group.

The disabled share with other minority groups the following characteristics and societal reactions:

1. Like many other "deviant" or "minority" groups, the disabled are granted a *separate* place in society in most countries, including industrialized nations such as the United States, England, and the Scandinavian countries. They are encouraged to interact with their fellow disabled who are afflicted with the same type of disability. This is done through the creation of clubs, schools, and even magazines serving one disability group only or persons with several types of disabilities. Even some industries which exclusively employ the disabled have been established.

2. Such segregation requires a majority which evaluates the characteristics of the "minority" group in such a way that its members are designated as inferior. The majority of the nondisabled consider the disabled to be inferior in many areas and use segregation as a means of keeping a considerable social (and even territorial) distance. Thus, they are safeguarded from extensive contacts with the disabled in employment and school situations, in social-recreational activities, and most crucial of all, from possibly close affective relationships and therefore from "intermarriage." The vocational (and educational) segregation is attributed by some to an unwillingness on the part of the nondisabled majority to compete on an equal basis with those they believe to be inferior.[32] Successful performance on the part of the disabled would constitute a significant threat to the nondisabled's self-concept.

3. The segregation imposed by the majority of the nondisabled is rationalized as "beneficial" for the disabled since they have a better chance to find happiness and acceptance among their "own kind" rather than within the larger society. The same segregational attitudes exist with respect to the aged, for whom separate retirement communities are built, blacks (at least up to now), and other ethnic groups who are usually forced to live in ghettos. Because the majority

of the nondisabled cannot completely accept the disabled on an equal footing, they wish to minimize trying and uneasy contacts with them. For this reason they encourage the disabled to "accept" their disability —that is, to accept the fact that they are different from the "normal" majority. A disabled individual is usually deemed "adjusted" if he performs his social roles (especially the vocational) to the best of his ability, but restricts the satisfaction of his emotional, social, and psychological (or even his vocational) needs to the segregated group of other disabled people.

4. The disabled—like all other minority groups—tend to be evaluated more on the basis of their categorical membership than on their individual characteristics. The disability trait overshadows and qualifies all other traits and abilities.[33] Thus, whether a blind person is a pianist or a lawyer, intelligent or dull, he is primarily a "blind" lawyer, a "blind" pianist, and so on. And the fact that he is disabled will color all his activities and potentialities in the eyes of the nondisabled in such a pervasive way that he will either be considered weak and inferior, incapable of doing anything, or possessed of exceptional capacities and abilities. Very seldom will he be evaluated objectively on the basis of his knowledge, abilities, skills, strengths, and weaknesses. And since stereotypes are often attached to categories of people singled out because of one "negative" attribute in common, those belonging to a category (to a minority group) are evaluated on the basis of these stereotypes. Thus, the disabled are assessed by the nondisabled on the basis of the overall stereotype attached to all disabled as well as on the basis of the particular stereotype attached to their specific type of disability. And since these stereotypes are usually negative, most of the time the disabled are discriminated against by the nondisabled because the assessment stops at the recognition of the presence of the disability. This process of stereotyping and using stereotypes as guidelines for behavior simplifies interaction for the nondisabled when they encounter disabled persons, but often leads to the unjust treatment of the latter.

Despite basic similarities between the disabled and other minority groups, some researchers find differences they consider valid and sufficient to challenge the conceptualization of the disabled as a minority group. These differences are:

1. Is the notion of a nondisabled majority completely valid?

The degree of temporary disability among this "healthy" majority is so frequent and so prevalent that it is questionable whether or not we can call this group "healthy" or "nondisabled." Health, nondisability, and disability are not a dichotomy such as man or woman, according to which a person is the one or the other, but rather a continuum along which we can make an arbitrary dichotomy. And the more "pure" the nondisability part of the continuum, the more drastically diminished is the numerical superiority of the nondisabled majority. The disability-nondisability continuum has much in common with the age continuum because all people grow older every day, at least chronologically, and the age limit above which people are considered "old" is quite arbitrary. For example, some people 40 years old may be much older physiologically and psychologically than some people 60 years old. And the lower the age limit above which people are considered to be old and discriminated against, the more the concept of majority group is questionable when applied to the "young." But of course arithmetical superiority has not been a necessary or sufficient condition for a group to become the "majority." The numerically superior (or at least equal) case of the female population illustrates this point. Another similarity between the continuums of nondisabled-disabled and young-old is the fact that all young people will eventually become old unless they die young, and each nondisabled person has a certain probability (higher in some groups) of becoming disabled. This possibility of stepping down from the majority to the minority group, involuntarily but more or less inescapably, distinguishes these continuums from mutually exclusive dichotomies such as the man-woman or the black-white.[34]

Another issue relates to the fact that the nondisabled majority (as well as most other majorities) is by no means uniform: it may include a great number of different minorities, such as nondisabled women, nondisabled blacks, nondisabled but elderly males, females, whites, blacks, and so on. We cannot, then, expect that this mixture of different types of minority groups, on the basis of a variety of criteria, will react in the same way to the disabled as will a small core of people who belong to majority groups in terms of age, sex, color, religion, social class, and ethnic origin. While there is some evidence that frustrated persons and disadvantaged groups experiencing prejudice and discriminatory behavior may demonstrate a higher degree of prejudice toward other minority groups than the corresponding majority, the findings are not consistent or conclusive. Thus, while lower class persons have been found more prejudiced than middle class persons[35] and downward-mobile individuals more prejudiced toward Jews than those in a stable social status,[36] no relationship has been found between age and acceptance of physical disability.[37] Furthermore, it has been found that nondisabled females show greater acceptance of physical disability than nondisabled males, but that there is no conclusive evidence about the influence of race, ethnic origin, or class on attitudes toward the disabled.[38] It is not clear to what extent and in what cases the minority status is conducive to greater or lesser prejudice and toward which other minority groups.

On the other hand, the disabled do not constitute a homogeneous "minority" group sharing the characteristics that bring about discrimination in the same way that blacks or women bear the discriminative characteristics. There is a continuum of severity, visibility, and stigmatization among the disabled that may determine the nature and intensity of discrimination by the nondisabled (and possibly by other types of the disabled) population. Thus, the whole problem of the relationship between the nondisabled and the disabled population should be investigated by means of a typology of the nondisabled (especially with respect to "minority" characteristics in subunits) and a typology of the disabled such as that suggested in the first section of this chapter.

2. While the disabled have been and are still discriminated against in the same way as other minority groups, there are some subtle differences in the manner in which discrimination is practiced in the case of the disabled and in the case of blacks. In the latter case as well as in the case of undesirable ethnic groups (for example, Southern Europeans), the stereotypes are so negative that discrimination can be as open as hostility or aversion. These groups are probably considered contemptible since their undesirable characteristics are stereotyped as being of a voluntary, moral character, such as laziness, shrewdness, manipulativeness, unreliability, corruptness, untrustworthiness, immorality or indecency. However, in the case of women, the old, and the disabled, discrimination is often camouflaged by protective legislation and is rationalized on the basis of biological and physiological limitations and weaknesses.[39] Thus, the current

official norms regulating individual as well as institutional behavior toward the latter three groups (women, the old, and the disabled) prescribe protection but not violence, aggression, or aversion, since their weaknesses and limitations "cannot be helped." Of course, if these groups attempt to break their protective chains and achieve equality on the basis of their individual real abilities, they may meet open aggression and rejection. And in liberal-humanitarian periods in different societies, special privileges are granted to these groups which further single them out and help perpetuate their being assessed on the basis of their categorical membership instead of their individual capacities.

The fact that cultural norms proscribe the release of tension on the part of the nondisabled interferes seriously with the quality of interpersonal relations the disabled are able to establish with the nondisabled. The final product in both the case of the disabled (or the women or the old) and the case of racial, ethnic, or religious groups is discrimination. If anything, it may be more difficult to break the vicious circle of discrimination directed against the former because it is cushioned by protective legislation and "sympathetic" attitudes.

3. Some writers have maintained that another difference between the disabled and a minority group is the fact that the latter is self-perpetuating. It is maintained that partly because of external segregatory pressures and partly because the group itself desires it, a minority group tends to remain self-contained, segregated, homogeneous, and closed, and to perpetuate its particular subcultural values and norms.[40] The disabled, on the contrary, are forced into segregation and never perpetuate their disability as an "ethnic" tradition. There are, however, several debatable points in this thesis. First, in the case of some disabled, their disability (or a predisposition toward it) is perpetuated in their children and their grandchildren not as an ethnic tradition, but unavoidably through genetic inheritance. Second, it is questionable whether a minority group ever seeks segregation and social isolation or wishes to remain segregated. Most probably what gives the impression of a seeking to keep the group boundaries closed is a defensive reaction to multiple rejections by the majority.

We think that the concept of the minority group can be applied in the case of the disabled despite minor differences. And as in the case of other minority groups, the position of the disabled in the larger society and the dynamics of their interaction with other disabled as well as with the nondisabled can be best analyzed and explained by means of the general theory of deviance. As with all other deviants, it is not so much their actual physical disability that is the key, but rather society's reaction to it. The disabled are not intrinsically deviant because of their disability, but because those around them label them "deviant" since they impute to them an undesirable difference.[41] Although it must be noted that when the nature and degree of the disability are such that mobility and/or functioning are seriously limited, a certain amount of deviance may also be due to the sheer presence of the disability. The resulting limitations render an individual more or less dependent—and therefore deviant—since he must break the norm of adult independence and self-reliance. But the existence of a physical disability does not always turn the individual into a deviant. Why then does the society of the nondisabled always label him as such? What societal rules have been transgressed that the disabled should be judged as deviant?[42] Every disabled does transgress one or more of the culturally valued norms concerning physical integrity, perfection, health, and beauty. Furthermore, a disabled person is a potential (if not an actual) threat to the rule of independence and self-reliance, since he may not be able to perform certain tasks because of his disability-imposed limitation and is thus legitimately exempted from them. Finally, the disabled (especially the men) may actually or potentially threaten to break the rule of financial independence or of remunerative work, for in a number of cases they may legitimately or semilegitimately be exempted from the occupational role.

Some issue, however, may be raised concerning the legitimacy of the concept "deviant" when applied to the disabled, since there seem to be some differences between the disabled and other categories of deviants. Some would claim that all impairments and disabilities are "unmotivated" conditions for which the afflicted individual cannot be held responsible. Others would claim that a considerable number of accidents and chronic illnesses are not random events totally "unmotivated" and beyond the individual's control. While the degree to which a disabled person may be held responsible for his physical disability may be debatable, the decision as to whether or not a disabled person will abandon the performance of social roles, especially the occupational one, and the performance of everyday tasks and activities may be much more within the realm of "voluntary" and motivated behavior. And it is exactly for this aspect of their deviance that the disabled are required to undergo vocational rehabilitation, the designated agency of social control. In the area of financial independence, we find that this type of deviance is much more frequent among lower class disabled, for which a "defect" in the social structure can be readily found to account at least partially for their deviance. This "defect" is the structural type of unemployment endemic for this category of workers as well as the workmen's compensation laws that to some extent foster compensable disabilities.

Another interesting distinction between the disabled and other deviants is that the former have already gone through an institution of social control—that of medical treatment—which has failed to eliminate their deviance. This fact diminishes even further the degree of responsibility that could be assigned to them for their present state of disability (although it could be argued that they could have been more or less motivated to profit from medical treatment and, therefore, to "get well").

Rehabilitation, then, becomes a peculiar type of institution, since it has the official function of a social control agency that must help the disabled overcome certain aspects of the deviance. But it also socializes the disabled to play the "deviant" role at the "social" level—that is, to "accept" a disabled status and its limitations as well as the societal segregation imposed because of disability. Society expects the disabled to correct the "vocational" and "dependency" aspects of their deviance but not their "social" deviance, which is assumed to be necessarily indefinite. The latter type of deviance, then, is not only tolerated and accepted, but even expected and fostered by society. No attempt is made to correct this deviance. On the contrary, those disabled who work and are fairly independent and are willing to accept the imposed social and emotional segregation are in a sense "rewarded" for remaining deviant.

It seems that the key to remaining "normal" (that is, nondisabled) is not the absolute state of health or ability but rather the lack of a societal label of deviance. A striking illustration has been provided by Josephson's and Scott's studies showing that people with the same degree of vision impairment may be labeled blind or not blind according to whether or not they have come to the attention of an agency for the blind.[43] Therefore, many disabled attempt at any price to avoid this label. Of course, this desperate attempt is open only to those whose disability is not severe or visible and can be detected only through repeated and intensive contacts with them. Despite a wide range of ingenious techniques that the disabled develop in order to guard their secret, "passing" is usually a stressful, complicated, and delicate process. It often meets with failure because of unpredictable or unmanageable "embarrassing incidents" through which the disability is revealed and the carefully and painfully woven cloak of normality torn apart.[44]

Those who cannot ever "pass" because their disability is visible or easily detectable may develop any one (or a combination) of the ego defenses Allport presents as reactions of discriminated individuals.[45] These ego defenses as applied to the disabled are: (1) *obsessive concern,* as in the case of those who are hypersensitive about their condition and the reactions of the others; (2) *denial of membership,* as in the case of those who reject their disabled status and try to go on living as if they were nondisabled; (3) *withdrawal and passivity,* as in the case of those who give in to their disability to an even greater degree than is necessary and even derive "secondary gains" from their disabled status; (4) *identification with dominant group: self-hate,* as in the case of the disabled who accept the majority evaluative criteria and feel diminished and inferior; (5) *aggression against own group,* as in the case of the disabled who discriminate negatively and become aggressive against other disabled with the same type of disability or with a more stigmatized disability than their own[46] or against those who derive sympathy, help, and love because of their disabled status; (6) *prejudice against out-groups,* that is, against other minority groups lower than themselves in the pecking order; (7) *sympathy toward other out-groups;* (8) *fighting back: militancy,* as in the case of those who embrace liberal ideologies which could advance their group and demand social action; (9) *strengthening in-group ties,* as in the case of those who develop an *esprit de corps,* a feeling that they all share a common lot, a group identification which is easier established when the disability is visible (if militancy and in-group identification were prevalent among the disabled, they could create a social movement); (10) *enhanced striving,* as in the case of a disabled individual who redoubles his efforts so that he has a chance to succeed in "normal" society by being much better than the nondisabled with whom he competes; (11) *symbolic status striving,* that is, compensation by substitution; (12) *clowning;* (13) *slyness and cunning;* (14) *neuroticism;* and (15) *self-fulfilling prophecy.*

The disabled may react differently to their being labeled "deviant" and consequently discriminated against; they may move from one to another of the categories depending upon the reaction of the nondisabled (especially their significant others) to their disability and their postdisability stage (grief phase, rehabilitation phase, plateau reached in rehabilitation, and so forth). But regardless of the disabled's reaction to their being discriminated against, the majority group of the nondisabled goes on discriminating against them and segregating them as much as possible. For example, society has erected architectural and psychological barriers than encourage and impose social segregation. Also the increasing specialization of social institutions (for example, education) finally results in the social segregation of the disabled in a socially acceptable manner.[47]

Paul Hunt's collection of disabled's autobiographical essays is probably the most eloquent and serious protest against the segregation of the disabled voiced by the disabled themselves.[48] All those included wanted for themselves as well as for other disabled a full societal integration which would permit disabled children to attend school with "normal" children, disabled teenagers to have "normal" teenagers as friends, disabled adults to work in regular jobs (and not only some second-class occupations reserved for them) with "normal" co-workers, and disabled individuals to be loved by "normals" and sometimes to marry a "normal." Love and marriage are not explicit in all the stories in Hunt's book, but they are certainly implicit in many of their comments.[49] The disabled are desperately trying to diminish the social distance that separates them from the nondisabled. And while the nondisabled tend to be cooperative and understanding when it comes to the occupational world, they close their ears to the disabled's attempts to gain social acceptance and marriage eligibility.

Intermarriage between the disabled and the nondisabled is undoubtedly the best index of societal integration. Interestingly enough, an intensive study of mental retardates showed that in effect these retarded men and women used marriage with a normal as the utmost criterion of definitive success in societal integration and adjustment. Here it seems that the disabled woman fares better than the disabled man in likelihood of marrying a normal person, probably because the disabled status is more compatible with the traditional, more passive role of the woman who does not have to support the family. Also, the dependent status of the disabled woman may inspire some insecure man who can then comfortably play the protective role of an "adequate" and "strong" male. However, it is interesting to note that all the mentally retarded who married "normal" men married "marginal" and in other ways deviant nondisabled, a pattern that has been found to hold also in the case of "mixed" marriages between blacks and whites or between "undesirable" foreigners and Americans.[50]

Of course, up to now the chances for most disabled, especially those afflicted with visible disabilities, to marry a nondisabled have been very small (unless married prior to onset of disability). So if such an individual desires to have heterosexual relations and to look for a mate, he must search for a field of eligibles among other disabled, who are probably also visibly disabled. That this situation represents a strain for the visibly disabled person who is caught in a dilemma has been well formulated by Weinberg. Generalized, his formulation could read as follows: The wider a visibly disabled person's *social* space (that is, the interactive network with those other than "his own kind"), the narrower his sociable space (that is, his field of intimate primary relationships—eligible dates and mates).[51]

Under the pressure of social and psychological isolation, the disabled have to create clubs or organizations that cater only to "their own kind" for social and recreational purposes. Weinberg's study of the Little People of America (LPA) organization showed that besides the rather secondary educative and practical purposes it serves for its members (information about the special problems encountered by midgets and dwarfs in everyday life and employment assistance), its principal attraction is the opportunity to meet eligible dates and mates during the monthly and annual conventions.[52] Some of the mentally retarded studied by Edgerton also went to a social club for the handicapped although this was by no means their first choice.[53] Generally, it seems that the disabled who do not join such clubs or organizations are those who have not accepted their disabled status and consider satisfactory intimate relations, especially marriage, with a nondisabled the only acceptable criterion of successful adjustment. They refuse to join such clubs and organizations and instead, go on trying to join the "normal" society.[54]

The issue of segregation versus integration of the disabled in society represents a difficult and complicated dilemma. While segregation sounds inhuman, integration is not always the most desirable choice either. For a disabled to become integrated in the "normal" society, he must compete on an equal footing with the nondisabled (and usually prove he is better than the average nondisabled) without the society making any accommodating change, any adjustment in the technological, cultural or social milieu.[55] Not only must the disabled be able to adapt to a world made for the nondisabled, but they must do so on nondisabled terms. Some of the disabled themselves have started realizing that integration too has been interpreted from the point of view of the nondisabled and is therefore not totally advantageous to them. And some of the most verbal among them are saying that integration cannot be one-sided.[56] Not only must the disabled adopt and adapt to some of the values and norms of the nondisabled, but the nondisabled must also adopt and adapt some of the values and norms of the disabled. Each group must partially accommodate the other; there must be a more or less equal mutual exchange. Otherwise it is not possible for the disabled ever to be really accepted on an equal basis in their own right and to contribute to the formation of societal values and norms. Why should they accept and adopt norms of efficiency and productivity that are sometimes unsuited to their abilities and disabilities? Why cannot they propose as equally acceptable norms those prescribing reflection, self-actualization, and humanitarianism? A truly modern society is a society that offers as many options as possible to *all* individuals, (regardless of age, sex, health status, social class, racial or ethnic background), a society in which this range of options is equally socially acceptable and desirable, and a society in which people are socialized so as to be truly free to take any of these options without having later to pay a social or psychological price. Ideally, the disabled should be accepted as "different but equal."[57]

Let us now move to the microsocietal level and examine the interaction between a disabled and another disabled as well as between a disabled and a nondisabled. Interaction with other disabled persons usually seems to present no problems to a disabled person but is, on the contrary, quite helpful in making it easier for him to accept his predicament. The "positive" influence of such interaction seems to occur either through identification with another disabled afflicted with the same type and degree of disability or through a comparison of his disability with that of a more seriously incapacitated disabled which produces a feeling of being "much better off."[58] In the latter case, however, we do not know the psychological mechanism operating within the disabled person which permits him to feel that his affliction is the lesser, and it would be important to assess whether or not he feels better because his morale has been boosted by considering the more severely disabled as inferior to himself. It has been found, for example, that some of the visibly but not severely disabled who can hold a regular job, interact successfully with normals, and marry a normal are sometimes making a distinction between themselves and the severely disabled for whom they think that segregated services, activities, and a generally segregated place in society would be most appropriate.[59] Whatever the psychological mechanisms operating, it has been seen repeatedly that a disabled person who is quite threatened and "paralyzed" by his affliction or feeling quite devaluated by it may finally find the strength to "accept" his disability after having met another disabled whom he can esteem and admire as a human and social being regardless of his disability.[60] Through his social acceptance and approval of another disabled and through his identifying with this well-functioning and otherwise "normal" person, he may eventually accept himself and his disability and continue his life with all the capacities that he has.

However, the most crucial social interaction usually is with the nondisabled. For an individual's reaction to his disability is dependent not only upon his predisability self-concept and social position, but upon the reaction toward his disability on the part of his significant others and the nature of the changes brought about in their usual mode of interaction. Changes in the mode of interaction with all other people in primary or formalized encounters will also influence the disabled's adjustment to his disability, that is, the extent and pervasiveness with which the change in body image will become incorporated into his self-concept. It is not usually enough for a disabled person to cope with the problem of his disability within himself. Throughout the process of trying to cope with it and after it has been provisionally settled internally, he continuously tests out his mode of reacting with others in order to validate it socially through their acceptance and approval. Only through such consistent and continuous social approval does the disabled's mode of adjustment to his disability become crystallized and permanent.

It is unfortunate for the disabled, in the light of the importance it has for them, that their interaction with the nondisabled is usually strained by ambiguities and emotional reactions. The nondisabled are very uncertain as to how they should behave toward the disabled and may vacillate between ignoring the disability altogether to treating the disabled individual as a total invalid.[61] There is also evidence that the nondisabled (as well as the disabled) have significantly greater difficulty in predicting the behavior of disabled than of nondisabled persons. The disabled, on the other hand, may not know either exactly how they want to be treated by the nondisabled, what amount of help they would welcome, and to what extent they want to play "normal" or "handicapped." Because of ambiguities in the role of definitions and role expectations of both disabled and nondisabled, there may develop role "synchronies" or "asynchronies," depending upon whether or not both the interacting disabled and nondisabled persons agree as to how the disabled should behave.[62]

Psychological and sociopsychological research has also shown that interactions between physically disabled and physically normal persons are anxiety-laden, tend to cause emotional discomfort, and usually take on the form of "stereotyped, inhibited, and over-controlled" experiences.[63] The disabled tries very hard to secure an easy and natural interaction pattern with a nondisabled beyond the often easily granted "fictional acceptance," and he is reported to be forced to develop an entire gamut of necessary behavioral manipulations in order to achieve this. The reason why the establishment of a "normal" interaction with the nondisabled is of crucial importance to many (but not all) disabled is the fact that such an interaction would reassure the involved disabled that he can be socially accepted despite his disability. If he fails to break through the stiff, conventional interaction pattern, he will tend to feel like a social deviant—a deviance assigned to him by the nondisabled simply on the basis of his disability. Thus, the disabled is made to feel that his efforts to localize the handicapping effects of his disability, to make maximum use of his capacities, and to avoid self-devaluation are futile, since the majority of the nondisabled will not easily permit him such a "localization" and will tend to see him through the effect of psychological "spread."[64]

Through the "spread" phenomenon of perceptional association, the nondisabled tend to create consistently and on the whole usually negative impressions about the disabled person, who is then necessarily viewed as inferior in terms of all possible attributes simply on the basis of his visible or known but nonvisible disability.[65] Thus, the nondisabled tend to talk down to a physically disabled person as if he were also mentally retarded and sometimes even as if he were deaf or blind, and they tend to be surprised at discovering that the disabled person may be quite intelligent and competent. In short, they behave as if there were a natural incompatibility between the presence of a physical disability and "positive" traits and qualities.[66] Available research studies have shown that "normal" children five to twelve years old express more rejecting attitudes toward amputee than toward nonamputee classmates by designating them as liked the least by both the entire class and themselves.[67] They also tend to consider amputee children as not being nice looking, the least fun to play with, as well as the saddest children in the class. The last attribute implies pity and suggests a particularistic and special treatment that can be as discriminatory as rejection.

Another sociometric study among high school students showed that disabled adolescents of both sexes are rated significantly lower than physically normal adolescents as friends, co-workers, and leaders. Moreover, visibly disabled adolescents received more extreme ratings than those afflicted with nonvisible disabilities. Teachers were found to rate female disabled students significantly higher than male disabled students regardless of the type and degree of disability.[68]

The question as to whether or not disabled subjects sociometrically reject other disabled subjects in a fashion similar to that of the nondisabled has also been studied using student populations.

The findings of these studies suggest that disabled students preferred nondisabled students as often as did the nondisabled students sampled.[69] It has also been found that children, handicapped or non-handicapped, prefer a nonhandicapped child over children afflicted with different types of handicaps.[70] Similar findings have resulted in studies of adult laymen as well as of trained rehabilitation personnel.[71] Thus, it seems that the presence of a visible physical disability (including obesity) is a serious deterrent to the formation of friendships with the nondisabled to an even greater degree than race or color.[72]

The influence of the age at the onset of disability on the nature of interpersonal relations with the disabled but especially with nondisabled individuals has not been systematically studied. We do not know, for example, whether or not the congenitally disabled and those afflicted with a disability in early childhood tend to develop better or poorer interpersonal relationships with the nondisabled. Arguments can be found for both sides. Those with a congenital or early childhood disability have had a better chance to develop a self-concept in which the disability is most probably completely incorporated and an appropriate range of techniques that increase their interpersonal skills. Possibly because they have "accepted" (or at least "adjusted" to) their disability, they feel more at ease in encounters with the nondisabled and are able to interpret openly and accurately the extent of their ability and disability so as to put the nondisabled at ease. Or is it possible that because they were disabled so early in childhood they have become socially isolated, and since there is evidence that they are rejected by their peers from an early age, they may have never established close or intimate relations with anyone? One study has shown that persons with a longstanding disability were more satisfied with themselves and more similar sociometrically to the nondisabled, a finding which has been interpreted as an indication of more developed personal relationships with others.[73] However, the available studies do not permit us to answer this question in a conclusive fashion.

The last issue of interest relates to an applied question. How can discrimination diminish and the strained, superficial interpersonal relations between the disabled and the nondisabled be changed so that the two groups can form warm, personal relationships? We find that even the social scientists who have written "sympathetically" about the disabled have tended to emphasize the need to educate the disabled about how to put the "noninjured persons with whom he associates at ease" and thus avoid "the discomfort of encountering their ambivalent attitudes."[74] It is true that such learning would be useful for the disabled person, especially because it would help him clarify in his mind how he wants to be treated by the nondisabled and also how he himself wants to behave consistently with relation to them. However, the entire burden of coping with negative responses to their "stigma" cannot lie entirely upon the shoulders of the disabled, who are in a disadvantaged position to handle them. There is evidence that the disabled are poorer than the nondisabled in social perception and that they have poor resources for dealing with the nondisabled.[75] They do not have the opportunity to develop interpersonal skills because they have few friendships and little social experience. Therefore, the nondisabled should also be educated to learn to cope with the fears and anxieties that the disabled arouse in them. They would then be able to act naturally toward the disabled, and interaction would accordingly be less strained and rigid.

Some writers have mentioned that exposure to disabled individuals and extensive contact with them would tend to diminish the nondisabled's degree of prejudice and resulting discrimination and ease interpersonal relations between the disabled and the nondisabled. Not all types of contact, however, produce this effect. It seems that Allport's typology of contact holds true, since the results depend upon the frequency, duration, variety, and especially the type of contact that the nondisabled have with the disabled.[76] Only contacts in which the minority group has equal status with the majority group and which are voluntary and "real" represent the best conditions for the breakdown of discrimination and the formation of close relationships.[77] Thus, practitioner-client relationships are ineffective, whereas contacts through friendship represent the ideal. This conclusion unfortunately leads us to a vicious circle, since those who have been once able to have warm and meaningful contacts with the disabled can do so again in the future.

The Disability at the Cultural Level

In this section we shall examine those values and norms concerning physical strength and integrity and physical appearance which seem to be universal so that they produce uniform reactions to disability and those values and norms which are culture- or subculture-specific and responsible for observed variations. Unfortunately, there are very few data available about other cultures, and this research gap will necessarily limit our discussion.

Physical strength, physical integrity, and attractiveness are probably valued and admired in all cultures, although the standards for strength, integrity, and beauty may vary widely from culture to culture and subculture to subculture. For example, obesity in women is greatly admired in most African tribes as a characteristic of beauty and distinction, while it is stigmatized in the United States among middle class men and women.[78] In some cultures more than others, these values and norms may be sex-differentiated. For example, in the American culture (especially in the middle class), it seems that physical strength and physical integrity are much more important for the male than for the female, while beauty is considered much more important for the female. This is probably due to the sex-typing of roles prevalent in the middle class, according to which men are responsible for the occupational-breadwinner role and women are sexual-decorative status symbols.[79] There are, of course, also differences in the degree of intensity with which these values are held and the degree of deviance from the desirable standard that is accepted and tolerated from country to country. In some countries only extreme deviations from the desirable standard may be stigmatized, while in others even slight deviations may be singled out and stigmatized. For instance, there are indications that the standards for physical integrity and perfection as well as for beauty are very strict in Anglo-Saxon countries (especially among the middle classes), and any deviation from the highly admired state of perfection is punished by social stigmatization.[80] Not only physical deformities or chronic invalidating illnesses, but also obesity (or even overweight), pimples, oily hair, "bad" breath or sweating odors are considered intolerable and label the "afflicted" individuals as deviants.[81] This labeling brings about devaluation, social isolation, and a more or less potent social stigma according to the nature and the degree of the deviation.

The higher the stage of industrialization and socioeconomic development in a country, the greater the tendency to value intelligence and all the qualities that are conducive to high achievement, productivity, competitiveness, and efficiency. Thus, stupidity is strongly stigmatized, since people with a low IQ have little chance of earning any kind of social status in societies in which one's personal ability and achievement determine his social standing practically to the exclusion of all other criteria. Such exaggerated emphasis on intelligence in societies such as the American is not always defensible, for several types of occupations and activities require but a minimum level of intelligence.[82]

Furthermore, in industrialized societies in which high productivity and efficiency are highly valued, smooth interpersonal relations in the work setting are desired, if not required, since they are conducive to efficiency and steady overall high rate of production. Because of this, there is very little tolerance of behavioral deviations that tend to disrupt the smooth functioning and easy flow of interpersonal relations. Even slight mental deviations get singled out very quickly if they interfere in any way with an individual's performance of the occupational role either in terms of actual productivity and efficiency or in terms of the nature of the interpersonal relations he establishes. Tolerance of mental illness is much lower in industrialized societies than in developing societies. For example, in a developing country like Greece, in which the values and norms of industrialization have not yet been wholeheartedly adopted, a wide range of mentally deviant behavior interfering with the quality of interpersonal relations at work is tolerated.[83] In an industrialized country, the same range of mentally deviant behavior would have led to the individual's being labeled as "deviant" or "mentally ill" and to his seeking (or being forced to undergo) psychiatric treatment.

Within each culture there are usually considerable differences between classes and cultural subgroups. For example, it has been found that lower class men, in contrast to those in the middle class, think that debility (for instance blindness) is more undesirable than mutilation in their wives, probably because they tend to consider them primarily as possible economic contributors rather than beautiful status symbols. =Lower class females tend to dread facial disfigurement more than do middle class women, probably because alternative sources of self-evaluation, such as intellectual or artistic attainments, are not usually available to them.[84]

With the exception of societies in which some types of disabilities have been connected with supernatural powers, the disabled are discriminated against. There are, however, strong moral-social norms which forbid the nondisabled from openly rejecting or mistreating the disabled.[85] The question that may then be raised is: Why do the nondisabled want to reject and mistreat the disabled and yet fear showing their negative feelings?

Sociopsychological research has shown that because the nondisabled live in perpetual fear of losing their physical integrity, contact with the disabled tends to arouse anxiety. Hebb has also found evidence that both chimpanzees and humans show intense fear responses to mutilated bodies.[86] Moreover, psychological investigations relating to the nature of the anxiety, discomfort, and aversion the nondisabled feel have indicated that the main type of aversion is "esthetic-sexual." Clear-cut feelings of repulsion and discomfort are felt by the nondisabled but never communicated to the disabled. The degree of aversion felt seems to be much greater in reaction to certain disabilities, such as skin disorders, amputation, body deformation and cerebral palsy, than to deafness, blindness, and paralysis.[87] Also, among all types of visible disabilities facial disfigurements seem to be the least liked, least tolerated, and the most anxiety- and aversion-provoking disabilities in children and adults.[88] Barker et al. also found that in a content analysis of jokes, the most frequently deprecated persons were those with an unattractive face, with obesity coming second.[89] Other studies have shown that blindness is the most feared disability and the one considered to be most severe. Interestingly, although blindness is considered to be the most severe disability, blind people do not provoke strong aversion as do those marked with facial disfigurements.[90]

Other investigators attribute the fear felt by the nondisabled and the resulting avoidance of the disabled to deep, unconscious mechanisms. They are: (a) the belief that the disabled are evil and dangerous and were therefore punished with their disability (especially in the case of visible disabilities); (b) the belief that the disabled person, unjustly punished and aware of the injustice, is vindictive, aggressive, and dangerous; and (c) the projection of aggressive and destructive desires upon the disabled and hence the belief that the disabled is dangerous.[91] Some suggest that childhood fairy tales and, later on, novels, plays, movies, and jokes may fit a reinforcement learning theory model through which negative, fearful characteristics and tendencies become associated with the disabled.[92]

Regardless of the degree of aversion felt toward the disabled, the nondisabled are normatively not permitted to show these negative feelings in any way, and their fear of making a verbal or nonverbal "slip" indicating their emotions renders the interaction quite formal and rigid.[93] The reason for this proscription, which also makes the nondisabled feel guilty for having felt "unacceptable" emotions toward an innocent human being, is perhaps the cultural belief that the disabled are "inferior" and it is therefore inhuman and cruel for their "superiors" to reject or mistreat them. At the individual level, this normative proscription is probably reinforced by "magical thinking" suggesting that the rejection or mistreatment of the disabled could result in the nondisabled being punished with a similar affliction.

Factor analytic studies of beliefs and feelings about different illnesses have shown that there are three dimensions which are relevant and crucial in the perception of these diseases. These dimensions are: the human mastery dimension, that is, the completeness of human understanding (of the disease) and the effectiveness of human intervention; the social acceptability–social stigma dimension; and the personal involvement dimension. The dimension of social acceptability–social stigma is underscored in the case of highly stigmatized illnesses, such as mental illness, under the influence of operating desirability bias.[94] This bias is very difficult to remove because of the prevailing social norms which forbid the open expression (verbal or behavioral) of negative feelings. It intervenes in all studies attempting to measure the attitudes toward the disabled of different groups with different characteristics and decreases the validity of the findings. Thus, while some studies have shown that there is an inverse relationship between level of education and unfavorable attitudes toward the disabled, as is true for other minority groups, we cannot be sure if this finding reflects a true pattern or is an artifact created by a social desirability bias.[95] This bias would tend to be much

stronger among highly educated individuals because the norm for-
bidding open expression of negative feelings is much more prevalent
and potent among them and because they would be in a better position to recognize the purpose of survey questions.

Despite this methodological difficulty, a considerable number
of studies exist which show that the disabled are subject to atti-
tudinal and behavioral prejudices similar to those exhibited toward
ethnic, racial, and religious minorities.[96] The degree of prejudice
varies with a number of sociopsychological and psychological characteristics—for example, the degree of authoritarianism or dogmatism,
the nature of the self-concept, the need for intraception, and the
degree of anxiety.[97]

We have seen that there are deep-seated fears and aversions
in the nondisabled about most types of disabilities—visible and nonvisible, stigmatized and nonstigmatized. These fears and aversions
are most probably at the heart of the prejudice against the disabled,
who share with other minority groups similar types of discrimination
and isolation. Moreover, the disabled are labeled "deviant" by society, and under their multiple social and physical handicaps, encounter serious difficulties in adjusting to their disability. They
usually have poor interpersonal relationships, especially with the
nondisabled, an additional factor that impedes their acceptance of
the disability and their real reintegration into society.

In the next chapter we shall see what role the institution of rehabilitation plays in reintegrating the disabled individual into society, how this role is performed and by whom, to what extent it
succeeds, and for what reasons the effort leads to success or failure.

NOTES

1. For interesting and detailed psychological-psychoanalytic discussions of body image and changes brought about by illness
   or other disabilities, see Paul Schilder *Image and Appearance
   of the Human Body* (New York: Wiley, 1964), especially pp.
   15, 63–74, 181–87; Karl A. Menninger, "Psychiatric Aspects

of Physical Disability," in James F. Garrett (ed.), *Psychological Aspects of Physical Disability*, Rehabilitation Service Series, no. 210 (Washington, D.C.: Office of Vocational Rehabilitation, 1960), pp. 10–12; Harry Prosen, "Physical Disability and Motivation," *Canadian Medical Association Journal*, 92 (June 12, 1965), 1262; and Beatrice A. Wright, *Physical Disability—A Psychological Approach* (New York: Harper & Row, 1960), pp. 138–53.

2. Schilder and others report many cases of patients who deny that an arm or a leg is paralyzed. See Schilder, *op. cit.*, pp. 17–24, 29–62; also David Starrett, "Psychiatric Mechanisms in Servere Disability," *Rocky Mountain Medical Journal*, 58, 1 (January 1961), 42–44.

3. F. C. MacGregor, T. M. Abel, A. Bryt, E. Lauer, and S. Weissman, *Facial Deformities and Plastic Surgery* (Springfield, Ill.: Thomas, 1953), p. 199.

4. Schilder, *op. cit.*, pp. 63–70; also Marianne L. Simmel, "The Body Percept in Physical Medicine and Rehabilitation," *Journal of Health and Human Behavior*, 8, 1 (March 1967), 60–64. The experience of "phantom limb" is not related to the overall adjustment of the disabled to their disability, since it seems to appear equally as often among those well adjusted as those maladjusted. See Victor D. Sanua, "Sociocultural Factors in Responses to Stressful Life Situations: Aged Amputees as an Example," *Journal of Health and Human Behavior*, 1, 1 (Spring 1960), 23; and Samuel Hirschenfang and Joseph G. Benton, "Assessment of Phantom Limb Sensation Among Patients With Lower Extremity Amputation," *The Journal of Psychology*, 63, second half (July 1966), 197–99. The latter study also found that the duration of the phantom limb postoperatively was directly related to the length of illness before the amputation.

5. Tamara Dembo, Gloria Ladieu-Leviton, and Beatrice A. Wright, "Adjustment to Misfortune—A Problem of Socio-Psychological Rehabilitation," *Artificial Limbs,* 3, 2 (Autumn 1956), 33–42, especially 36–39.

6. Irving Shelsky, "The Effect of Disability on Self-Concept" (unpublished Ph.D. dissertation, Columbia University, 1957).

7. Dembo, Ladieu-Leviton, and Wright, *op. cit.*, pp. 33–36; Constantina Safilios-Rothschild, "The Reactions to Disability in Rehabilitation" (unpublished Ph.D. dissertation, Ohio State University, 1963).

8. Theodor J. Litman, "The Influence of Self-conception and Life Orientation Factors in the Rehabilitation of the Orthopedically Disabled," *Journal of Health and Human Behavior*, 3, 4 (Winter 1962), 252; and Tamara Dembo, Gloria Ladieu-

Leviton, and Beatrice A. Wright, "Acceptance of Loss Amputations," in Garrett, *op. cit.*, pp. 91–93.

9. Theodor J. Litman, "Self-conception and Physical Rehabilitation," in Arnold M. Rose (ed.), *Human Behavior and Social Processes* (Boston: Houghton Mifflin, 1962), p. 566.

10. One study has shown this pattern very clearly in the case of the blind who still hope their sight will return and therefore do not accept the white cane, cannot travel independently, have not brought about any modification in their self-concept, and are poorly adjusted in the vocational area. See Lee Thume and Oddist D. Murphree, "Acceptance of the White Cane and Hope for the Restoration of Sight in Blind Persons as an Indicator of Adjustment," *Journal of Clinical Psychology*, 17, 2 (April 1961), 208–9.

11. Dembo, Ladieu-Leviton, and Wright, "Adjustment to Misfortune —A Problem of Socio-Psychological Rehabilitation, *op. cit.*, pp. 36–41.

12. Robert A. Scott, *The Making of Blind Men: A Study of Adult Socialization* (New York: Russell Sage Foundation, 1969), pp. 7–8, 75, 108–10; and Eric Josephson, *The Social Life of Blind People*, Research Series no. 19 (New York: American Foundation for the Blind, 1968), p. 18.

13. Harold J. Wershow, "The Balance of Mental Health and Regression as Expressed in the Literature on Chronic Illness and Disability," *The Social Service Review*, 37, 2 (June 1963), 193–200.

14. Shibutani, for example, writes that the face, because of its highly individualized features, has great symbolic significance for a person's self-concept. This would explain the reported extreme depression of persons who have been disfigured through accidents or illnesses. See Tomatsu Shibutani, *Society and Personality* (Englewood Cliffs, N. J.: Prentice-Hall, 1961), pp. 237–38; and Frances Cooke MacGregor, "Some Psycho-Social Problems Associated With Facial Deformities," *American Sociological Review*, 16, 5 (October 1951), 629–38.

15. John R. P. French, Jr., and Robert L. Kaln, "A Programmatic Approach to Studying the Industrial Environment and Mental Health," *The Journal of Social Issues*, 18, 3 (July 1962),17–22, especially 19.

16. In this typology, it is assumed that the body image before disability was positive as well as all the emotions with which it was invested. Authoritarian persons with a rigid personality structure may also predominantly choose this reaction to disability because it saves them from active soul-searching and having to take a deep look at themselves and the world about them.

17. Safilios-Rothschild, *op. cit.*
18. Shibutani, *op. cit.*, pp. 230–31; and Anselm Strauss, "Transformations of Identity," in Rose, *op. cit.*, pp. 63–85.
19. Psychotherapy evaluations have shown much greater success in enabling patients to see themselves and their lives in a new light and to alter their behavioral patterns when their self-concept was negative. Here the very fact of undergoing psychotherapy means that the patient is more willing to seek change. It seems, then, that a negative self-concept is often conducive to change, especially if this change will help the individual conceive of himself in a more acceptable manner.
20. The derivation of secondary gains (such as the escaping from impossible situations or finding excuses and reasons for failures and shortcomings) from illness or disability has been discussed in Safilios-Rothschild, *op. cit.*; see also E. Weiss and O. S. English, *Psychosomatic Medicine* (Philadelphia: W. B. Saunders, 1957), p. 112; and Leo W. Simmons and Harold G. Wolff, *Social Science in Medicine* (New York: Russell Sage Foundation, 1954), pp. 186–87.
21. Safilios-Rothschild, *op. cit.*
22. Gene G. Kassebaum and Barbara O. Baumann, "Dimensions of the Sick Role in Chronic Illness," *Journal of Health and Human Behavior*, 6, 1 (Spring 1965), 21–25.
23. Mary K. Bauman and Norman M. Yoder, *Adjustment to Blindness Reviewed* (Springfield, Ill.: Thomas, 1966), p. 157; and H. R. Myklebust, *The Psychology of Deafness* (New York: Grune & Stratton, 1960).
24. Barney G. Glaser and Anselm L. Strauss, *Awareness of Dying* (Chicago: Aldine, 1965).
25. *Ibid.* The only pattern reported in this study is that lower class patients are often disliked by physicians and other personnel who do not give them enough information about their own condition. And since such individuals seldom ask direct questions and cannot usually evaluate and interpret cues concerning their condition, they often are quite unaware of their imminent death. Thus, they react only to a serious and uncertain illness but not to death.
26. *Ibid.*; and Renee C. Fox, *Experiment Perilous* (New York: Free Press, 1959).
27. Stanley James Smits, *Reactions of Self and Others to the Obviousness and Severity of Physical Disability* (Ph.D. dissertation, University of Missouri, 1964; University Microfilms, Inc., Ann Arbor, Mich.), pp. 78–80, 88. Another study concluded that men more often than women emphasized denial as a reaction to disability. See Kassebaum and Baumann, *op. cit.*, p. 26.
28. Wright, *op. cit.*, pp. 153–57. Kassebaum and Baumann found,

for example, that older people more often than younger ones emphasized denial as reaction to disability. See Kassebaum and Baumann, *op. cit.*, p. 26.

29. It has been found, however, that educated persons emphasize denial less than uneducated disabled persons. See Kassebaum and Baumann, *op. cit.*, p. 26.

30. Saad Z. Nagi, "Status Profile and Reactions to Status Threats," *American Sociological Review*, 28, 3 (June 1963), 440–43.

31. Wright, *op. cit.*; R. G. Barker, "The Social Psychology of Physical Disability," *Journal of Social Issues*, 4, 4 (Fall 1948), 28–38; H. Chevigny and S. Braverman, *The Adjustment of the Blind* (New Haven: Yale University Press, 1950); P. H. Mussen and R. G. Barker, "Attitudes Toward Cripples," *Journal of Abnormal and Social Psychology*, 39, 3 (July 1944), 351–55; L. Myerson, "Physical Disability as a Social Psychological Problem," *Journal of Social Issues*, 4, 4 (Fall 1948), 2–10; H. Rusalem "The Environmental Supports of Public Attitudes Toward the Blind," *The New Outlook for the Blind,* 44, 10 (December 1950), 277–88; and Sidney Jordan, "The Disadvantaged Group: A Concept Applicable to the Handicapped," *The Jounral of Psychology*, 55, second half (1963), 313–22.

32. Gowman's entire book is an excellent treatment of the position of the blind in American society. See Alan G. Gowman, *The War Blind in the American Social Structure* (New York: American Foundation for the Blind, 1957).

33. *Ibid.*, p. 46; and Beatrice Wright, "Spread in Adjustment to Disability," *Bulletin of the Menninger Clinic,* 28, (July 1964), 198–208.

34. Gowman, *op. cit.*, p. 51. He also mentions as another difference the fact that stereotypes against the disabled seem to be sex-linked, since blind women are less discriminated against than blind men.

35. Frank R. Westie, "Negro-White Status Differentials and Social Distance," *American Sociological Review,* 17, 5 (October 1952), 550–58. The negative relationship between socioeconomic status and prejudice held true whether years of education or income were used; see T. W. Adorno, Else Frenkel-Brunswick, D. J. Levinson, and R. N. Sanford, *The Authoritarian Personality* (New York: Harper & Row, 1950); R. Brown, *Social Psychology* (New York: Free Press, 1965); R. L. French, "Social Psychology and Group Processes," in P. R. Farnsworth and Q. McNemar (eds.), *Annual Review of Psychology,* vol. 7 (Stanford, Calif.: Annual Reviews, Inc., 1956), pp. 63–94; and Gowman, *op. cit.*, pp. 64–96.

36. Bruno Bettleheim and Morris Janowitz, *Dynamics of Prejudice:*

A Psychological and Sociological Study of Veterans (New York: Harper & Row, 1950), p. 59.

37. Harold E. Yuker, J. R. Block, and Janet H. Younng, *The Measurement of Attitudes Toward Disabled Persons*, Human Resources Study no. 7 (Albertson, N.Y.: Human Resources Center, 1966), pp. 44–58.

38. *Ibid.*

39. Jordan, *op. cit.*; and Jacobus tenBroek and Floyd W. Matson, *Hope Deferred: Public Welfare and the Blind* (Berkeley and Los Angeles: University of California Press, 1959).

40. Jordan, *op. cit.*

41. Eliot Freidson, "Disability as Social Deviance," in Marvin B. Sussman (ed.), *Sociology and Rehabilitation* (Washington, D.C.: American Sociological Association, 1965), p. 72; Edwin M. Lemert, *Social Pathology* (New York: Free Press, 1963); John I. Kitsuse, "Societal Reaction to Deviant Behavior: Problems of Theory and Method," *Social Problems*, 9, 3 (Winter 1962), 247–56; and Werner J. Cahnman, "The Stigma of Obesity," *The Sociological Quarterly*, 9, 3 (Summer 1968), especially 293–96.

42. Kai T. Erikson, "Notes on the Sociology of Deviance," in Howard S. Becker (ed.), *The Other Side: Perspectives on Deviance* (New York: Free Press, 1964), pp. 9–21.

43. Scott, *op. cit.*, pp. 71–75; and Josephson, *op. cit.*

44. Erving Goffman, *Stigma: Notes on the Management of Spoiled Identity* (Englewood Cliffs, N. J.: Prentice-Hall, 1963), pp. 73–91; and Robert B. Edgerton, *The Cloak of Competence: Stigma in the Lives of the Mentally Retarded* (Berkeley and Los Angeles: University of California Press, 1967).

45. Allport's typology has been applied in the case of the disabled. See Gordon W. Allport, *The Nature of Prejudice* (Cambridge, Mass.: Addison-Wesley, 1954), pp. 143–60.

46. H. Harbauer, "Social Prejudice Against the Mentally Disabled," in *Industrial Society and Rehabilitation—Problems and Solutions, Proceedings of the Tenth World Congress, International Society for Rehabilitation of the Disabled* (Heidelberg: Deutsche Vereinigung fur die Rehabilitation Behinderter e.v., 1967), p. 35.

47. Claude Veil, *Handicap et Société* (Paris: Flammarion, 1968), pp. 58–60.

48. Paul Hunt (ed.), *Stigma: The Experience of Disability* (London: Chapman, 1966).

49. Louis Battye and Judith Thunem, two of the contributing disabled, discussed much more explicitly and in detail the problems of affective relations between the disabled and the nondisabled than did any of the others. See Louis Battye, "The

Chatterley Syndrome," in Hunt, *op. cit.*, pp. 3–16; and Judith Thunem, "The Invalid Mind," in Hunt, *op. cit.*, pp. 50–51.
50. Edgerton, *op. cit.*, pp. 112, 119–26, 153–54. Ten out of the sixteen retarded women who married normal men married much older men (on the average, seventeen years older than their wives) who were divorced or widowed. The remaining six husbands were marginal wage earners with a history of one or more of the following: narcotics addiction, alcoholism, criminal conduct, or mental illness. Interestingly enough, the older husbands admitted they married their wives because they were "dependent, submissive and appreciative." If the conclusions from other types of "mixed" marriages are applicable here, we could expect that when a disabled person is able to hold a prestigious job successfully he will be able to marry a "normal" woman of a lower socioeconomic status than his or a not very attractive and desirable nondisabled one.
51. Martin S. Weinberg, "The Problems of Midgets and Dwarfs and Organizational Remedies: A Study of the Little People of America," *Journal of Health and Social Behavior,* 9, 1 (March 1968), 65–71.
52. *Ibid.,* pp. 67–70.
53. Edgerton, *op. cit.*, pp. 52–53.
54. Weinberg, *op. cit.*, pp. 70–71.
55. M. François Block-Lainé, *Etude du problème général de l'inadaptation des personnes handicapées* (report presented to the Prime Minister, Paris, December 1967), pp. 68–73.
56. This point of view came through in discussions with Mr. Jules La France, a doctoral student of sociology attending the author's seminar on Medical Sociology at the University of Montreal.
57. Veil, *op. cit.*, p. 136.
58. It is known from disaster theory that when people who have undergone similar catastrophic experiences are brought together in the same locale and discover that they are among many who have suffered as much or even more than themselves, the widespread sharing of loss makes them able to more easily overcome their personal mourning and adjust to their misfortune. See Charles E. Fritz, "Disaster," in Robert K. Merton and Robert A. Nisbet (eds.), *Contemporary Social Problems,* 1st ed. (New York: Harcourt, Brace & World, 1961), pp. 651–694; also I. Silone, in R. Crossman (ed.), *The God That Failed* (New York: Bantam, 1952), chap. 2; and W. James "On Some Mental Effects of the Earthquake," in *Memories and Studies* (London: Longmans, Green, 1911). Similarly, the stress resulting from a disabling injury or illness is more easily absorbed by the afflicted individual when it is not an unshared

experience, probably because then the disabled person no longer feels singled out by his misfortune. The rehabilitation setting is the ideal locale for the disabled to feel that their experience is by no means unique and that others with similar or more serious disabilities carry on remarkably well. See Stephen L. Fink, Rainette Fantz, and Joseph Zinker, "The Growth Beyond Adjustment: Another Look at Motivation" (mimeographed paper, Cleveland, n.d.); also Joseph John Raymond Grau, "Permissive Treatment of Disabled Persons: A Sociological Study" (unpublished Ph.D. dissertation, University of Pittsburgh, 1963); and Veil, *op. cit.*, p. 165.

59. Margaret Gill, "No Small Miracle," in Hunt, *op. cit.*, pp. 102–3.
60. H. Shands, "An Outline of the Process of Recovery From Severe ⸳Trauma," *A.M.A. Archives of Neurology and Psychiatry*, 73 (1955), 403–9; also Sidney Fishman, "Amputee Needs, Frustrations, and Behavior," *Rehabilitation Literature*, 20, 11 (November 1959), 328; and Grau, *op. cit.*
61. It is well known, for example, that heart specialists do not always agree with each other regarding the degree of necessary inactivity dictated by heart disease; some will frighten their patients and force upon them almost a total incapacity "unless they wish to die," while others may encourage their patients to continue their "normal" lives with or without adjustments and with only certain precautions. The definition of the disability by the treating specialist has great influence upon the disabled person who, of course, is greatly concerned with the development of his disability. See *Final Report of the Cardiac Rehabilitation Project* (Syracuse, N.Y.: Syracuse University and Upstate Medical Center, 1966). The parent of the disabled may also, because of his own needs and motivations, define the disabled as totally incapacitated and force or precipitate such a definition upon the disabled. See Eleanor S. Reid, "Helping Parents of Handicapped Children," *Children*, 5 (January–February 1958), 15–19. See also Lawrence E. Schlesinger, "Disruptions in the Personal-Social System Resulting From Traumatic Disability," *Journal of Health and Human Behavior*, 6, 2 (Summer 1965), 95–98; and Scott, *op. cit.*, pp. 20–38.
62. Richard H. Ingwell, Richard W. Thoreson, and Stanley J. Smits, "Accuracy of Social Perception of Physically Handicapped and Non-handicapped Persons," *The Journal of Social Psychology*, 72, first half (June 1967), 107–16, especially 113; Edwin J. Thomas, "Problems of Disability From the Perspective of Role Theory," *Journal of Health and Human Behavior*, 7, 1 (Spring 1966), 7–13. Thomas developed an interesting typology based on the degree of congruency and incongruency

between the way roles are defined by the disabled and by the nondisabled.

63. Robert Kleck, "Emotional Arousal in Interactions With Stigmatized Persons," *Psychological Reports,* 19 (1966), 1226; also Fred Davis, "Deviance Disavowal: The Management of Strained Interaction by the Visibly Handicapped," *Social Problems,* 9, 2 (Fall 1961), 120–32; also Robert Kleck, Hiroshi Ono, and Arbert H. Hastorf, "The Effects of Physical Deviance and Face-to-Face Interaction," *Human Relations,* 19, 4 (1966), 425–36; Goffman, *op. cit.*; and Thomas, *op. cit.*, pp. 2–14.

64. As Davis has pointed out, some handicapped persons intentionally undermine sociable relations by flaunting their handicap in such a way that "fictional acceptance" becomes untenable. See Davis, *op. cit.*, pp. 122–25, 127, 128. The perceptional phenomenon of "spread" has been expounded in detail by Wright in "Spread in Adjustment to Disability," *op. cit.*

65. While most authors have emphasized the strain that visible disabilities place upon social interaction, the author of this book believes that a similar effect could be produced when the nonvisible disability is known to the nondisabled actors. Because the disabling illness is not visible, the interacting actors may go to even greater extremes of "overnormalizing" the disabled or of seeing their disability as all-pervasive and totally incapacitating.

66. Hunt, *op. cit.* Actually, this is a posture not unlike that accorded different types of minority group members.

67. Louise Centers and Richard Centers, "Peer Group Attitudes Toward the Amputee Child," *The Journal of Social Psychology,* 61, first half (October 1963), 127–32.

68. Smits, *op. cit.*

69. Ingwell, Thoreson, and Smits, *op. cit.,* pp. 107–16; and Eileen G. Potter and Fred E. Fiedler, "Physical Disability and Interpersonal Perception," *Perceptual and Motor Skills,* 8, 3 (September 1958), 241–42.

70. S. A. Richardson *et al.,* "Cultural Uniformity in Reaction to Physical Disability," *American Sociological Review,* 26, 2 (April 1961), 241.

71. Ari De-Levie, "Attitudes of Laymen and Professionals Toward Physical and Social Disability" (unpublished Ph.D. dissertation, Columbia University, 1966).

72. S. A. Richardson and Jacqueline Royce, "Race and Physical Handicap in Children's Perference for Other Children," *Child Development,* 39, 2 (June 1968), 467–80.

73. Potter and Fiedler, *op. cit.*

74. Schlesinger, *op. cit.*, p. 98.

75. Ingwell *et al.*, *op. cit.* See also the review of the literature in Stephen A. Richardson, "Some Social Psychological Consequences of Handicapping," *Pediatrics,* 32, 2 (August 1963), 291–97.
76. Allport, *op. cit.*, pp. 262–63.
77. For a review of contradictory findings as to whether or not and what type of contact can favorably change the nondisabled's attitudes toward the disabled, see Eugene L. Gaier, Donald C. Linkowski, and Marceline E. Jacques, "Contact as a Variable in the Perception of Disability," *The Journal of Social Psychology,* 74, first half (February 1968), 117–26.
78. Cahnman, *op. cit.*, pp. 283–99.
79. Gowman, *op. cit.*, pp. 71–75, 93–96.
80. William Gellman, "Attitudes Toward Rehabilitation of the Disabled," *American Journal of Occupational Therapy,* 14, 4 (1960), 188; also Peter Townsend, "Foreword," in Hunt, *op. cit.*, p. vi; and Paul Hunt, "A Critical Condition," in Hunt, *op. cit.*, pp. 150–52.
81. Goffman, *op. cit.*, and Barker *et al.* report that in 80% of the jokes referring to the physically disabled, the disabled were clearly deprecated. See Roger G. Barker *et al., Adjustment to Physical Handicap and Illness: A Survey of the Social Psychology of Physique and Disability,* Bulletin 55, revised (New York: Social Science Research Council, 1953), pp. 75–76; and MacGregor, *op. cit.*, pp. 631–32.
82. Townsend, *op. cit.*; Lewis Anthony Dexter, "On the Politics and Sociology of Stupidity in Our Society," in Howard S. Becker (ed.), *The Other Side: Perspectives on Deviance* (New York: Free Press, 1964), pp. 37–49, especially pp. 42–44. See also Edgerton, *op. cit.*, pp. 205–19.
83. Constantina Safilios-Rothschild, "Prejudice Against the Disabled and Some Means to Combat It," *International Rehabilitation Review,* 19, 4 (October 1968), 8–10.
84. Gowman, *op. cit.*, pp. 71–75.
85. Jordan, *op. cit.*, pp. 316–17.
86. Gellman, *op. cit.*, p. 188; Kleck, *op. cit.*; Kleck, Ono, and Hastorf, *op. cit.*, pp. 425–36; see also D. O. Hebb, "On the Nature of Fear," *Psychological Review,* 53, 5 (September 1946), 259–76.
87. Jerome Siller and Abram Chipman, "Perceptions of Physical Disability by the Non-disabled" (paper presented at the American Psychological Association meetings, Los Angeles, September 1964).
88. Richardson *et al., op. cit.*, p. 241.
89. Barker *et al., op. cit.*, p. 75.
90. Gowman, *op cit.*, pp. 67–70; Martin Whiteman and Irving F.

Lukoff, "Attitudes Toward Blindness and Other Physical Handicaps," *The Journal of Social Psychology*, 66 (June 1965), 135–45; Marceline E. Jacques, Eugene L. Gaier, and Donald C. Linkowski, "Coping-Succumbing Attitudes Toward Physical and Mental Disabilities," *The Journal of Social Psychology*, 71 (April 1967), 295–307. See also Donald C. Linkowski, Marceline E. Jacques, and Eugene L. Gaier, "Reactions to Disability: A Thematic Analysis" (mimeographed, State University of New York at Buffalo, n.d.).

91. Meng's findings as reported in Barker *et al.*, *op. cit.*, p. 76; also Hunt, *op. cit.*, pp. 155–57.

92. Siller and Chipman, *op. cit.*

93. It has been reported that another basic element in rejecting attitudes is the nondisabled's fear of what to do in interactions with the disabled or his fear that his feelings or curiosity will show and will offend the disabled. See *ibid.*

94. C. David Jenkins and Stephen J. Lyzanski, "Dimensions of Beliefs and Feelings Concerning Three Diseases—Poliomyelitis, Cancer, and Mental Illness: A Factor Analytic Study," *Behavioral Science*, 13, 5 (September 1968), 372–81.

95. Yuker, Block, and Younng, *op. cit.*, p. 58.

96. See the review of the literature, as well as the article itself, in Mark Chesler, "Ethnocentrism and Attitudes Toward the Physically Disabled," *Journal of Personality and Social Psychology*, 2, 6 (December 1965), 877–92.

97. For example, high dogmatism has been found to be related (but not significantly so) to more favorable attitudes toward the disabled in Jack K. Genskow and Frank D. Maglione, "Familiarity, Dogmatism, and Reported Student Attitudes Toward the Disabled," *The Journal of Social Psychology*, 67, second half (December 1965), 329–41. See also Yuker, Block, and Younng, *op. cit.*, pp. 78–81, where all relevant studies are reviewed and it is reported that "while these results are conflicting, there is some support for the hypothesis that the acceptance of the disabled tends to be somewhat greater in non-authoritarian samples." See also pp. 59–70 for a discussion of findings on the other sociopsychological and psychological characteristics.

CHAPTER 4

The Sociology and Social Psychology of Rehabilitation

Although the analytical separation of the concept of disability from the concept of rehabilitation is to some extent artificial, it has some
merit since not all the disabled necessarily
adopt the rehabilitant role. Throughout our discussion, however, we will be relating rehabilitation to disability so that our theoretical
framework is more complete.

Using the Parsonian analytical schema, we
shall examine rehabilitation at three different
levels: the personality, the social system, and
the cultural. Here again, although the theoretical discussion at each level cannot be completely isolated from that of another level, the
schema has been adopted for the sake of
analytical clarity.

Rehabilitation at the Personality Level

Probably the most central concept to be examined in connection with rehabilitation at this level of analysis is *motivation*. Regardless of the many possible theoretical definitions of the term, the usual operational definition found in rehabilitation literature refers to the disabled's ability and willingness to mobilize physical and psychological resources to cope with his disability; that is, his desire for and cooperativeness in rehabilitation and, more specifically, in the prescribed goals which he must realize in order to be successfully rehabilitated. Furthermore, since in all rehabilitation settings, but especially the vocational settings, central to the staff-determined rehabilitation goals is the return to work, rehabilitation motivation may often be used interchangeably with motivation to work.[1]

The operational criteria for assessing the degree of motivation in prospective or actual rehabilitants vary considerably and usually depend upon the therapist's professional membership as well as his values and sociopsychological background; the stage in the rehabilitation process as well as the rehabilitants' ages, socioeconomic status, and sociopsychological backgrounds. At the time of evaluation for admission, verbal expression of motivation tends to influence rehabilitation personnel favorably. However, once the disabled is admitted to a rehabilitation facility, verbal expression of motivation, while not totally discarded (even when it is contradicted by his actions), is not always taken at face value.[2] Three major operational criteria are usually employed by the rehabilitation staff in categorizing rehabilitants as either "motivated" or "unmotivated." The labeling of "unmotivated" is given to a rehabilitant when he fails to perform adequately in terms of any of these criteria: (a) when he refuses to perform the prescribed therapeutic tasks; (b) when he tries but gives up quickly at the first discouragement or failure or at the first sensation of pain, discomfort, or fatigue; (c) when he keeps trying but fails to learn;[3] and (d) when he is not "insightful"; that is, when he does not accept the rehabilitation workers' definitions and interpretations of his "problem" and of the required and appropriate solutions.[4]

Psychological research indicates, however, that motivation is not a unitary force either present or not present in an individual. The disabled simply cannot be dichotomized into "motivated" and "unmotivated." Factor analytic studies of the disabled's motivational patterns have isolated some factors that may be viewed as neutral, some that contribute to, and some that impede different kinds of rehabilitation efforts. These factors are: (a) reality orientation, that is, the extent to which the patient recognizes the nature and degree of his disability (or in other terms, the degree to which he accepts his disability); (b) energy level, that is, the degree to which the patient engages in spontaneous physical activity; (c) cooperativeness, that is, the extent to which he is willing to go along with the formal demands and regulations of the institution; (d) breadth of motivation; and (e) ultimate social requirement, that is, the patient's ultimate realistic goals (especially vocational goals).[5] Each disabled person may possess some of these factors, but to varying degrees. Seldom will he have only those factors which facilitate rehabilitation or only those which impede all rehabilitation efforts. A "motivated" disabled person is not necessarily willing to cooperate with all rehabilitation goals, and an "unmotivated" one is not always a "vegetable" unwilling to do anything. Instead, disabled people may be more fruitfully conceptualized as being situated on a continuum ranging from "high" to "low" motivation, since everyone may be motivated to some extent to perform at least certain tasks. Since a disabled's type and strength of motivational factors play a very important role in his rehabilitation outcome, the significant question is: What factors in the disabled's personality, in the rules and regulations of the rehabilitation center, in the demands made upon the disabled, and in the behavior of the rehabilitation staff and their relations with the disabled are responsible for a more or less effective motivational make-up?

In order to understand how the disabled's personality may affect his motivation, we must examine the meaning that disability has for him. By using the theoretical typology of disability effects upon self-concept developed in Chapter 3, we can explain some of the motivation differentials. First, those who have been able to accept their disability favorably, localize it in only a few self-images, and still think of themselves as basically the same person as before are probably the most motivated and cooperative rehabilitants. Since disability has not lowered their self-esteem or discontinued their identity, they tend to be quite willing to cooperate with the rehabilitation personnel in order to limit the effects of the disability and to capitalize on their abilities for achieving greater independence—emotional, social, and financial.

However, in order for a disabled to be able to accept his disability and restrict its emotional impact, he must first know its exact extent. But since not all disabled are told the extent of their physical limitations and ability, it is often difficult to reach such a level of motivation. This lack of sufficient and specific information becomes greater the greater the social class gap between therapist and patient. Rehabilitants of low socioeconomic status often have a hazy idea about the nature and degree of their disability as well as about the purpose of the different rehabilitation tasks.[6] Thus, without being reassured by anyone about the efficacy of the rehabilitation tasks and without understanding the purpose of such tasks, the disabled may indeed be very little motivated to participate in painful physical therapy, especially when visible improvement does not follow quickly. Sometimes, then, "uncooperativeness" represents a motivation for self-preservation and a way of coping with a little-understood and threatening environment.[7] Fears and uncertainty interfere with the ability to learn and profit from the rehabilitation services. If these "uncooperative" rehabilitants were told the exact nature and extent of their disability and the purpose of and connection between each therapeutic task and eventual improvement, some at least would become motivated and cooperative.

Physicians themselves sometimes cannot accurately evaluate the degree of disability present or predict the extent of possible improvement. They may set rehabilitation goals too high. This failure and the physical stress and pain experienced frustrates the rehabilitant and renders him "poorly motivated" and "uncooperative" in pursuing the rehabilitation program.[8]

It is also conceivable that motivated rehabilitants who have accepted their disability and are willing to limit its effects as much as possible may lose the drive to achieve some of the rehabilitation goals if they perceive them as threatening to their self-esteem. For example, if a disabled worker who because of his physical limitations cannot return to his previous job is discouraged by the vocational counselor and the social worker from establishing a small business and is instead urged to accept a light service job with low prestige and pay, he may stop cooperating with the vocational rehabilitation aspects of his program.[9] Could we label this disabled person "unmotivated" just because he rejects a goal that is unacceptable to his self-esteem? In terms of Shontz's five motivational components, he has reality orientation, energy level, breadth of motivation, and he may cooperate with all other aspects of rehabilitation except those that prepare him for the suggested service jobs.[10] Whether his goals are "realistic" or not is not a matter that cannot be easily assessed. Maybe they seem extremely unrealistic to the vocational counselor or the placement specialist because he knows that the probability of success in such an undertaking is quite low. But ways might be found in some instances to help the person so that his chance of success increases. Some case studies have indicated, for example, that it is the disabled's family which sometimes makes it difficult for him to "make a go" out of a particular venture such as a small repair shop.[11] Through discussions with the disabled's family, the vocational counselor or the social worker could first assess the family's attitude toward his "unrealistic" goals as well as the reasons for any negative attitudes and the likelihood of influencing them toward acceptance.

Second, there are those who cannot accept the fact of their disablement because their body image and the emotions attached to it have a prominent place in their self-concept. For them, the incorporation of the disability would necessitate such drastic and self-diminishing overall changes that the continuity of their identity would be threatened. These persons may be extremely motivated to cooperate with any effort or procedure aimed at improving their physical condition. Thus, the disabled who cannot tolerate their disability often appear to be extremely motivated, "model" rehabilitants—at least in the first stages of rehabilitation, when they may believe that by doing everything they are told they may get rid of the disability. When, however, they reach a plateau in their physical progress and have to face the fact that the remaining amount of disability cannot be made to disappear, they may suddenly become "uncooperative."[12] They may either leave the rehabilitation center in search of further treatment and cure, scientific or not, or they may return to their previous employment (if the job is still open to them) regardless of whether or not they are physically able to carry out the tasks. The return to the previous job, even when too strenuous for their physical state, is necessary to make them feel that nothing has changed in their lives and that they are "as good as ever."

Finally, the disabled who welcome their disability because it helps them become reconciled with a negative self-image, with experiences of failure, or with socially undesirable needs (such as intense dependency) usually tend to be uncooperative with some or all rehabilitation efforts. If their negative self-concept refers only to their occupational failures and maladjustments, they may appear motivated during physical therapy but not during occupational therapy (which they may even refuse altogether). If, however, they always had strong unmet dependency needs and a negative self-concept about their family role as well as their occupational role, they may be unmotivated toward both physical and occupational rehabilitation. Or, if the "secondary gains" derived from the disability are represented by the amount of workmen's compensation that can be obtained, the disabled may be motivated not to admit any improvement in physical status even when they have improved considerably. They may never miss physical or occupational therapy and perform all the necessary tasks but still talk about their aches and pains, complaining that nothing has been done for them in rehabilitation. Thus, we find that even this category of disabled with some kind of vested interest in the temporary or permanent preservation of their disability (and who could be expected to approach the model of the "unmotivated" rehabilitant) are not necessarily uncooperative in all rehabilitation efforts and do not always or totally waste the rehabilitation personnel's time.

Besides the type of the rehabilitant's self-concept and mode of incorporating the disability in it, their significant others' level of motivation and the goals they have set for them often play a very important role in determining the disabled's own level of motivation (see Chapter 7, section on The Family). Thus, it is important that the rehabilitation staff take into consideration the significant others' goals in setting the rehabilitants' programs and objectives in order to maximize motivation and rehabilitation success.[13]

Because of an overall prevailing tendency toward adjusting the

disabled to the social structure of rehabilitation setting and its requirements rather than the other way around, the rehabilitants' lack of
motivation and uncooperativeness has been often regarded as "something arising entirely from within" themselves rather than from the
type of institution and relationships with rehabilitation staff.[14] We
shall now turn to the examination of the latter possibility; that is, the
effect the types of demands made upon rehabilitants, the degree to
which permissive or authoritarian norms pervade the rehabilitation
milieu, and the type of patient-to-patient relationships have upon the
rehabilitants' level of motivation. All these factors interacting with
the individual personalities of the rehabilitants and the meaning that
disability has for them produce different types of motivational make-
ups.[15]

Some rehabilitation centers require their rehabilitants to behave
as regular hospital patients and to abide by a number of more or less
strict rules which do not foster ideal rehabilitation goals but make
the life of custodial personnel considerably easier. The rehabilitation
staff usually decides what the rehabilitation goals should be, often
without consulting the rehabilitant (or after having rejected as "unrealistic" whatever goals he considers desirable).[16] One study suggests that the lack of motivation on the part of some rehabilitants
may be due to the fact that often rehabilitaion programs concentrate
mostly on the disabled's physiological needs and not adequately on
his safety, love, esteem, and self-actualization needs.[17] This unbal-
anced emphasis may render rehabilitation activities and the required
effort meaningless for the disabled. Thus, when rehabilitants have
to conform to staff expectations and goals which may be irrelevant,
unimportant, or secondary in terms of the rehabilitant's particular
values and needs hierarchy, family and social life, vocational perspectives and personality structure, they may appear to be "unmotivated"
and "uncooperative."[18] The degree of irrelevancy of goals is often
greater the greater the social distance between the staff and the
rehabilitant.[19] This atmosphere tends to be less conducive to motivated
behavior than one in which rehabilitants are encouraged to participate
on an almost equal basis with rehabilitation personnel in the determination of rules and rehabilitation goals.[20] It may be possible,
however, that even when patient participation is encouraged, those
who participate most are those who think that the rehabilitation

personnel approve of them, their approval being related to level of income, social class, vertical mobility, family harmony, stability of residence, and race.[21] That is, the less the rehabilitant is like the "model" middle class staff, the less he may feel like participating. He may withdraw instead and passively accept the staff-determined goals.

The type of patient-to-patient relationship and its effect on the disabled's motivation for rehabilitation has been well documented. Since in the rehabilitation center each disabled usually has the opportunity to observe and talk with others afflicted with the same or more severe types and degrees of disability, it may be easier for him to accept his disability and become motivated to do well in rehabilitation if other disabled whom he admires and identifies with are motivated and progressing well in their rehabilitation.[22] While it is possible that some "uncooperative" rehabilitants may have a negative effect upon the motivational mechanisms of other disabled, generally the realization that others are also stigmatized by a disability tends to have a positive and encouraging effect. There is, however, hardly any research indicating the psychological mechanism that permits some disabled to accept their disability and become motivated when in a community with other disabled or what types of patient-to-patient relationships can enhance or inhibit this effect.

The type of prevailing staff-to-staff relationships and their effect upon the rehabilitants' motivational makeup is probably one of the most important factors after the disabled's personality in determining motivation. It is also the least studied factor. Several very good studies of this kind have been conducted about mental hospitals,[23] but only very few about rehabilitation centers[24] despite the presence of many new and self-asserting professions in the latter that increase the chance for conflicts and dissatisfactions. Rehabilitation centers, like all other therapeutic settings, cannot avoid a basic split between the custodial and the therapeutic staff, but in the case of rehabilitation this split is even more accentuated and may have far-reaching effects. A study comparing the attitudes of nursing and therapeutic rehabilitation staffs has indicated, for example, that the former view the severely disabled as helpless while the latter do not.[25]

In practice, custodial personnel are more concerned with the efficient completion of their routine tasks than with the rehabilitation progress of the disabled. Thus, the attempts of physical therapists to gradually make a disabled independent in the activities of daily living may be seriously jeopardized by the nursing aide's doing everything for the disabled because this is the easiest and neatest thing to do. And since physical therapists do not have the time (or necessarily the authority) to supervise the custodial personnel's treatment of the disabled, the same rehabilitant may be sometimes subject to two different pressures: one toward independence and the other toward dependence.[26] There is actually some evidence that patients perceive the custodial personnel differently from the therapeutic personnel, their perception being reciprocal to the type of perception the personnel have of them. Thus, patients tend to see nurses and other custodial personnel as symbols of their dependency state, while they perceive the physicians and the therapeutic staff as symbols of their "hope" to become "normal" again.[27] Under such conflicting messages and pressures, the disabled's motivation may weaken, and he may take the road of least resistance for most of the time he spends at the center—that of dependence—and therefore appear uncooperative and unmotivated to the therapeutic staff.

Furthermore, despite the ideal of a rehabilitation team working closely together, each rehabilitation profession, anxious to establish its own importance and professional identity, tends to accentuate the narrow goals pertaining to its specialty rather than the overall rehabilitation goals. Thus, much rivalry, interdepartmental friction, timing and scheduling conflicts, and conflicts in evaluation and rehabilitation philosophy occur with greater or fewer repercussions for the rehabilitants' morale and motivation.[28] When the rehabilitant senses that the therapeutic staff cannot agree on the extent of his permanent disability, on what the rehabilitation goals ought to be, or on whether he is improving or not, he may become hostile and uncooperative or become depressed and regress physically. He may either leave the center discouraged or choose to "hang on" to the therapist who thinks he can still improve his physical state and be motivated to follow only what this therapist tells him to do.

The weekly conferences of the rehabilitation team and their discussions of individual cases sometimes become a battleground for the members of rival professions in their fight for professional recognition, power, and prestige. It is within this context that we can

better understand the significance of a disabled's "good" relationship
with a member of the rehabilitation team, since this staff person is
willing to listen sympathetically to the needs and goals the r habilitant
considers important and to introduce them for consideration in team
discussions. This team member usually lends support to the rehabilitant's goals and needs whenever he can, for by adopting them he can
present them as evidence of his faithful adherence to truly rehabilitative and humanitarian principles. A therapist may fight vigorously
over a case because he would score highly in professional power and
prestige if his opinion prevails. To the extent that the rehabilitant's
needs and goals are included in his program, he will tend to be more
willing to accomplish painful and unpleasant tasks—especially if he
feels he is reaching for the goals he, rather than another, has set for
himself. Roth and Eddy's study is probably the most illuminating in
this area. They point out that patients who had managed to become
"sponsored" by a physician (or a social worker, or a physical
therapist)—one who "bought" their rehabilitation goals and needs
and then tried to influence the remaining staff in this direction—
appeared to be "motivated" and usually achieved a considerable level
of rehabilitation success.[29]

The disabled's "good" relationship with one or more therapists
may be reciprocally functional in that the therapist(s) may be inclined
to make a greater therapeutic effort which in turn may encourage and
motivate the disabled to try harder and reward the therapists's efforts.
Thus, there seems to be a circle, according to which the disabled
initially most motivated and sympathetic to the therapists receive
most of the attention and effort while those less motivated do not
inspire the therapists to try as hard.[30] In this way, the motivated
usually become more so and are helped to achieve rehabilitation
success, while the unmotivated become more discouraged and bitter
during their stay at the rehabilitation center and often improve very
little.

At this point it is interesting to note that some of the more
astute disabled who for some reason wish to be admitted or stay
on at the rehabilitation center can successfully play the "motivated"
role so as to impress rehabilitation personnel.[31] They have correctly
perceived that the magic key to the rehabilitation center is motivation
and can successfully "play" the institutional rules and requirements

to their advantage. They pretend to accept the institutional philosophy and goals in order to receive the benefits they consider relevant and important. A typical case are those disabled who are not planning to return to work but wish to improve their physical condition and therefore skillfully pretend they are anxious to return to work.[32] During rehabilitation the pretense is more difficult, but some disabled are quite successful at keeping it up until the moment that they think (or are told) that they have achieved the maximum level of physical rehabilitation.

Relatively little research has been carried out on the possible intervention methods and techniques that could modify the motivational makeup of the disabled. While several articles have discussed specific inducements and rewards, the main motivating method described in the literature is the so-called programmed therapy, according to which the rehabilitant's behavior can be remotivated in the desired direction by giving him rewards (such as recognition, approval, or esteem) after he has behaved in an appropriate manner.[33] Kerr and Meyerson applied a similar technique (which they call "operant conditioning principle of positive reinforcement"), using as reinforcements social attention and a resting period. The antagonistic behavior of the involved disabled gradually changed because the psychological and social rehabilitation environment had changed for them. It has been suggested that "some impediments to rehabilitation can be removed more easily and economically by staff education than by intensive counseling with individual clients."[34] Other suggested remotivating techniques refer entirely to the reeducation of the rehabilitation staff so that they truly function as a coordinated team. This reeducation aims at making the rehabilitation team willing to (a) explain simply and clearly to rehabilitants the nature and extent of their disability as well as the purpose of each rehabilitative task; and (b) determine the rehabilitation goals as well as modifications that must be brought about in the rehabilitation program together with the rehabilitants.[35]

Both these major orientations have been applied sporadically and have not been adequately evaluated. Probably, a combination of the two would bring better results for the rehabilitants. Reliance upon the first method of "programmed therapy" should necessarily assume the second; otherwise it would be senseless to force and condition the rehabilitants to accept irrelevant rehabilitation goals or to perform painful rehabilitative tasks whose purpose they cannot understand. But one point is clear: "Unmotivated" rehabilitants should not be left to their fate after being unfavorably labeled. Instead, the factors responsible for this inadequate motivational make-up must be located and then changed to the fullest extent possible. This "remotivational" process should actually become the core of rehabilitation programs if rehabilitation is to fulfill its promise.

Rehabilitation at the Social System Level

The rehabilitation center, whether administratively independent or part of a larger hospital complex, is a social system made up of personnel and rehabilitants in a variety of reciprocal relations. We could further divide the rehabilitation social system into the sub-systems of the hierarchy of staff, the interacting rehabilitants, and the interacting dyads, triads, etc., of staff and rehabilitants. An even further differentiation of subsystems is possible if we distinguish be-tween the subsystem of custodial personnel and that of the pro-fessional staff, or between the particular cliques that groups of rehabilitants tend to form.

Whether we consider the entire rehabilitation setting or only a portion of it as a social system (with the possible exception of rehabil-itants' cliques), we will inevitably find a number of tensions and adaptations to these tensions in order for the subsystem, or more im-portant, the entire social system, to be maintained. In this section we shall examine the nature and possible causes of tension in the entire rehabilitation social system and in each of its subsystems as well as the nature of the adaptations taking place between and within subsystems.

Some rehabilitation facilities are organized in such a manner and abide by such norms, rules, and values as to constitute a truly thera-peutic community. Some tend to be more rigidly organized as hospitals rather than as institutions whose only purpose is rehabilitation. Despite the fact that the rules in the latter type of setting are quite strict and institution- rather than client-oriented and that some fea-tures of "total institutions" permeate a certain number of decisions, policies, and procedures, it seems that it is almost impossible for a rehabilitation center to be a truly "total institution." Because the ideal of the rehabilitation philosophy is quite prevalent and well-known, a particular therapist will at least give it lip service even if he does not entirely accept it. He will have to act more or less according to its principles whenever another staff member or rehabilitant deems a particular action or procedure necessary for these principles to be followed. Even in the most totally institution-like rehabilitation facility, at least some therapists abide to varying degrees by the rehabilitation philosophy and principles, interpreting them in a variety of ways congruent with their personalities and sociopsychological backgrounds. Thus the rehabilitants are allowed to show at least some initiative about their program. Of course, some of the rehabilitants are themselves perceptive enough to remind staff members of the expected ideal rehabilitative behavior, thereby bringing the rehabilitation staff "into line"; that is, convincing them to go along with their goals and wishes.[36]

In the available literature two different rehabilitation facilities have been described in some detail: the Harmarville Rehabilitation Center[37] and the rehabilitation wards of the Farewell Hospital.[38] Grau has described the permissive therapeutic milieu of the former setting, which emphasizes self-help on the part of the disabled, gives rehabilitants a great amount of initiative in making up their own therapy program and the freedom not to follow scheduled therapeutic activities without incurring any kind of penalty. He found that this kind of permissiveness had both positive and negative effects upon the rehabilitation success of disabled individuals. The main negative effects were: (a) the occasional confusion of patients (as well as of staff members) as to what exactly their role was vis-à-vis their own rehabilitation efforts as well as in their relationships with the other disabled; and (b) poor adjustment at the interpersonal level because they often chose the way of least resistance, that of social withdrawal, because they felt they should not get too involved with people from whom they would soon be separated, because they were too preoccupied with overcoming their disability, or because they did not find anybody particularly congenial.[39]

The first of the negative effects of total permissiveness and minimum guidance often tends to deter the disabled from doing their utmost to help themselves, especially if they have been accustomed to following directions rather than setting and fulfilling their own goals. In this "noninterventive," "nonpunitive" therapeutic method no effort is made to increase the degree of motivation in the case of those who—frozen by fears, apprehensions, and self-depreciating evaluations—cannot benefit from the open therapeutic milieu without some previous special psychological guidance and help. Also because of the permissive philosophy, staff members often contradict each other or hesitate to give the patient their opinion of his present state or a prognosis of his condition.[40] Finally, the fact that many of the disabled withdraw does not necessarily mean that they did not benefit from the fact that other disabled at the center were trying to overcome their handicaps or imply that they will be less competent in their postrehabilitation adjustment. It may simply mean that they are concentrating on improving their level of ability and leaving the center as soon as possible instead of getting attached to people and places. In this sense, it may represent a "functional" adaptation to the center.

Despite the negative effects, which could easily be eliminated with a higher degree of guidance and supervision when necessary and through the use of group therapy, the overall positive results of a more permissive, self-oriented therapeutic milieu in rehabilitation seem to outweigh the adverse ones. Probably the most important positive result is that the disabled, by being able to take an active part in planning or modifying their rehabilitation goals, are generally more motivated to fulfill goals which tend to reflect their own needs and wishes rather than externally imposed ones.[41] As we have seen, when goals are determined by the rehabilitation team, there is a greater chance that they will not coincide with the rehabilitants' expectations and goals. And the incongruency of rehabilitation goals set by the rehabilitation team and those set by the rehabilitant himself is usually much greater when the rehabilitant belongs to the lower class. In such cases, success in rehabilitation entails espousal of middle class values and goals.[42] Refusal to comply is often labeled "lack of motivation" or "uncooperativeness," and the disabled may either be denied rehabilitation services after the initial evaluation period or soon discharged.[43] A permissive milieu helps avoid such pitfalls and improves the chances for rehabilitation success since the rehabilitants can more or less pursue their own goals even when they are unrealistically high. The frustration of failure could in many cases be managed through counseling, especially since the rehabilitant has usually made considerable headway even though it is not as much as he would have wished.

Roth and Eddy have described the rehabilitation wards at Farewell Hospital as a facility coming close to a "total institution." They have analyzed the ongoing processes and the rehabilitants' modes of adaptation in the light of Goffman's theoretical framework concerning total institutions.[44] The rehabilitants were mostly aged disabled persons without social position, truly "unwanted" by the larger society as well as by their own families, despite the rehabilitation staff's deliberate efforts to choose younger persons, especially those with "desirable" disabilities.[45] Probably because of the extremely unfavorable social condition of the rehabilitants and the poor prognosis for true social rehabilitation (including social reintegration into familial and/or occupational or friendship roles), the main emphasis of the rehabilitation services is upon improving the degree of independence in activities of daily living (ADL)—a goal functional for the institution—and on long-term custodial maintenance of the disabled patients. These goals are imposed on the rehabilitant without any margin of choice, and while he is expected to follow diligently and spiritedly all the prescribed therapeutic tasks as well as to comply with hospital rules and regulations, he improves his rehabilitation chances if he is also "willing and able to act as a coordinator and promoter of his own program of therapy and care."[46] Despite the presence of several features of a total institution, there were a variety of mechanisms and conditions that permitted the rehabilitants to enjoy a greater degree of permissiveness and to control their fate to a certain extent. As we have mentioned, it is probably impossible for a rehabilitation facility to truly become a total institution.

Most rehabilitation centers tend to combine some elements of a therapeutic milieu and some elements of a total institution in varying proportions. Some of the staff abiding by more permissive norms tend to treat rehabilitants as co-equals, while others, adhering to stricter and more rigid norms, tend to treat the rehabilitants as subordinates. Sometimes deep cleavages may exist between individual staff members or between categories of rehabilitation personnel such as between the custodial and the therapeutic staff (see the first section of this chapter). Such cleavages may create tensions and conflict that more or less seriously affect the rehabilitants. But interprofessional rivalries often create conflicts and tensions either because one staff member feels belittled by a professional in another field or because he (or she) feels that another staff member is interfering with his work by suggesting an alternative method or by disputing the appropriateness and effectiveness of a particular therapeutic philosophy or technique.[47] In order to better understand the nature and causes of these interprofessional rivalries and conflicts, we must now examine the different rehabilitation professions in detail.

Rehabilitation became a multidisciplinary field after World War II. Consequently, both new professions as well as newly developed specialties of already existing professions have not yet always established clearly delineated goals or professional identities. In a typical rehabilitation agency there are eight professional members of the rehabilitation team: nurses, occupational therapists, physical therapists, physiatrists, vocational counselors, psychologists, social workers, and speech therapists. Sometimes a sociologist is added to the list. However, some people argue that rehabilitation administrators and managers should constitute a separate occupational specialty rather than being drawn from the rehabilitation team, where they most frequently function as rehabilitation counselors.[48]

The presence of all these professionals with their own vested interests as well as differing professional codes may in a way defeat the rehabilitation ideal. Extremely serious problems of communication are frequently reported, as well as conflicting treatment and patient management philosophies which negatively affect the disabled's rehabilitation progress and outcome.[49] And because practically all rehabilitation professions are new, the individual professionals exhibit great zeal in noting the particular contributions of their discipline to the rehabilitation process and outcome. Because they are involved in acute status-striving and because their professional status tends to be enhanced by a clearly delineated professional identity and specialization, they may be ambivalent toward participating in a truly interdisciplinary collaboration. As would be expected, this "professionalism" often tends to defeat the ideal of a unified rehabilitation team. The question has been raised as to whether or not all these different professionals are necessary. It is feasible and meaningful to explore the possibilities of consolidating, redistributing, or eliminating the functions performed by the eight or more rehabilitation professions.[50] Such an idea implies that a retrenchment would help unify the rehabilitation team and alleviate the ever-increasing health manpower shortage.

The nature of the manpower shortages in the rehabilitation professions is in large measure due to the fact that most of these professions are "feminine"; for example, nursing, physical therapy, occupational therapy, and social work. They are therefore beset by all the major problems of professions that are entered by a large number of women: great turnover and withdrawal from work for at least twelve to thirteen years while children are growing up. However, in predominantly masculine occupations such as physiatry, the projected shortages are also quite serious. There have been several proposals to alleviate the problem, among them, the use of automation, the use of subprofessionals, and reorganization of the structures and organizations related to rehabilitation so that manpower can be utilized more efficiently.[51]

The use of subprofessionals is especially promising, since this solution may also contribute to the solution of another problem, that of communication between medical and paramedical personnel and patients. The use of disabled subprofessionals would be an extremely fruitful and ingenious idea that would bring to the disabled a feeling of being understood and helped while motivating them through the effective use of the "model" disabled. The fact that these subprofessionals would be disabled and of lower socioeconomic status than the medical and paramedical personnel might give them a greater degree of empathy with the rehabilitants. Physicians seem to be extremely reluctant to relegate any function that could be defined as "medical" to either paramedical personnel or subprofessionals, and especially to the latter. They act this way mainly out of conservatism, economic self-interest, protectiveness for their specialization, and an antiquated position on the issue of "final medical responsibility."[52] In fact, however, many medical tasks are assumed by subprofessionals by default.

Let us now examine some of the rehabilitation professions for which information is available. Physiatrists, the new rehabilitation specialists among physicians, still tend to have a rather marginal position within medicine. Professional antagonism exists between them and the orthopedic surgeons who initially dominated the medical rehabilitation arena and whom they have somewhat displaced. The fact that physiatrists must work in close cooperation with paramedical personnel and social scientists and not necessarily in a position of power but theoretically, at least, as just another team member makes them suspect in the eyes of their medical colleagues. The physiatrists, on the other hand, in their effort to prove that they "run the show" in rehabilitation, have tried, although not always successfully, to domin te the rehabilitation scene. Sometimes, because of the bureaucratic processes involved in vocational rehabilitation programs funded by the state and the federal government, the vocational rehabilitation counselor may hold the money strings and thus be able to exercise considerable control over rehabilitation decisions.[53]

One aspect of the rehabilitation team has not been examined to determine its potential effect upon the power structure of the team; namely, its sex composition. Since most of the rehabilitation professions are to a considerable extent "feminine" occupations, it may be that the physiatrist has only the vocational counselor as a male opponent in the quest for leadership. What happens, however, when several of the team members are men? Is there more conflict, or do they manage to operate as a team of equals rather than as a group of "second-rate" female professionals under the leadership of the male physician? Does the presence of male professionals in the different rehabilitation professions facilitate both their acceptance as equals and the smoother functioning of the team? Or does it produce more professional friction and antithesis? Research on the rehabilitation team could answer these and other relevant questions.

A rehabilitation team ideal as it may be conceptualized in terms of multidisciplinary equality almost never works out in practice. Physicians are not trained to work with others (possibly with other physicians but not with other professionals), and their tendency is to give orders and to treat other professionals as helpers. Physicians are traditionally trained to treat patients as helpless, ignorant children who must be told what to do and who must faithfully comply with their orders. How can they accept the rehabilitation ideal which classifies the physiatrist or the orthopedic surgeon as just another team member who must consider and respect other professional opinions even when they contradict his own? And how can they shift to a different doctor-patient relationship in which the patient has (and should have) a considerable say in his fate?[54] Rehabilitation physicians have to accept a different model of physician-patient relationship in which the patient participates almost as much as the medical and paramedical personnel in his treatment, goal determination, and eventual rehabilitation success. In order to achieve this, physicians as well as paramedical personnel have to be willing to teach others the medical procedures, the medical explanation of the physical condition, the reason for each medical procedure, and a simple diagnosis.[55] They must also be flexible so that medical programs and recommendations are feasible in terms of the life conditions of disabled individuals. And they must be able to socialize the disabled into the specifications and norms of their new role as disabled. Only very thorough changes in medical education can make the rehabilitation ideals reconcilable with the attitudes of the physicians who participate in rehabilitation programs.

Many of the physicians writing on rehabilitation have been urging all physicians to include rehabilitation in their definition of medical responsibilities.[56] But if every physician accepted this "logical" advice and carried it out with a reasonable degree of success, would there be any justification for physiatrists to exist as a separate specialty? Other rehabilitation professionals such as physical therapists, occupational therapists, rehabilitation counselors, and the orthopedic surgeon would still be needed. But the physiatrist would no longer be necessary. Could it be that the established medical profession wishes to absorb the functions of the emerging profession of physiatry within the already established medical specialties? It could be argued, of course, that such an integration of rehabilitation into medical practice could be quite beneficial to the individual patients, who would probably receive rehabilitation services at a much earlier stage and as an integral part of medical treatment. Whether or not physicians of different specialties could be trained adequately and quickly enough to provide satisfactory rehabilitation services is an open question. But the issue still remains: Why this relative reluctance to accept this new medical specialty as easily as all other new medical specialties which have similarly monopolized functions and roles diffused in the past?

Another fairly new medical specialty which is involved in the rehabilitation of industrial workers and often significantly determines the direction of its outcome is industrial medicine. Although by now a recognized specialty, it is still "marginal" in that it enjoys relatively low prestige. Industrial doctors, who constitute 1 percent of all physicians, are looked down upon by their medical colleagues. In general, they are young doctors using the industrial setting as a stepping stone to a more important clientele. Only 1 out of 4 work full-time.[57] There are many possible reasons for their low prestige: (a) industrial doctors are employees of a nonmedical third party; (b) they serve mostly working and lower class patients; and (c) they have a structural advantage in the competition for patients (since most of the ailing workers at least temporarily become their patients).[58] Because industrial doctors are employed by the company, they cannot represent the patient. Whenever there is a showdown between a worker and the company, they must represent the company. This compromises their role as physicians and could potentially create serious conflicts were they at times inclined to take the ailing worker's side. The industrial physicians' problem of divided loyalty has several points in common with the dilemmas of all those in "dependent" practice who must balance the needs and demands of the client, as well as those of the medical profession, with those of the organization which employs them. In such cases it is not uncommon for their obligations to their organization and their profession to be given precedence over the clients' preferences or convenience.[59]

A recent study showed that although industrial doctors identified with management, they did not consider this a hindrance in providing workers with adequate and ethical medical care. This belief may be due to the fact that those physicians willing to work in an industrial setting tend to be more conservative and authoritarian than the average physician and may therefore rarely experience conflict. Instead, they tend to see the workers and their ailments in terms of management's values, which coincide with their own. When a worker is hurt or sick they will treat him. However, when his illness or accident may have financial consequences for the company because of compensation or because of the risk involved in hiring a handicapped individual—instances in which the doctor's responsibility and degree of identification with his patient are not clearly prescribed by the medical ethical code—the industrial doctor sides with management and may even share its hostility toward a worker claiming compensation. It is interesting to note that industrial doctors often tend to have strained relationships with physicians in private practice who treat workers. The central cause of their mutual suspicion and disaccord is the fact that a private physician in a controversial case exclusively represents the "interest" of his patient, while the industrial physician represents the company.[60] One could almost be cynical and conclude that physicians seem to represent the interests of the party who pays the bill, at least in controversial cases.

Industrial doctors are involved in the determination of a difficult and inadequately defined problem: the question of when an illness or a disability legitimately warrants the withdrawal of the afflicted person from social and occupational obligations. The timing of such legitimation may vary with the type of social system to which the disabled person belongs and with the nature of the negative sanctions that his withdrawal from his usual obligations will entail.[61] Thus, while the disabled's family may consider his withdrawal from the occupational role legitimate because of the expected compensation check not being lower than his customary salary, his employer may not because of the high compensation he has to pay. Or, his family may not accept withdrawal from the occupational role despite its legitimation on the part of employer and physicians because of the great loss of income and the need for familial restructuring and reorganization. Industrial doctors loyal to their employer usually attempt to solve this problem by considering which solution will be least costly to the company. This type of solution, while expedient for the company, may be far from just for the individuals disabled and their families. Probably, industrial doctors should be partly paid by the employees or by the government so that they might act in a more equitable manner.

Perhaps the most studied rehabilitation profession is that of vocational rehabilitation counseling. In 1965, the 4,559 persons engaged in rehabilitation counseling or supervision had very heterogeneous educational backgrounds, ranging from a bachelor's degree to a Ph.D. in psychology.[62] The actual performance of their job also varied considerably from setting to setting, especially among the three major types—Veterans Administration, private agencies, and state vocational rehabilitation offices. In the first setting the rehabilitation counselors were called "counseling psychologists," had doctorates in psychology, were highly professional, and tended to be disengaged from the rehabilitation label and to identify instead with the psychologists. Rehabilitation counselors in state vocational rehabilitation offices were the least trained (60 percent having only a B.A. or a few graduate courses), were more often disabled (25 percent), or had a disabled person in their immediate family. They were the least "professional." Private agency counselors fell between the other two categories, their unique feature being the high percentage of female staff (47.9 percent). The differences are so great in terms of training, pay, actual work orientation, and professional identity that some researchers have been led to ask if in fact all vocational rehabilitation counselors regardless of work setting can be considered as belonging to the same profession.[63]

Rehabilitation counselors themselves are not sure and often disagree as to what constitutes their primary function in the rehabilitation team: Should they be coordinators, vocational counselors and placement experts, or counselors whose main role is psychotherapeutic? A recent study indicated that most rehabilitation counselors prefer the psychotherapeutic role, probably because this activity is in their eyes (and in the eyes of professional "significant others") the most prestigious.[64] Some researchers have analyzed the marginal profession of vocational rehabilitation counseling in terms of the structured strains produced by: (a) the materialistic orientation of the role toward "product," that is, placement of the handicapped; (b) the caseload size; (c) the time restrictions; (d) the pressures for quantitative production, that is, the pressure to constantly increase the number of rehabilitation successes (disabled people placed in employment); and (e) the cultural barrier against success posited by employers' attitudes toward hiring the handicapped.[65]

The counselors tend to solve these strains in a variety of ways: by (a) aggressive acting out of their frustration; (b) exhibiting a variety of deviant withdrawal patterns; (c) "adjusting" to the situation by idealizing, for example, their role as coordinator of all services; and (d) actively attempting to change their role definitions.[66] Recent data show that the higher the educational achievement of vocational rehabilitation counselors, the better they may be able to cope with some of the strains of their profession, since they accept a higher percentage of disabled applicants for rehabilitation.[67] Of course, we do not know whether or not they are able to accept a greater percentage of "poor risk" disabled applicants with "undesirable motivational inadequacies," and we cannot therefore be sure at this point of the influence of education upon the screening process.

An extremely interesting and relevant characteristic of rehabilitation counselors working in state vocational rehabilitation offices is their high rate of disability (25 percent of them had some disability versus 3 percent of the entire population). Furthermore, Sussman found that among those for whom rehabilitation counseling was a second career, one-third were disabled (most often afflicted with blindness or neuromuscular disorders), and 40 percent had a disabled person in their immediate family. He also found that 65 percent of those formerly in routine white or blue collar jobs were themselves disabled compared to only 25 percent of those in business or professional occupations.[68] Unfortunately, there are no data relating the age, previous socioeconomic background, and disability status of rehabilitation counselors to the criteria they use in selecting those cases to be closed before rehabilitation is complete and those rehabilitants who will be denied vocational training. Rehabilitants often verbalize a preference for disabled rehabilitation staff "because they can understand us better." The older the age and the lower the socioeconomic background of second-career rehabilitation counselors, the greater the probability (at least theoretically) that they more than other rehabilitation counselors will be able to develop good empathy with all rehabilitants, especially with the "hard core" older, semi-skilled and unskilled and seriously disabled ones.

The question remains open, however, since we do not know to what extent rehabilitation counselors of working class origin do in fact identify with and relate well to the "hard core" lower class rehabilitants or to what extent their social origin makes them feel socially insecure and anxious to place as much social distance as possible between themselves and the rehabilitants of low socioeconomic status. Since they are upward-mobile and ambitious, their adoption of those success standards for rehabilitation counselors which stress serving only those with a reasonable possibility of vocational placement would inhibit them from bothering with the "hard core" who are a "bad professional investment."[69]

Recent data have shown that 76 of the 90 state vocational rehabilitation agencies have persons on their staff with disabilities that could qualify them for vocational rehabilitation services if they became unemployed.[70] However, we do not know which rehabilitation occupations tend to have the greater number of disabled persons and what types of disabilities are most prevalent. One is led to ask to what extent the disabled status, seemingly more prevalent among physiatrists as compared to other rehabilitation professions, affects their occupational status and prestige.

Among other new rehabilitation occupations are the rehabilitation nurse, the disability adjudicator, and the network manager. The disability adjudicator evaluates medical and nonmedical evidence that a claimant presents when he applies for disability and decides whether or not such benefits should be granted.[71] He is in actuality a vocational rehabilitation counselor with quasijudicial duties.

The network manager is emerging as a new rehabilitation occupation because of a recognized need to coordinate, integrate, and simply be aware of the many health, welfare, and community rehabilitation agencies which are available and in frequent competition with each other.[72] Ideally, the network manager could represent the client, organizing his "career" by buying him, or making available to him, the best services.[73] He could function best at this role as a better representative of his client's interests if he were not tied to an institutional establishment. But this free and powerful position has not been secured, since there is no one willing to pay his salary without attaching strings. On the other hand, there are those who see the role of the network manager as an interorganizational coordinator without any particular function as a representative of the client.

Given this background on the different rehabilitation professions and their professional problems, we can return to an examination of their interaction with each other and with the patients. Since each discipline has a never-ending need to prove that it alone is the most useful and the most needed, therapeutic staff members may sometimes compete with one another over the superiority of their discipline for a particular patient's disability. Such a zealous commitment to one's professional field may sometimes have beneficial results for the treated rehabilitants. More often than not, however, it tends to have discouraging results, because the therapist's enthusiasm and professional faith have given him unrealistically high hopes. There is also some evidence that occupational groups or professionals within an occupational group higher in professional striving than others tend to be much more interested in serving high rather than low status clients.[74] Since practically all rehabilitation professions seem to be high in professional striving, the lower class rehabilitant is quite undesirable to most of their members, a fact that explains the frequent rejection of lower class disabled persons. It also explains why vocational counselors who constitute probably the most "professionalizing" rehabilitation occupational group are often found to be unwilling to serve lower class patients. Of course, the degree of reluctance to serve lower class rehabilitants will vary with the individual's degree of professional striving, being minimal when serving clients has become a more important consideration than professional status.

Few if any controlled evaluative studies exist about the relative effectiveness of the different techniques used by therapists in the same or different fields. Thus it is very difficult to judge either success or failure in an objective way and aside from the influence of other techniques and treatments given simultaneously. In this way, it is easy for any therapist to keep believing in the greater effectiveness of his particular type of therapy. Thus, the battle among at least three major categories of physical therapists, the "corrective" therapists, the "Kenny" therapists, and the physical therapists, goes on. Each school presents its proof—some dramatically improved case which may or may not have improved even without any physical therapy modalities. And, of course, any failures can be conveniently labeled "uncooperative" or "unmotivated." Clinical records, interestingly enough, often indicate wide discrepancies in the staff's labeling of a rehabilitant as motivated or unmotivated, depending on whether or not he has responded to the particular treatment for which they are responsible.[75] If a physical therapist says the rehabilitant is unmotivated and the occupational therapist says he is motivated, does this mean that the rehabilitant is more motivated to get back to work than to improve himself physically? Or does it indicate that the occupational therapist has developed a close relation-

ship with the rehabilitant and is able to adapt the therapeutic tasks
to his personality and interests? Or, finally, is it an indication that
the rehabilitant is not responding because the applied physical
therapy modalities are not effective with his type of disability, while
the contrary is true in the case of the occupational therapy modalities?

In recent rehabilitation literature there is an increasing recognition that a variety of interdepartmental, inter- and intraprofessional
conflicts and rivalries exist and are often acutely felt within rehabilitation settings and seem to affect the rehabilitants' level of motivation
and rehabilitation success. However, with the exception of the Roth
and Eddy study, there is little concrete and systematically gathered
information on which to build some theoretical conclusions and
generalizations.

There is also a lack of systematic studies of patient cliques in
different types of rehabilitation settings that would permit the de-
lineation of relationships between modes of interaction and level of
motivation or modes of interaction and degree of physical improvement.[76] Thus, it seems that the entire area of the rehabilitation
social system (or any of the subsystems) requires a great number of
additional research studies before it becomes a substantial area of
knowledge.

Rehabilitation at the Culture Level

We can now examine why the idea of rehabilitation came about
in its present form; what dominant cultural values directly or indirectly
stimulated the development of the institution; and how a different set
of cultural values gave the rehabilitation institution its present form.

It is difficult and even rather meaningless to single out one or two
cultural values or events and attribute to them a causal relation with
rehabilitation. What seems to be the most plausible explanation is
that rehabilitation resulted from the interplay of a variety of factors
which happened to become apparent at about the same time. The fact
that a greater number of disabled veterans survived World War II
than had ever survived a war before and that an advanced medical
knowhow had been developing, combined with the prevalent Ameri-

can value of "mastery" of the environment (in this case of the disability), spelled out a need for an organized way of handling and controlling the challenging problem of disability. From this beginning, the idea spread to increasingly more categories of civilians for a variety of reasons.

First, while rehabilitation in the larger sense of the word had always been the traditional responsibility of physicians, it had been put aside because of the contemporary emphasis on clinical findings and the estrangement of the doctor from his patient, since he had become more interested in the disease than in the "whole" person.[77] Despite a recent return to the treatment of the whole person (leading to the concept of comprehensive medicine, of which rehabilitation is theoretically an essential part), the medical profession has undergone such basic changes within the last ten years that the principle of comprehensive medicine cannot easily be put into practice.[78] One trend which has gone hand in hand with the trend toward treating symptoms and disease entities instead of "whole" people has been a businesslike orientation which probably brought about or reinforced the tendency to treat specific symptoms and syndromes to facilitate the efficient operation of medical practice. This businesslike orientation is present not only in the practice of general practitioners (although it may be more accentuated in their case), but also in that of specialists in private practice or in a hospital setting. Thus, not only have general practitioners decreased in number (38 percent of all physicians in 1960, but only 25 percent in 1966), but their relationship with their patients has radically changed.[79] Although patients assume that their doctor will have the ability and interest to consider their illness in terms of their total life situation, these expectations are infrequently met because the physicians have changed the definition of their role.

American physicians have delineated a very narrow role for themselves, that of treating the physical symptoms of disease, and feel quite uncomfortable when patients relate life experiences "apparently" not directly related to their symptoms or ask for advice about preventive or rehabilitative measures. Such patient expectations are considered peripheral in the physician's role definitions. As long as such role definitions on the part of the physician facilitate the operation of his medical practice on the basis of efficient business principles (in a society in which business principles have permeated all institutions, even welfare agencies, as we shall see later), it is doubtful that medicine will revert back to an individualized, comprehensive medicine in which profit will have only secondary importance.[80] Because modern medicine failed to cope successfully with any other illness factor but the strictly "acute" physical one and to extend the physician's responsibility beyond the limitations of the accorded treatment or consultation period, people became increasingly unhappy with the quality of medical care received and with its restricted nature. And since the value of health is another prevalent American value, some kind of solution was eagerly welcomed. Rehabilitation, promising to be such a solution, was greatly favored and aided to develop.

Second, physical disability in the past usually gave the afflicted person a semilegitimate excuse to stop working and become financially dependent on some family member or on governmental or private aid. As long as this opportunity to abandon the occupational role was taken by only a small percentage of the population (since only a few people survived serious illnesses or accidents), the situation was tolerated by society. In many cultures those individuals who did not make use of this opportunity but continued to work despite their disability were generally admired and cited as examples. When, however, the incidence of disability rose considerably, especially among men in their productive years, the entire issue of whether or not its presence could in any way legitimize withdrawal from an occupational role had to be reexamined. The potential existence of a large number of men of working age who would not work because of their disability and would be federally or privately supported started taking the form of a serious social problem. In addition, because of the fact that tradition, stereotyped beliefs, and "humanitarian-like" beliefs would give a considerable degree of social acceptance to the unemployed when disabled, such cherished "core" values of the American culture as work and financial independence would be both weakened and questioned. The fact that able-bodied family members, including wives, would be expected to work and support the disabled one could have a disorganizing influence on family life. The presence, then, of large numbers of unemployed, disabled men would become a threat to the "normal" American way of living and a potentially undermining influence on the entire social structure.[81]

Third, a variety of new and developing occupations such as social work, vocational counseling, nursing, or "marginal" medical specialities such as orthopedics held very interesting potentials for professional advancement and growth through the establishment of a new type of sociomedical agency represented by rehabilitation. Of course, other occupations, such as the medical establishment represented by the American Medical Association, fought (and to some extent is still fighting) rehabilitation because of the added responsibility it demands of the physician. According to Wessen's typology, when a new institution is being developed that touches upon other fields, the more established the field, the more it will fight the new institution, and the newer the field, the greater will be its support since those in the new fields have more to gain than to lose from new occupational developments.[82]

Despite some opposition, rehabilitation was finally accepted and is growing not only because it "defends" basic American values, but also because it is vested with noble humanitarian concerns and ideals. Among them are the lessening of human suffering and the physical, social, and emotional restoration of the disabled so that they can compete with the nondisabled on as equal a basis as possible. The societal benefit comes from the fact that rehabilitation is an institution of social control aimed at the correction of the deviance present in disabled people.[83] Their deviance is, as we have seen, potentially double. It may be only a deviation from the desirable standards of physical appearance and/or physical strength—but it may also be a potential deviation from the prescribed vocational role and economic independence, as in the case of men. Rehabilitation has, then, as a basic function the resocialization of the disabled; that is, making them able and willing to enact their "normal" social roles as effectively as possible despite the presence of the disability. Thus, it aims to minimize the degree of disruption that disability could bring about in the functioning of different social systems. This combination of ideals and practical aims made and still makes rehabilitation especially "salable" to all categories of people.

Some of the reasons why rehabilitation became a new social agency rather than an extension of a related preexisting institution may be the following: (a) The medical institution—probably the most relevant institution—was failing to extend its members' responsibility beyond the treatment of acute conditions and the strictly medical management of episodes in the case of chronic ones. In addition, it was resisting innovations in the mode of administering medical care and was hostile to the ideal of rehabilitation. Probably a considerable part of this hostility may have been due to the fact that rehabilitation required an interdisciplinary collaboration which may have been interpreted as an attempt on the part of nonmedical people to usurp absolute medical authority over a patient.[84] (b) It follows the usual American tendency to develop a new social agency to cope with the failure of an existing one rather than expand or modify the one which failed to accomplish its functions.

Once rehabilitation was established as a separate institution (sometimes administratively independent, other times an adjunct to a hospital), its fate was not much different from a variety of other social agencies in the United States. Success being a dominant preoccupation and the only acceptable measure of worth, any social agency must show a striking and impressive record of success if it is to receive federal, state, municipal, or private support—or even prestige and recognition. Therefore, only the "good risks" can be accepted as cases, since the others would not be likely to contribute to the necessary success statistics. No chances can be taken in experimenting with new methods of successfully rehabilitating the somewhat more difficult cases except on special grants and projects where financing is not contingent upon "success statistics." Because all social agencies, including rehabilitation agencies, must give proof of their efficacy and productivity in concrete numbers, they are often turned into business undertakings operating on a short-range profit interest which defeats the purposes for which they were established. Not only does the very existence of the institution come to depend upon the enumeration of success cases, but the promotion and professional recognition of its rehabilitation personnel as well. Thus, the number of successful cases completed rather than the degree of skill involved in rehabilitating "difficult" cases becomes the major object.

Another clear-cut illustration of the profit orientation in rehabilitation is provided by the gradual changes that took place in the organization and goals of sheltered workshops. Scott has traced the gradual shift in operative policies of workshops for the blind from an originally predominant "social service" orientation to a "business" and then to a "big business" value orientation.[85] Thus, although they were originally set up to provide employment for the severely disabled who cannot be placed in regular competitive employment, as a result of the economic and occupational adversities in the Depression, they were organized and run as efficient business undertakings in order to survive. The purposes for which the sheltered workshops were originally set up were defeated, since they kept only those blind who were competent, efficient, and capable of industrial work, and systematically rejected the incompetent. Subsequently, because they had a vested interest in keeping such competent employees within their "business structure," they discouraged their vocational placement in "outside industries" even when the industries came asking for such workers (as was the case during World War II). Moreover, despite the fact that the excess profits from the efficient operation of the workshops were supposed to be used for the establishment of special "craft shops" for less skilled and competent workers which would not be totally self-supporting, they were rarely used in this way; instead, profits were usually used to extend the workshop and its operation.[86]

It seems that at least in the American society, it is extremely difficult for a social service organization to stay as such and to be supported morally and financially if no concrete evidence of profit can be provided. If proof of profit cannot be given, a variety of pressures will eventually arise from a profit-geared society demanding or obliging the financially "failing" social service organization to shift emphasis or perish. The main form of pressure is withdrawal of financial help or reluctance to subsidize the deficit, although other types of pressure in the form of criticism may also be present.

Because of the success orientation of rehabilitation therapists, administrators, and managers of sheltered workshops, some categories of disabled are seldom selected because they tend to be bad risks in terms of vocational rehabilitation or actual vocational performance. These disabled are usually the severely afflicted, the older (over 45), the blacks, the white lower class males, and generally, the women. Of course, the rehabilitation personnel's reluctance to accept lower class disabled persons for rehabilitation services may also be due to their inability or unwillingness to effectively treat lower class persons. But whichever reason operates more strongly in the case of different therapists, the fact remains that the greater number of disabled denied services or discharged after a short evaluation or period of rehabilitation treatment or not accepted in "profitable" sheltered workshops are lower class, unskilled individuals or severely disabled ones. And it is significant to note that it is the lower class disabled who must often after disablement assume the deviant role of the unemployed, since they prefer to live on the small but stable income of some type of disability pension. The reasons for their inclination toward the deviant alternative are many and will be discussed in detail in the next chapter. What is important in this context is the fact that the newly established institution of rehabilitation, like all other social agencies, is not effective in the case of socially marginal people, especially the lower class or the severely disabled. Lower class or severely disabled people tend to be helped least even when a social agency's purpose is to help them specifically.[87] And then another agency is developed to help the same type of problem in the "hard core" unemployed, and so on.

Despite the fact that the idea of rehabilitation defends the American values of work, financial independence, and "mastery," in practice it seems that it fails to inspire the disabled who least believe in their intrinsic importance. This failure has been rationalized by the concept of "motivation" which, as conceptualized by most therapists, comfortably places the entire blame upon the shoulders of the disabled themselves. Even this rationalization is consistent with the prevalent American belief which sees each person as entirely responsible for all his successes and all his failures—and therefore deserving "what he gets." Although the rehabilitation philosophy has had an activistic orientation and a "militancy against letting even the aged and chronically ill rest on their oars," in actual practice it has not accomplished this goal with those who need the most help in order to enact the ideals of rehabilitation (that is, the old, the severely disabled, and the socially disabled).

Although some writers have conceptualized rehabilitation as a social movement, it is doubtful whether such a conceptualization is valid. Rehabilitation is not a movement that came directly out of or was shaped by the interested disabled people themselves, but instead came about through people concerned with the social problem of the disabled. And while these unappointed "representatives" have tried to "do their best" for the disabled, their definition of what constitutes the best does not seem to always correspond with the one voiced by the disabled themselves. The disabled demand independence, integration into "normal" society, and acceptance as equals, but their "representatives" emphasize "protective" measures and tend to rationalize the purposefulness of social segregation in terms of its psychological "benefits."

Unless the disabled themselves unite, thus becoming a kind of "militant" group trying to shape their own destinies according to their own "needs" and demands, it is difficult to conceptualize the present state of the field of rehabilitation as representing a social movement. A militant movement of disabled would try to create a new image of man, that of man with a disability as equally acceptable and "normal" as man without a disability. Their effort would be similar to that of the militant blacks who are attempting to project the image of man as one with black skin. The disabled's present representatives are not presenting a new image of man; instead they are trying to maintain the status quo by placing the full responsibility for adjustment and compromise on the disabled rather than the society at large. Some writers suggest that the organization of the disabled in unions or a similar type of association would tend to foster group consciousness, communication with each other (outside of "agencies" *for* the disabled), and communication with the nondisabled as well as with those in power. Only in this way could the disabled possibly become successful in socializing rehabilitation legislators and practitioners in their conceptions of disability and rehabilitation and gain a strong voice in rehabilitation policies and programs.[88]

It is not very difficult to explain why the disabled have not as yet created a social movement. Some of the reasons are common to all "minority" groups which have been discriminated against for a long time. As in the case of the blacks, those disabled who can "pass" as "normals" or are successful in becoming integrated in and accepted by the "normal" society dissociate themselves almost completely from the disabled and are unwilling to represent them in the larger world. Thus, they lose the support of a potentially influential group that could help them to obtain what they all wish for—that which these

select individuals have succeeded in obtaining for themselves. Before
the voice of a discriminated group can be clearly and effectively
heard, at least a few of its members must be able to "make it" to a
place of prominence that will permit them to speak and act influen-
tially. But in order to be willing to do this, they must retain an identification with the discriminated group. The fact that blacks have
managed to reach this stage facilitates negotiations and adds to their
bargaining power.

The many types of disabilities may delay the awakening of the
disabled. Different categories of the disabled have different problems
specific to their disability and are subject to discriminatory practices
different in nature and intensity. In addition, some categories of
disabled may be prejudiced toward disabled in other categories for
exactly the same reasons that the nondisabled are prejudiced toward
the disabled. An amputee may be prejudiced toward a person with
a facial disfigurement or people with heart disease may be prejudiced
toward both amputees and those with facial disfigurements. Because
of this it may be difficult for each to identify with the other and to
present a unified front vis-à-vis the nondisabled.

Another reason why the disabled have not yet taken the offense
may be the fact that some disabled (those with nonvisible disabilities,
usually chronic illnesses) never accept the notion that they are disabled. Because of identity needs they go on identifying with the nondisabled and living as if their disability did not exist. A typical
example are those who after one or two heart attacks, and despite
doctors' admonitions, go on living and working at a pace that soon
kills them. This category of disabled represents a loss, since for them
a social movement is irrelevant.

In contrast, another category of the disabled, as we have already
seen, gladly and eagerly assumes the disabled status because of the
secondary gains it offers; namely, the semilegitimate excuse to withdraw from undesirable or stressful social responsibilities and unsuccessful social roles. These disabled have no reason and no motivation
to fight, to be accepted as "normal" people, since such an acceptance
would return them to their earlier problematic situations and the
failures from which they are now exempt. Instead of demanding to
be treated as equals by the nondisabled, they tend to emphasize and
sometimes exaggerate their limitations and "different" status in order
to safeguard the privileges and exemptions granted on the basis of

their disability.[89] Therefore, the only disabled interested in becoming integrated into "normal" society and accepted as equals by the non-disabled are those who accept their physical limitations but are willing to use their remaining abilities to perform their social roles and fulfill their responsibilities to the fullest extent possible. These are the disabled who, having accepted their disability, are trying to live as normal a life as possible. But they constitute only a segment of all the disabled.

A further fragmentation of the disabled comes about because of the degree of severity of the disability. It has been found that for the disabled to represent themselves and to influence the rehabilitation team, they must not be very severely afflicted. Because they must have a fairly good capacity for movement and communication, it may well be that in order for the disabled to unify and fight for their interests, they must meet certain criteria of "ability." Disabled whose survival is threatened by rapidly developing degenerative diseases or by diseases with poor prognosis may be so preoccupied and depressed by their affliction that any other thought or activity is unimportant. Also, severely disabled persons who are confined to their beds or who cannot communicate because of a multiple sensory disability could not identify with a social movement since they may to some extent realistically recognize that they could not profit from such a movement because of the severity of their affliction. Of course, the mere fact that the disabled seem to include different groups, some of which have little or no vested interest in becoming integrated, does not necessarily preclude their being able to create and successfully promote a social movement. The suffragette movement succeeded despite the fact that it probably represented the opinions and wishes of only a few women. It may be, however, that the reason the enacted legislative rights granted to women were not used by a large number is the fact that these few suffragettes were well ahead of the thinking and values of the majority of their sex.

Having discussed all the inhibiting factors that make the unification of the disabled and the formation of a genuine social movement so difficult, we have still this question: Will the disabled ever succeed in uniting and creating a social movement, and if so, under what conditions? The answer is yes, if: (1) they are permitted to enter prestigious occupations where they can ascend the occupational hierarchy to positions of power, especially in the rehabilitation and welfare fields; and (2) the image of the disabled is somewhat freed from at least a few of the stereotypes attached to it. Only then is there hope that the disabled will manage to unite and become self-defining "militants" of their rights and status in society.

In this chapter we have examined rehabilitation as a social system at different levels of analysis. Some social changes emerging in the last few years may gradually transform different aspects of rehabilitation and eventually reverse some of the present trends. In Chapter 8 we shall discuss in detail possible future trends in rehabilitation philosophy and programs as well as in the social status of the disabled in view of probable social changes and technological innovations. Now we shall turn our attention to the reasons for which some disabled more than others tend to become deviants in the vocational area with or without rehabilitation.

NOTES

1. Harry Prosen, "Physical Disability and Motivation," *Canadian Medical Association Journal,* 92 (June 12, 1965), 1261; Edward R. Schlesinger *et al.,* "Evalution of Rehabilitation Services for Disabled Welfare Recipients," *Public Health Reports,* 77, 5 (May 1962), 413. And as Nadler and Shontz say, "motivation" has sometimes been used to refer to the rehabilitants' moral character. See Eugene B. Nadler and Franklin C. Shontz, "A Factor Analytic Study of Motivational Patterns in a Sheltered Shop," *The Personnel and Guidance Journal,* 37, 6 (February 1959), 444; and Celia Benney, "Factors Affecting Motivation for Rehabilitation," *Psychiatric Quarterly Supplement,* 38–39 (1964–65), 205.
2. Benney, *op. cit.,* p. 209.
3. Manuel D. Zane and Milton Lowenthal, "Motivation in the Rehabilitation of the Physically Handicapped," *Archives of Physical Medicine and Rehabilitation,* 41 (January 1960), 400.
4. Robert A. Scott, *The Making of Blind Men: A Study of Adult Socialization* (New York: Russell Sage Foundation, 1969), pp. 72–76.
5. Nadler and Shontz, *op. cit.,* p. 448; Stephen L. Fink, Rainette

Fantz, and Joseph Zinker, "The Growth Beyond Adjustment: Another Look at Motivation" (mimeographed, Cleveland, Highland View Hospital); and Franklin C. Shontz, "Concept of Motivation in Physical Medicine," *Archives of Physical Medicine and Rehabilitation*, 38 (October 1957), 636–38.

6. The available literature indicates that physicians spend less time, explain less, and give less adequate medical care to lower class patients. See Lee Rainwater, "The Lower Class: Health, Illness, and Medical Institutions" (mimeographed; background paper prepared for a study of medical facilities planning conducted by Anselm L. Strauss for the Institute of Policy Studies, March 1965); *A Study of the Integration of Services of Industrial Medical Departments and a Rehabilitation Center: Final Report* (Pittsburgh: Harmarville Rehabilitation Center, June 1963); and Raymond S. Duff and August B. Hollingshead, *Sickness and Society* (New York: Harper & Row, 1968).

7. The rehabilitant is expected to "cooperate" by performing uncomfortable or often painful or meaningless tasks without any, clear-cut reassurance that some definite benefit will ensue. Lower class patients, because of less general knowledge and understanding of their condition and less information received from the rehabilitation staff, as well as because of a general life orientation, are badly equipped to perform under ambiguous rehabilitation conditions. See Irving Kenneth Zola, "A Social Scientist's Perspective on the Problem of 'Unmotivated' Clients," *Education for Social Work With Unmotivated Clients, Proceedings of an Institute*, Brandeis University Papers in Social Welfare, no. 9, (Fall 1965). See also Irene Mackintosh Hulicka, "Psychological Manifestations of Physical Disability," *Association for Physical and Mental Rehabilitation*, 17, 6 (November–December 1963), 160; Fink, Fantz, and Zinker, *op. cit.*

8. There is an abundance of literature—medical, sociological, and psychological—pointing out very clearly the great difficulty encountered in evaluating most disabilities or in making prognoses (see Chapters 6 and 7). See also Zane and Lowenthal, *op. cit.*, pp. 400–7.

9. Scott found that some blind prefer to beg rather than be trained and have to work in highly routinized, boring, and poorly paid jobs. See Scott, *op. cit.*, p. 111.

10. Shontz, *op. cit.*, pp. 636–38.

11. Constantina Safilios-Rothschild, "The Reaction to Disability in Rehabilitation" (unpublished Ph.D. dissertation, Ohio State University, 1963).

12. Actually, the typical behavior of the person who wants to deny the presence of a disability almost perfectly fits Litman's

description of the rehabilitation behavior of those harboring a negative self-concept coupled with resentment toward their disability. And there is no question that those who deny their disability are those whose extremely negative self-image *with* the disability makes the only tolerable solution one of denial. See Theodor J. Litman, "Self-Conception and Physical Rehabilitation," in Arnold M. Rose (ed.), *Human Behavior and Social Processes* (Boston: Houghton Mifflin, 1962), pp. 565–66. The fact that he refers to a postdisability self-concept and we, in the theoretical discussions, refer to a predisability self-concept explains why his findings only seemingly contradict our discussion. Of course, it is possible that 50% of those who view their postdisability selves negatively may accept their disability while the other 50% may not. And since rehabilitants were dichotomized and no such provision was made, we do not know how many of those with a negative postdisability self-concept who accept their disability do so because they derive secondary gains (see pp. 567–68).

13. John Barry, "Patient Motivation for Rehabilitation," *The Cleft Palate Journal*, 2, 1 (January 1965), 4.

14. Julius A. Roth, " 'Management Bias' in a Social Science Study of Medical Treatment," *Human Organization*, 21, 1 (Spring 1962), 47–50.

15. Lawrence E. Schlesinger, "Patient Motivation for Rehabilitation," *American Journal of Occupational Therapy*, 17, 1 (January–February 1963), 5–8.

16. The rehabilitation facility described by Roth and Eddy is such a place, although even within it some rehabilitants are able to communicate the rehabilitation goals they are interested in, or even have them adopted by the staff, through a "sponsoring" member of the rehabilitation team. See Julius A. Roth and Elizabeth M. Eddy, *Rehabilitation for the Unwanted* (New York: Atherton, 1967).

17. Fink, Fantz, and Zinker, *op. cit.*

18. Scott has described how rehabilitation workers ignore the rehabilitants' own views about their disability as well as about appropriate solutions as "uninsightful" and "maladjusted." See Scott, *op. cit.*, pp. 78–80.

19. Even when the rehabilitants are motivated to perform or learn tasks not deemed by the staff to be important, desirable, and "realistic," they are labeled "unmotivated" and "uncooperative" since they are not willing to go along with the staff's opinions. See Fink, Fantz, and Zinker, *op. cit.*; Zola, *op. cit.*; William Gellman, "Attitudes Toward Rehabilitation of the Disabled," *American Journal of Occupational Therapy*, 14, 4 (1960), 189; S. Bernstein, "Motivation in Rehabilitation," *Journal of*

the *Association of Physical and Mental Rehabilitation*, 18 (January–February 1964), 4–7. See also John R. Barry and Michael R. Malinovsky, *Client Motivation for Rehabilitation: A Review*, Rehabilitation Research Monograph Series, no. 1 (Gainesville, Fla.: Regional Rehabilitation Research Institute, University of Florida, February 1965), p. 20; M. Pilisuk, "Motivation for Therapy: The Gap Between Ego Skills and the Self-image," *American Journal of Occupational Therapy*, 17 (May–June 1963), 111–15; and Howard R. Kelman and Jonas N. Muller, "Rehabilitation of Nursing Home Residents," *Geriatrics*, 17 (June 1962), 410.

20. Several authors have explained and documented how the patient's participation and relative self-determination can increase motivation. See Lawrence E. Schlesinger, "Staff Authority and Patient Participation in Rehabilitation," *Rehabilitation Literature*, 24, 1, part 1 (January 1963), 248–49; Joseph John Raymond Grau, *Permissive Treatment of Disabled Persons: A Sociological Study* (Ph.D. dissertation, University of Pittsburgh, 1963; Ann Arbor, Mich.: University Microfilms, no. 63–7797); and S. Siegel, "Existentialist Aspects of the Vocational Rehabilitation Process," *Mental Hygiene*, 46 (October 1962), 533–42. Others have also documented that when the goals are "externally" imposed upon the rehabilitants, they feel less inclined to do their utmost to achieve them. See Herbert S. Rabinowitz and Spiro B. Mitsos, "Rehabilitation as Planned Social Change: A Conceptual Framework," *Journal of Health and Human Behavior*, 5, 1 (Spring 1964), 13; Roth and Eddy, *op. cit.*, p. 149; and Hulicka, *op. cit.*, p. 160.

21. Ray Elling, Ruth Whittemore, and Morris Green, "Patient Participation in a Pediatric Program," *Journal of Health and Human Behavior*, 1, 3 (Fall 1960), 183–91; and Gellman, *op. cit.*, p. 189.

22. Disaster theories indicate that when people become aware that others have also been singled out in a catastrophe, and have been similarly or more severely afflicted, they are helped to accept their affliction. What is more, they feel encouraged to live and struggle and even feel optimistic since they have been hit less severely. Case studies of rehabilitants abound in statements indicating that very similar mechanisms operate when the disabled interact with other disabled in a rehabilitation center. The author has such unpublished data in the case studies that served as a basis for her dissertation. See also Theodor J. Litman, "Physical Rehabilitation: A Social Psychological Approach," in E. G. Jaco (ed.), *Patients, Physicians, and Illness*, 2nd ed. (New York: Free Press, 1968); and Fink, Fantz, and Zinker, *op. cit.*

180   DISABILITY AND REHABILITATION

23. Alfred H. Stanton and Morris S. Schwartz, *The Mental Hospital*
(New York: Basic Books, 1954); Maxwell H.
Jones, *The Therapeutic Community* (New York: Basic Books, 1953);
Milton Greenblatt, Richard H. York, and Esther L.
Brown, *From Custodial to Therapeutic Care in Mental Hospitals* (New
York: Russell Sage Foundation, 1955); Charlotte Green
Schwartz, *Rehabilitation of Mental Hospital Patients,* Public
Health Monograph 17(Washington, D.C.: U.S. Public Health
Service, 1953). But see also Bernard Kutner, "Modes of
Treating the Chronically Ill," *The Gerontologist,* 4, part 2
(June 1964), 44–48.
24. Franziska W. Racker, Edward F. Delagi, and Arthur S. Abram-
son, "The Therapeutic Community: An Approach to a Medical
Community," *Archives of Physical Medicine and Rehabilitation,*
44, 5 (May 1963), 257–61; P. Rosenberg and R. Berger,
"Methods and Measurements of a Therapeutic Community
in Physical Rehabilitation" (paper delivered at the New York
Psychological Association meetings, May 1962); and R. Coser,
"A Home Away From Home," in Dorian Apple (ed.), *Sociological Studies of Health and Sickness* (New York: McGraw-
Hill, 1960).
25. Judith A. Goldston and Cynthia P. Deutch, "Comparison of
Attitudes of Hospital Staff, Disabled Patients, and Families
Toward Basic Concepts of Physical Disability" (paper presented
at the American Psychological Association meetings, Cincinnati,
September 4, 1959).
26. Lawrence E. Schlesinger, "Staff Tensions and Needed Skills
in Staff-Patient Interaction," *Rehabilitation Literature,* 24, 1,
part I (January 1963), 363; Roth and Eddy, *op. cit.,* chap. 4,
"Patients and Their Caretakers," pp. 41–61. Of course, the
custodial personnel prefer that a disabled is independent in all
the activities of daily living, but cannot tolerate the intermediate
stage during which the disabled must gradually reach independence goals because it is taxing in terms of time and
effort. See Roth and Eddy, *op. cit.,* pp. 41–61.
27. Theodor J. Litman, "The Influence of Concept of Self and Life
Orientation Factors Upon the Rehabilitation of Orthopedic
Patients," (unpublished Ph.D. dissertation, University of Minnesota, 1961). Also written communication by Theodor J.
Litman included in his comments on the second draft of this
chapter.
28. Schlesinger, "Patient Motivation for Rehabilitation," *op. cit.,*
pp. 6–7; and Schlesinger, "Staff Tensions and Needed Skills in
Staff-Patient Interaction," *op. cit.,* pp. 363–64.
29. Roth and Eddy, *op. cit.,* pp. 91–92, 168–69. Those sponsored
by a rehabilitation staff would also tend to get higher quality

as well as generally more intensive and coordinated treatment.
30. *Ibid.*, pp. 113–15.
31. *Ibid.*, pp. 114, 117–18, 185–86, especially p. 192; the author also has relevant unpublished data from the rehabilitants' case studies used for her dissertation. See also Scott, *op. cit.*, p. 79.
32. Unpublished data from the author's dissertation material.
33. Benney, *op. cit.*, pp. 212–19; Prosen, *op. cit.*, pp. 1262–65. Some articles mention the use of competition and/or monetary inducements to increase the rehabilitant's motivation to participate in occupational therapy and/or training leading to his eventual return to work. However, in the case of some rehabilitants, such techniques may have the opposite result. See J. Howard Moes, "VR Workshops Attack Psychological Barriers," *Journal of Rehabilitation*, 28, 2 (March–April 1962), 12; Prosen, *op. cit.*, p. 1264; H. A. Storrow. "Money s a Motivator," *Public Welfare*, 20, 4 (October 1962), 199–204. See also Schlesinger, "Staff Tensions and Needed Skills in Staff-Patient Interaction," *op. cit.*, p. 364. Barry and Malinovsky, *op. cit.*, p. 9, also mention the work on reinforcement techniques by L. Meyerson, J. L. Michael, O. H. Mowrer, C. E. Osgood, and A. W. Staats, "Learning Behavior and Rehabilitation," in L. H. Lofquist (ed.), *Psychological Research and Rehabilitation* (Washington, D.C.: American Psychological Association, 1963), pp. 68–111; and by R. N. Filer and D. D. O'Connell, "Motivation of Aging Persons," *Journal of Gerontology*, 19 (January 1964), 15–22.
34. Nancy Kerr and Lee Meyerson, "From Malingerers to Eager Beavers," *Rehabilitation Record*, 6, 2 (March–April 1965), 28–29. Linde points out that motivation can be increased through operant conditioning procedures; see T. Linde, "Techniques for Establishing Motivation Through Operant Conditioning," *American Journal of Mental Deficiency*, 67 (November 1962), 437–40. Another application of the learning theory is found in H. L. Madison and Marjorie Herring, "An Experimental Study of Motivation," *American Journal of Occupational Therapy*, 14, 5 (September–October 1960), 253–55.
35. Racker *et al.*, *op. cit.*, pp. 258–60; and Leo Shatin, Paula Brown, and Marian Loizeaux, "Psychological Remotivation of the Chronically Ill Medical Patient: A Quantitative Study in Rehabilitation Methodology," *Journal of Chronic Diseases*, 14, 4 (October 1961), 452–68.
36. Roth and Eddy, *op. cit.*
37. Grau, *op. cit.*
38. Roth and Eddy, *op. cit.*

39. Grau, *op. cit.*,
40. *Ibid.*
41. *Ibid.*
42. Rabinowitz and Mitsos, *op. cit.*, p. 13.
43. Fanshel found an association between socioeconomic status and caseworker estimates of the potentiality of cases at the Family and Children's Service in Pittsburgh. See David Fanshel, "A Study of Caseworkers' Perceptions of Their Clients," *Social Casework*, 39, 10 (October 1958), 543–51. Similarly, the author of the present book found a significant positive correlation of .81 between the rehabilitants' socioeconomic status and the degree to which they were judged to be "motivated" and "cooperative." (Finding not included in author's doctoral dissertation, "The Reactions to Disability in Rehabilitation," *op. cit.*)
44. Roth and Eddy, *op. cit.*, pp. 100–43.
45. While in the case of most of these rehabilitants desertion by their families was extreme and clear-cut, we do not know the exact role the family plays in the disabled's assuming the rehabilitant role. Perhaps a similar process (although not always as intensively negative and rejecting) is often behind the assumption of the rehabilitant role, in that the disabled's family may not be willing to accept the limitations and inconveniences resulting from the physical disability and is largely instrumental in his having entered the rehabilitation center. The center is expected to accomplish what the hospitals and the physicians have failed to do: to make the disability go away or to compensate for it in such a way that the disability will finally be an asset rather than a liability. The "right" disabilities were: hemiplegia, amputations, spinal cord injuries, multiple sclerosis, arthritis, muscular dystrophy, or an improperly healed fracture.
46. Roth and Eddy, *op. cit.*, p. 183.
47. Probably one of the most beautiful illustrations of such rivalries is included in the following article: Mieczyslaw Peszczynski, "Rehabilitation of the Adult Hemiplegic," *Fourth Annual Volume of Physiology and Experimental Medical Sciences, 1962–1963*, rehabilitation issue (Calcutta: The Physiological Society of India and the Society of Experimental Medical Sciences, 1963). See also Fred Davis, *Passage Through Crisis* (Indianapolis: Bobbs-Merrill, 1963), pp. 100–1.
48. Reuben J. Margolin and Alan B. Sostek, "Professional Development and Training in Rehabilitation Administration and Supervision," *Journal of Rehabilitation*, 34, 3 (May–June 1968), 18–20.
49. Paul M. Elmwood, Jr., "Can We Afford So Many Rehabilitation Professions?" *Journal of Rehabilitation*, 34, 2 (May–June 1968), 22.

50. Richard M. Titmuss, "The Welfare Complex in a Changing Society," *The Milbank Memorial Fund Quarterly*, 45, 1 (January 1967), 9, 21.
51. In response to these manpower shortages, the American Scholarship Association carried out a pilot demonstration study in order to find the most effective way to contact and motivate high school students to enter the different health and rehabilitation professions. See *Pilot Demonstration Report: Student Recruitment for Health and Rehabilitation Professions* (New York: American Scholarship Association, 1967), p. 21.
52. Leo Levy, "Factors Which Facilitate or Impede Transfer of Medical Functions From Physicians to Paramedical Personnel," *Journal of Health and Human Behavior*, 7, 1 (Spring 1966), 50–54.
53. C. H. Patterson, "Is the Team Concept Obsolete?" *Journal of Rehabilitation*, 25, 2 (March–April 1959), 9–10, 27–28; Elliot A. Krause, "After the Rehabilitation Center," *Social Problems*, 14, 2 (Fall 1966), 199–200.
54. Per G. Stensland, "The Health Profession and the Changing Community," *The Milbank Memorial Fund Quarterly*, 43, 4, part I (October 1964), 445–49.
55. Betty E. Cogswell and Donald D. Weir, "A Role in Process: The Development of Medical Professionals' Role in Long-term Care of Chronically Diseased Patients," *Journal of Health and Human Behavior*, 5 (Summer–Fall 1964), 95–103.
56. J. A. L. Vaughan Jones, "Rehabilitation: Concept and Practice," *British Journal of Industrial Medicine*, 18, 4 (October 1961), 241–49; Howard A. Rusk, "The Philosophy of Rehabilitation," *Connecticut Medicine*, 25, 11 (November 1961), 678–79; and W. A. Spencer *et al.*, "Rehabilitation in Concept and Practice," *Southern Medical Journal*, 55 (July 1962), 721–28.
57. Bernard Goldstein, Lawrence G. Northwood, and Rhoda L. Goldstein, "Medicine in Industry: Problems of Administrators and Practitioners," *Journal of Health and Human Behavior*, 1, 4 (Winter 1960), 259–60.
58. Rhoda L. Goldstein and Bernard Goldstein, *Doctors and Nurses in Industry* (New Brunswick, N.J.: Rutgers University Press 1967), pp. 5–19.
59. See Eliot Freidson, *Patients' Views of Medical Practice* (New York: Russell Sage Foundation, 1961), pp. 218–20; also Mark G. Field, *Doctor and Patient in Soviet Russia* (Cambridge, Mass.: Harvard University Press, 1957).
60. Goldstein and Goldstein, *op. cit.*, pp. 35–64.
61. Mechanic makes this point in David Mechanic, "The Sociology of Medicine: Viewpoints and Perspectives," *Journal of Health and Human Behavior*, 7, 4 (Winter 1966), 239–40.

62. Marvin B. Sussman, Marie R. Haug, and Gloria A. Krupnick, *Professional Associations and Memberships in Rehabilitation Counseling*, Working Paper no. 2 (Cleveland, O.: Western Reserve University, 1966).
63. Marie R. Haug and Marvin B. Sussman, "The Impact of Organizational Characteristics on Occupational Change" (paper read at the Ohio Valley Sociological Society meetings, Detroit, May 2–4, 1968).
64. George J. Goldin, "Some Rehabilitation Counselor Attitudes Toward Their Professional Role," *Rehabilitation Literature*, 27, 12 (December 1966), 360–64.
65. Elliot A. Krause, "Structured Strain in a Marginal Profession: Rehabilitation Counseling," *Journal of Health and Human Behavior*, 6, 1 (Spring 1965), 55–59.
66. *Ibid.*, pp. 59–61.
67. *Highlights of National Studies at 90 State Vocational Rehabilitation Agencies by the Patterns of Rehabilitation Services Project* (Washington, D.C.: National Rehabilitation Association, 1964).
68. Marie R. Haug and Marvin B. Sussman, "The Second Career— Variant of a Sociological Concept," *Journal of Gerontology*, 22, 4, part I (October 1967), 441–42.
69. Krause, "After the Rehabilitation Center," *op. cit.*, p. 201.
70. *Patterns of Rehabilitation Services Provided by the 90 State Vocational Rehabilitation Agencies of the United States* (Washington, D.C.: National Rehabilitation Association, 1964), pp. 105–6.
71. A. Arthur Rosse, Joseph L. Marra, and Frederick W. Novis, "The Disability Adjudicator: Identification of Duties and Qualifications," *Journal of Rehabilitation*, 28, 2 (March–April 1962), 29–30.
72. Alexander Ropchan, "The Need of Integrating the Community Rehabilitation Agency and Disciplines," *Journal of Rehabilitation*, 26, 3 (May–June 1960), 4–7, 45–47; also William P. Richardson, "Inter-agency Coordination: A Basic Need in Serving Handicapped Children," *Rehabilitation Literature*, 27, 7 (July 1966), 196.
73. Marvin Sussman, "Emerging Relationships and Roles in Health and Welfare" (presentation at the Eastern Sociological Society meetings, Boston, April 5–7, 1968).
74. James Leo Walsh and Ray H. Elling, "Professionalism and the Poor—Structural Effects and Professional Behavior," *Journal of Health and Social Behavior*, 9, 1 (March 1968), 16–28.
75. From unpublished data analyzed by the author while preparing her dissertation at the Ohio Rehabilitation Center, Columbus, Ohio.

76. Again, with the exception of the Roth and Eddy book, most other studies are about the mentally ill. See, for example, Stanton and Schwartz, *op. cit.*; and Barry S. Brown and William Flynn, "Sociometric Choice in a Mental Hospital Population," *Journal of Health and Human Behavior*, 7, 4 (Winter 1964), 309–12.

77. Herman A. Dickel, "The Philosophy of Rehabilitation," *Western Journal of Surgery, Obstetrics and Gynecology*, 71, 2 (March–April 1963), 100–2.

78. William A. Steiger, Francis H. Hoffman, A. Victor Hanse, and H. Niebuhr, "A Definition of Comprehensive Medicine," *Journal of Health and Human Behavior*, 1, 2 (Summer 1960), 83–86; and Joseph D. Matarazzo, "Comprehensive Medicine: A New Era in Medical Education," *Human Organization*, 14, 1 (Spring 1955), 4–9.

79. John Eisele David, "Rehabilitation and the Great Society," *Journal of the Association for Physical and Mental Rehabilitation*, 20, 5 (September–October 1966), 168. Slightly different statistics have been reported for 1965 elsewhere; see *Medical Economics*, 42, 25 (December 13, 1965), 84.

80. Some physicians have voiced the existing dilemma in medical education: Basic medical research is emphasized as well as limited aspects of health services, while the community increasingly expects comprehensive health care and "that physicians accept responsibility for an increasingly wide range of problems related to health." Thus, medical students during their training are gradually detached from and lose interest in the total health needs of the community, and the incorporation of rehabilitation in academic medicine meets serious and probably insurmountable barriers. See John L. Caughley, "The Academic Capabilities of Rehabilitation," *New England Journal of Medicine*, 268, 26 (June 1963), 1447–50.

81. The behavior of disabled men who probably could work if they received special services and training but who choose not to work is deviant, since it violates the institutionalized expectation of work. As a result, the behavior of these men is organized into a deviant role. See Eliot Freidson, "Disability as Social Deviance," in Marvin B. Sussman (ed.), *Sociology and Rehabilitation* (Washington, D.C.: American Sociological Association, 1965), p. 73. However, as Freidson also points out, the creation of rehabilitation agencies serves to classify these men as deviant if they do not avail themselves of whatever services they need (all presumably to be found within the rehabilitation agency) and return to work. The availability of rehabilitation services (despite the fact that in reality they are not available equally to all) tends to define this behavior more

clearly as deviant; otherwise, semilegitimate excuses could be found which would make the behavior acceptable to society. See *ibid.*, pp. 82–86. See also Robert D. Wright, "Rehabilitation's Wave of the Future," *Archives of Physical Medicine and Rehabilitation*, 43 (August 1962), 395–400. In the latest amendments to the Rehabilitation Acts (1965 and 1966), which attempted to encourage the rehabilitation of even the disabled who would never be able to work, their needing physical rehabilitation was justified because their physical independence would release other members of the family for full-time employment. Strauss also mentions the remark made by a congressman during hearings before a special subcommittee that another goal of rehabilitation was to save "the children of a half-million families from growing up in the psychology of living at public expense." See Robert Strauss, "Social Change and the Rehabilitation Concept," in Sussman, *op. cit.*, pp. 19, 21, 30. For a discussion of prominent American values, see Robin M. Williams, Jr., *American Society* (New York: Knopf, 1954), pp. 390–428.

82. Albert Wessen, "The Apparatus of Rehabilitation: An Organizational Analysis," in Sussman, *op. cit.*, pp. 153–60.

83. Rabinowitz and Mitsos, *op. cit.*, pp. 2–14.

84. The American Medical Association and individual physicians did not like the implications of failure to accomplish what was needed for the patient, but they also did not like the idea of spending more time on each patient. The rehabilitation team concept was not entirely welcome since it removed the patient from the exclusively important dyadic relationship with the physician to a multiple relationship with several medical and paramedical staff members. Once rehabilitation became accepted and a medical speciality—physical medicine or physiatry—was developed, however, the medical association made sure that the physician would be the "captain" of the team and started making appeals to physicians to become interested in rehabilitation so that the field would be dominated and controlled by the medical profession. See Wessen, *op. cit.*, pp. 153–160; also Jones, *op. cit.*, p. 245.

85. Robert A. Scott, "The Factory as a Social Service Organization: Goal Displacement in Workshops for the Blind," *Social Problems*, 15, 2 (Fall 1967), 160–75.

86. Of course, we do not claim that it is undesirable for a sheltered workshop to become self-supporting or even profitable if such an operational orientation does not entail the "negative" consequences for the severely disabled described above. Profit-making is desirable only to the extent that it is compatible with the primary function of sheltered workshops: the provision of employment for severely disabled workers.

87. Martin Rein, "The Strange Case of Public Dependency," *Transaction* 2, 3 (March–April 1965), 16–23.
88. Claude Veil, *Handicap et Société* (Paris: Flammarion, 1968), pp. 184–85.
89. There is an interesting parallel here between the disabled and a particular category of women—those who emphasize the fact that they are female and, therefore, cannot be expected to have any work commitment (or to work at all) or to carry on any strenuous or responsible activity. Thus, they are able to use their "inherently different feminine nature" as a socially acceptable excuse for laziness or incompetence.

CHAPTER 5

Disability and Work

In this chapter we shall examine the interrelationships between disability and work, since work is an important independent as well as dependent variable in relation to disability. The type of work determines to a considerable extent the type of disabling illness or accident an individual has a significantly high probability of incurring. Furthermore, since the occupational role is the most important role for American men, the degree of satisfaction from work and the meaning that work has for every individual are crucial for the type of definition that will be attached to an incurred disability. The more a person has experienced frustrations and maladjustments at work, the more he may be inclined to see disability as precluding his being able to work any longer. And finally, an individual's self-definition of a disability as a more or less serious vocational handicap as well as the prevailing demand for people with his particular skills will determine whether or not he will in fact stay unemployed "because of his disability." The work experiences of some occupational groups are consistently so negative and meaningless and the demand for that level of skill so low and fluctuating that they most often become vocationally handicapped after even a not too severe physical disability. These occupational groups are the unskilled and most of the semiskilled workers who make up the lower class. It is, then, important to understand the life conditions, the values and attitudes of lower class men, as well as the social structure features that create a low demand for their level of skill, if we wish to understand why there is a "hard core" of disabled that makes up the rejects and the failure statistics of vocational rehabilitation programs.

Finally, we will take a brief look at the variety of federal programs which have been established in order to diminish the social handicaps of the core disadvantaged segment of the population. For as long as the existing programs and agencies are not successful in rehabilitating socially handicapped persons, the rehabilitation agencies will be faced with the very difficult (and often insurmountable) problem of having to rehabilitate physically *and* socially handicapped persons.

Work and Incidence of Disability

Disability is not a randomly distributed phenomenon among workers in different occupational categories: Evidence exists that certain types of disabilities are much more frequent among particular occupational groups while other occupational groups are more often besieged by a variety of disabilities. For example, a relationship has been demonstrated between lung cancer and the occupation of asbestos mining in Quebec, mesothelioma and asbestos mining in South Africa, and between coal mining and bronchitis and tuberculosis.[1] However, besides the occupational environment, the influence of other variables such as social class or stress situations has been found to be of equal importance.[2] Thus, although empirical data exist associating disease rates or disability rates with specific occupations, other possibly intervening variables have seldom been controlled, so that the association has not been firmly and conclusively established.

The larger number of accidents occur among blue collar workers (that is, "craftsmen, foremen and kindred workers" and "operatives and kindred workers"), and more than half of these accidents happen at work (of the 346.8 persons injured per 1,000 blue collar workers, 206.7 were injured while at work). Health statistics similarly indicate that private household workers and farm workers show a high frequency of chronic conditions more often than do those in other occupational categories (61 percent of private household workers and 64 percent of farmers, only 53 percent of the "craftsmen and foremen, and service workers," and 49.5 percent of operatives, with similar frequencies for the white collar workers).[3]

The relationship observed between some occupational categories and a higher frequency of accidental injuries and chronic conditions may not necessarily mean that these have been caused by either the nature of the work performed or the working conditions themselves. Sometimes this is true, as in the cases of silicosis among coal miners or accidents among construction workers.[4] But in other cases, for example, the high incidence of chronic conditions among farm workers, the higher incidence may be largely a reflection of the prevalence in the group of persons over 45 years of age.[5] Or, as in the case of high incidence of chronic conditions among private household workers, the incidence may reflect the predominance of nonwhite females over 45 years of age who generally have a higher prevalence of chronic conditions than white men under 45 (although not equally in the different occupational categories). Definitions of illnesses in general, that is, the sick role conceptions, seem to vary significantly with age, sex, and race. Moreover, it has been found that workers over 45 years of age and females on the average show a greater degree of absenteeism than do males under 44 years of age.[6] According to Enterline, however, the higher sickness absence rate among women is true only for married, divorced, or widowed women (not for single women, who, on the contrary, show a lower sick leave absence rate than do men of the same age group), probably because of their responsibility for child rearing.[7]

Generally, then, a chronic illness or an accident may or may not be defined as a disabling condition depending upon the type and degree of physical disability, the type of occupation, age, sex, race, education, and a number of other sociopsychological characteristics. The same type and degree of disability may constitute a vocational handicap for people engaged in one occupation (or belonging to one occupational category) but not for those engaged in another. For example, the loss of a left arm may be a serious vocational handicap for some unskilled workers whose customary work requires the use of two strong arms (for lifting), but may be no more than an inconvenience for a secure university professor. Furthermore, workers in different occupational groups, under the influence of varying motivations, work experiences and satisfactions, values concerning work, and nature of "secondary gains" derived from work incapacity, may be more or less driven to maximize or minimize the extent of work limitations resulting from an existing chronic condition.

The examination by occupational category of the distribution of work limitations resulting from a chronic condition indicates that while 7.3 percent of all persons 17 years of age and over are limited in their ability to work, 5.3 percent of the white collar workers are thus limited, 7.2 percent of the blue collar workers, 9.8 percent of the service workers, and 17.0 percent of the farm workers. And these differences become much more accentuated with advancing age, especially after 45 (see Table 1, Chapter 3). Among white collar workers, professionals and clerical and sales people show the smallest incidence of work limitations. And when income and level of educational attainment were examined, it was found that a high incidence of work limitations due to chronic conditions was associated with low income and education.[8]

These trends could be explained both in terms of the differential nature of tasks and requirements in these occupational groups and in terms of the greater societal demand for highly skilled and educated persons in view of their relative scarcity. Most of the chronic conditions, with the exception of those resulting in mental, intellectual, or speech impairment, do not usually seriously interfere with the work activities of professionals, clerical workers, and salespeople.[9] On the contrary, the presence of most chronic conditions interferes seriously with the performance of the usual tasks involved in blue collar work. The demand for semiskilled and unskilled workers is also low, a fact that renders their work potential very problematic when disability has been added to their lack of skill. Furthermore, people of low income and education do not usually have enough money to spare for curing or controlling a disabling condition; what is more, they often receive inadequate or second-rate medical care even when they seek it. They tend not to follow medical suggestions regarding the long-term care of chronic diseases or disabling injuries either because the nature of their condition and the required care have not been adequately explained to them or because their life conditions do not permit them to do so.[10]

It is rather striking that, according to statistics, the percentage of nonwhite, female, and white unskilled (and to a lesser extent white semiskilled) workers with a work limitation is considerably lower than that of white skilled workers and not much different from that of white professionals, clerical workers, and salespeople. The reason for this seems to be that these national statistics exclude the "physically handicapped unable to work" as not belonging to the labor force. However, statistics from another source have shown that women and black men (especially those over 55) have a higher reported incidence of severe disability (that makes it impossible for them to work altogether or to work regularly) than have white men of all age groups. Probably, the same trend holds true for unskilled white men in comparison to more skilled ones.[11] Also while 4 percent of the severely disabled men and 72 percent of those with a major occupational disability are employed full-time, only less than one-half of 1 percent of the severely disabled women and 16 percent of those with a major occupational disability are working full-time.[12] Is it that women, blacks, and unskilled workers tend to define as seriously disabling conditions, warranting withdrawal from work, those physical impairments that would be defined only as "work limitations" by most white men? Or, are women, black males, and unskilled workers, who even when able-bodied encounter discrimination and difficulties in finding jobs, more easily rendered seriously handicapped in the vocational area by even a slight or moderate degree of physical disability?

An often-measured consequence of limitations in the ability to work has been the "days of work loss." It seems, however, that this tends to vary with the type of occupation and degree of work commitment as well as with the sick-leave privileges and cash sickness benefits granted to workers in different occupational categories. Thus, white collar workers—who reputedly have a higher work commitment than blue collar workers and whose satisfaction from work is based on more intrinsic factors than money—also show the lowest rate of work loss in all types of employment. Furthermore, blue collar workers and service workers show a considerably higher degree of work loss when employed by federal or local governments.[13] One possible explanation for this may be that blue collar workers (and especially service workers for whom money is often the main job satisfaction and rationale for working) tend to adopt the sick role more often when actual loss of income does not result from absence due to sickness. Gordon's empirical validation of the sick role also showed that the lower the educational level, the greater the tendency to foster dependency in case of illness and disability.[14] This tendency finds freer expression when actual income is not affected by work loss, as in the case of the federal government, which grants workers generous sick-leave privileges.

It seems, then, that type of occupation determines, on the one hand, the meaning that work has and, on the other hand, the level of societal demand for particular skills. Whether or not a particular disability will become a vocational handicap depends upon the individual's type of occupation as well as upon his sociopsychological characteristics, some of which are also highly related to the type of job he holds (for example, level of education and social class). We shall first examine how occupation determines to a large extent the meaning that work has and then we shall see how the impact of a disability may be very different depending upon occupation, work history, and sociopsychological makeup. (This discussion will be limited to men, since only men are required by society to work in all cases.)

The Meaning of Work: Work and Identity

Work has a different meaning for different occupational groups: The vocational identity is not equally central in the self-concept of men in different occupations and with different vocational experiences. The degree to which a physical impairment becomes a vocational handicap depends partially upon the nature of the disability, partially upon the nature of the work performed in the usual occupation, and partially upon the symbolic significance invested in the vocational role. More specifically, whether or not a physical disability will lead to the discontinuity of the working role largely depends (except in the case of terminal conditions) upon the importance of the working role for the self-concept. We shall now see how type of occupation and work experience influence the importance that work will have for identity and how these differences lead to a differential mode of disability definition as well as mode of reacting to the disability. This in turn determines whether or not an individual needs or receives rehabilitation services, whether or not he benefits from these services, and whether or not and to what degree he will finally remain physically or vocationally handicapped.

In our century work is probably valued more than ever before, and this seems to be true all over the world. However, work seems still to be more stressed in American culture for a larger segment of the population and over a more extended life cycle.[15] Single women and all men between 18 and 65 are expected to work regardless of socioeconomic status.[16] The only exceptions to this rule are college students (until they have either left school or acquired their degree) and the obligatory exemption granted to those who are so severely incapacitated that they are institutionalized and usually federally or state supported.[17] Work is valued not only for its instrumental usefulness, that is, as a means to sustenance or financial prosperity, but also for the psychological "side effects" which such economic independence gives. It is valued for its "intrinsic" importance for a person's psychological and moral makeup. Work is thought to play a crucial role in the formation of the core identity, in self-esteem, in overall organization of life, and in family life, as well as in mental and physical health.[18]

However, despite the fact that work is an overall societal value, it may acquire a different meaning and importance for different individuals who do not share the same social status, sociopsychological background, and work experiences. Patterns of similarities in the meaning that work may have for different people are usually determined by level of education and degree of skill, as well as by the nature of the work and its external and intrinsic rewards. Also involved are values about achievement and success, plus level of performance and definitions of such roles as the occupational, the familial, the social, the political, and the "masculine" or "feminine" role. For the purposes of this book, the patterns of similarities in the meaning of and the importance attached to work will be examined mainly by occupational category and social class.

For most professionals, their work constitutes the very essence of their lives, it is their raison d'être, the basic dimension in their core identity. Success is highly valued among all middle and upper middle class males, and work is usually instrumental in obtaining it. These men are able to establish a valid identity because their working status permits them to have access to a "career success."[19] Nothing else can ever substitute for work, even partially; they are deeply attached not only to work but often to their particular jobs so that they would not even be inclined to interrupt their careers.[20] A number of studies have shown that in the case of white collar workers (particularly those in professional and managerial occupations), both the motivation to work as well as a sense of satisfaction are derived from the existence of such conditions of personal growth as promotions, challenging work assignments, and type of work performed.[21] Because of this strong occupational attachment, disabling accidents or diseases do not usually affect their employability very seriously except when the disability affects their mental faculties or when it is extremely severe and threatens sheer survival. These people have too much of themselves invested in their work and have usually been satisfactorily rewarded so that their withdrawing from the labor force would penalize them too acutely from a financial, social, and psychological point of view. Even from the financial point of view alone, workmen's compensation could not in most cases come anywhere near the salaries they would be earning if they were to continue working after the occurrence of a disability. Of course, they are able to return to gainful employment because there is usually a considerable demand for their skills so that they are sought after despite their disability. But also from the sociopsychological point of view, disability does not seem to seriously affect their self-concepts, probably because they tend to define themselves basically in terms of abilities and traits other than physical strength. One notable exception would be when physical appearance or the performance of the sexual role was quite central in their self-concept and the disability seriously affected the former or the latter.

Unless their self-definition as intellectually capable and achieving individuals is affected by the nature of the disability, they are able to more or less insulate the effects of the disability on a few directly affected self-images. Their continuing to work helps them maintain continuity in their identity and therefore serves a valuable psychological function. In the case of all disabled men, we could apply Merton's model of adaptation to deviance[22] and use as variables the disabled individual's level of work morale and his attitude toward the disability (see Table 3). According to this table, we could say

TABLE 3.
Modes of Adaptation to the Potential Vocational Deviance Created by Disability*

Work Morale	Attitude	Toward	Disability
	Accepted	*Rejected*	*Secondary Gains*
High	*Conformism* Return to gainful employment	*Ritualism* Return to same job or type of job	*Innovation* Vocational training or small business
Low	*Favorable* physical but not vocational rehabilitation	*Continuous* treatments to get cured & return to normal	*Retreatism* Retiring on compensation check

* This table is a modified version of the typology developed by the author in "The Reactions to Disability in Rehabilitation" (unpublished Ph.D. dissertation, Ohio State University, 1963).

that the most usual adaptation of professionals to their disability is that of conformism. In the case of other white collar workers (salesmen or clerical workers), their adaptation may be ritualistic whenever they no longer believe that their work is a career.[23] If they are older people and have experienced work maladjustments and disenchantments, they may be willing to improve physically but be uninterested in or ambivalent toward vocational rehabilitation.

For blue collar workers, on the other hand, the meaning of work seems to be quite different and to provide a quite different set of satisfactions. To the blue collar worker, work represents a valued continuous activity, often a very strenuous activity, giving him a sense of well-being and sustaining his sense of worth and self-respect.[24] Work, furthermore, seems to mean different things to the skilled and the stably employed semiskilled workers and to the unskilled and semiskilled workers who for a variety of reasons experience unemployment quite frequently. In essence, then, the distinction will be made between working class (that is, skilled and stable semiskilled workers) and lower class males (that is, the unskilled and the periodically working semiskilled workers) throughout this discussion concerning the meaning of work and the impact of disability upon actual employability as well as the desire to continue working.

For most working class males, that is, those with skilled jobs or in-demand semiskilled and service jobs, it may be possible to build an identity as a "good provider" who can give his family the "good American life" because of usually steady wages and the occasional small wage increases which sustain this identity.[25] Because of this emphasis on "respectability" and on being self-supporting, affliction caused by a disability can be quite threatening to the self-concept. The most effective way to handle this threat is by returning to gainful employment (preferably the predisability type) and thus reestablishing as soon as possible the predisability equilibrium. Because of this need for continuity in their threatened self-concept, working class males may have a great tendency to deny the disability, their mode of adaptation being predominantly ritualistic (see Table 3). When, however, these working class men (and especially the skilled workers) are over 40 or 45 years of age, they may have a tendency to want to get out of their employee status and, if their disability is compensable, to want to use a lump-sum compensation for the establishment of a small business, usually a small repair shop.[26] This may be partly because the compensation sum represents an opportunity to realize a lifelong dream, but a more important factor is probably their reduced chance of finding another job because of advancing age. These workers are the "innovators," since they use their disability in order to change their lives as they had always desired (see Table 3). Finally, if their work morale has been low because of a series of maladjustments, they might, when 50 or over, decide to retire, especially when their family

198   DISABILITY AND REHABILITATION

is opposed to plans for establishing a small business and the wife (or children) is willing to be the breadwinner.

Some studies have shown that for semiskilled and unskilled workers, the motivation to work as well as work satisfaction are largely determined on the basis of the salary level and the nature of the working conditions—for example, good supervision, good group relations, and being able to rely on others.[27] This pattern seems to be even more accentuated in the case of all black blue collar workers.[28] The fact that their satisfaction lies in these aspects of the job rather than in the more intrinsic ones probably can be explained in terms of the failure of the jobs to provide these elementary conditions. The very nature of these jobs does not permit advancement or demand high work commitment—they are just accessible since they require no education or special skills. Lower class people hold jobs at the bottom of the occupational ladder which offer no psychological rewards and often involve unpleasant, humiliating or completely routinized tasks, as well as marginal financial rewards which do not even suffice for family support.[29] Even the best jobs among those available (such as construction work) are seasonal and extremely influenced by business fluctuations. For example, assembly line work, probably the most highly paid of blue collar jobs, depends on the state of business and has high unemployment rates when business is bad.

Employers do not place any particular value upon the usual lower class jobs and hire people when and for as long as they need their services. They view these workers as completely expendable. In turn, lower class workers, even when they start with high hopes of becoming good providers and raising a family, have fears that the working experiences of their fathers, brothers, and friends may be repeated. And after a few years their fears almost inevitably materialize as they begin to periodically experience unemployment and are unable to find a meaning in their jobs.[30] They usually become quite detached from their jobs, which they have come to view as expendable since they do not see them as providing any adequate psychological or financial rewards. They are therefore inclined to quit for a variety of reasons, not all of them serious. And because they have often met with frustrating work experiences, they may appear "unmotivated" to work. Their detachment leads to their being willing to change employment whenever they have the opportunity, especially if there is promise of some financial improvement.[31] The continuous or at least frequent economic deprivation which undermines their marriages and their social relationships leads to a resignation to the fact that most of the jobs open to them are "hard, dirty, uninteresting, and underpaid." At the end they come to value only the size of the paycheck.

This final disillusionment with all working conditions may lead them, especially in their forties and fifties, to prefer the more secure source of income represented by the unemployment or welfare check. It is interesting to note that although some writers point to the unemployment check as being of only short duration and the welfare check not always so "secure" an income, such relatively "regular" and "predictable" checks represent security to some economically deprived lower class males—probably because a relatively steady income regardless of its source tends to have a stabilizing effect on their lives. There is even evidence that some other people may consider the person more reliable when he receives an unemployment or welfare check than when he is working.[32] When, therefore, lower class workers are afflicted with a compensable disability, the temptation is great to choose the regular compensation check instead of work wages which would most probably now be even more irregular than before. The temptation may be accentuated by the feeling that compensation is something owed them by society. Lower class disabled men therefore tend to react to their disability predominantly through "retreatism."

As we have already seen, the "good provider" role is shaky for lower class males because they work only occasionally—when there is a high demand for unskilled labor and they "feel like working"—and even when they work they often cannot earn enough to support their families. Consequently they are forced to seek a different type of identity, one which allows them to evaluate and respect themselves and to be evaluated and respected by the others. In such cases identity must be based on criteria at which one can excel regardless of his performance in the occupational role or his having or not having a definite occupational role. There is cross-cultural evidence which suggests that whenever the playing of the occupational role is uncertain, intermittent, unsatisfactory or provides low and unreliable wages, usually because of different types of structural unemployment, men have to revert to basic expressions of masculinity in their search for an identity. Moreover, depending upon general culture values, subcultural values, and modes of leisure and entertainment, men may also excel in terms of singing, dancing, playing musical instruments, drinking tolerance, the relating of jokes, and so forth, as in the case of the black and the lower class Greek.[33] Thus, "expressive" traits (indirectly attributable to the individual's "male soul") also contribute toward building and confirming the lower class identity.

In some developing countries in which urban lower class people have recently migrated from rural areas and still adhere to traditional values, men may also base their identity in terms of age and kinship positions. For example, in a developing country such as Greece, where unemployment has been quite frequent in all occupational groupings and low pay has made it very difficult for the large majority of Greek men to be good providers (in all classes except the upper and the upper middle classes), identity has been traditionally based on "masculinity" and "maleness." "Man is a man is a man is a man . . ." could be said about Greek men. Unless their "masculine" identity was in some way challenged, Greek men were by no means devalued in the eyes of others or self-devalued by unemployment, being fired, or other work maladjustments. Their wives did not challenge their authority when they were unemployed or underpaid; in short, they were still the "men" they always were.[34] In the last fifteen years unemployment and severe work maladjustments have been more acute among working and lower class Greeks, and it is among these that identity is presently based on "masculinity." Because for a long time following World War II unemployment plagued even the professionals, it has been easy for the working and lower class Greek to blame his occupational maladjustment on faulty governmental policies, corrupt politicians, or the ruined economy of the country. Similarly, in the United States black lower class men may still be able to largely externalize the blame for their work maladjustments because all blacks, regardless of education or skills, have been and still are being occupationally discriminated against.[35] The white lower class may "objectively" have less ground for externalizing their work failures, but they can often find scapegoats such as blacks, or ethnic or religious groups on which to shift the blame.

Another identity basis for which there is cross-cultural evidence whenever the road to achievement and success is blocked is "smartness," as defined by Miller. This is "the capacity to achieve a value entity—material goods, personal status—with a minimum use of physical effort."[36] Prestige is accorded to those who demonstrate they are competent in getting what they want by duping others, by pretending, by persuading somebody else to do work for which they will get credit, and most of all by working the least amount possible and preferably not at all. Thus, one may establish his identity as being "smart" in this sense in both the American lower class and the Greek middle, lower middle, working and lower class.

American lower class men cannot establish through any of the institutionally accepted means available a "valid" identity according to either of the two prevailing value complexes of *career success* or *good provider*. Thus, they must choose between using illegal means to reach the culturally valued goals or finding a new basis of identity in terms of which they can define themselves and be evaluated and accepted by others. Lower class males tend to define themselves in terms of physical prowess (usually measured by their fighting strength), sexual potency, and toughness, these being different expressions of their basic masculinity, and signs of a special brand of "smartness."[37] On these identity criteria they may excel to varying degrees without having to be occupationally or financially successful. By rating high on the basis of these criteria, lower class men are attempting to reassure themselves that they are worthwhile persons possessing more desirable characteristics than are possessed by others and that these characteristics are valid criteria according to which they will be evaluated by others.

There is controversy, however, as to whether or not American lower class men are able to establish a valid identity based on these critieria. Rainwater thinks it is possible. Liebow calls these "second hand" values, a "shadow system" of values that cannot make up in a real sense for lack of success in the occupational and husband roles. He does not accept the idea that through a "stretching" of values these people can establish a satisfactory and solid identity.[38] The latter view may be closer to the lower class males' reality (who all along may know they do not measure up to the socially acceptable criteria for a valid identity), so that the implications of this type of inadequate and probably semisatisfactory identity validation are quite significant for the impact of disability and the outcome of vocational rehabilitation in the case of lower class men.

Depending on the criterion used by the lower class man to establish a valid identity and depending on the degree to which the working role is nonessential, his reactions may vary considerably with regard to an incurred disability. If the working role was always considered marginal, when disabled he will not be concerned with becoming able to return to work. This aspect of rehabilitation will tend to be irrelevant, since the inability to work will in no way threaten the continuity of his self-concept. But depending on whether "smartness," physical prowess and toughness, or sexual potency was the basis for his identity, he may react differently to his disability to the extent to which the nature of the disability directly affects his self-concept in terms of these qualities. If, for example, his disability threatens the lower class man's basic self-concept as a sexually potent male or as a strong and tough male, he may deny his disability, with result that he may be accepted for rehabilitation since he will appear to be extremely "motivated." Depending upon how well he can "play" the rehabilitant role, that is, the extent to which he can pretend to be interested in vocational rehabilitation (although this aspect of rehabilitation does not concern him), he may be able to stay on in the rehabilitation center. Of course, when he reaches a plateau in noticeable improvement and is faced with the need to accept his psychologically intolerable disability, he usually loses all motivation and is either discharged or leaves before his discharge.

If, on the other hand, "smartness" as defined by lower class values is the basic element in the disabled man's identity, the disability will be used in order to derive "secondary gains," in this case money. The "smart" thing to do is to turn the disability into profit by making society pay you for the rest of your life so there is no necessity to work or to find means to support yourself and your family. These lower class men represent the classic "compensionitis" cases. Since, however, they do not understand the laws well and often establish strained relationships even with their lawyers, they may not necessarily be successful in obtaining substantial settlements for their disabilities (especially if they choose the lump sum type of settlement). They may eventually have to return to whatever unsatisfactory and unstable jobs they are able to obtain.

Finally, if the working role has not been completely marginal in a lower class man's self-concept prior to his disability and work is still valued as an activity, he will tend to have a negative self-concept, since he has met only vocational failure and frustration. In some cases, he may attempt to deny the disability and ritualistically return to a frustrating and disappointing job. If, however, the nature of the disability is such that he cannot perform the job tasks required, he may be fired or forced to quit because of extreme pain. He may then either continue working intermittently, whenever his physical condition permits, or revert to "retreatism" (see Table 3). In most cases, however, the advent of a disability may be a welcome opportunity to change the undesirable self-concept. This change may be brought about by means of at least two basic mechanisms. Either he may "use" the presence of the disability to be altogether excused from performing the usually disappointing vocational role (see Table 3), or he may try to use vocational training to improve his skills and therefore his vocational career regardless of ability to perform the tasks involved in the previously held job and the possibility of a return to it (see Table 3). Both reactions represent attempts to alter significantly the vocational role so that the sustained self-concept can become more tolerably positive. Besides the importance of work for the self-concept, age also seems to be an important variable in determining which of the two reactions will be acted upon by the disabled lower class worker in this category.[39]

It must be acknowledged, however, that even moderate disability quite seriously affects those who have always been "marginal" workers because of low education, lack of vocational skills, advanced age (over 40 or 45), and undesirable race or ethnic membership. The addition of disability to such social handicaps makes these individuals even less in demand in the labor market and definitely places them in the category of the "hard core" unemployable.

Furthermore, as we have seen, disabled lower-class persons referred to vocational rehabilitation facilities are most often rejected before any services are offered or before such services are completed —allegedly because they are not "motivated" or "cooperative."[40] This is the socially accepted terminology which says that they are bad placement risks and therefore bad for the success statistics of the rehabilitation facility. If accepted for rehabilitation, they are often refused vocational training because it is believed they would not profit from it, would not complete it, or would not even use it. It is rather ironic that those who were always marginally employable because of "unfavorable" sociopsychological characteristics, when further burdened by the social stigma of disability, are seldom given the benefit of vocational training or are seldom successful in completing it. Of course, vocational training is not always adapted to the labor market so that it may not necessarily help these marginal workers break through the vicious circle and may have the same shortcomings for them as formal education has had in the past. It is, however, their only chance: a chance most often denied to them or made so unattractive and purposeless that they are not motivated to pursue it. Furthermore, the lower class disabled with many dependents do not feel they can afford the uncertain results of vocational training or the economic hardship on their families. Depending on a variety of factors, they prefer either to look for a job, even one that is low-paying and unstable, or to stay on the stable workmen's compensation payroll.

Existing and Suggested Solutions
to Help Lower Class Disabled

As we have seen up to now, the most serious and frequent consequences of disability for the performance of the working role occur among lower class workers who have always had difficulties in finding and keeping a job. While it is difficult to estimate exactly the percentage of male workers who are lower class, the 1960 labor force statistics showed that semiskilled and unskilled workers comprise 35.3 percent of the total male labor force.[41] Unskilled workers comprise 14 percent of the male labor force; of the operatives (which represent 21.2 percent), at least half experience wide unemployment swings as a result of technological change and cyclical variations. Thus, we could estimate that at least 25 percent of all males are lower class. There is no convincing evidence that the percentage of lower class males will diminish in the future, since the number of school dropouts is not decreasing and we have not been too successful in changing the conditions which account for a lack of interest in education on the part of lower class adolescents. A variety of solutions have been discussed or tried during the last few years in an effort to break the vicious circle in which these people are trapped. It is important for us to examine briefly some of these solutions, their promises, and their shortcomings, because if satisfactory solutions can be found and operationalized, the most serious and difficult cases for vocational rehabilitation programs could be made easier or completely eliminated. Rehabilitation agencies could then concentrate on the handicapping effects of a physical and/or psychological disability without the added complication of having to deal with socially caused handicaps.

Some of these solutions are *preventive* in that they aim to decrease the number of poorly educated and unskilled persons by intervening with the socialization process of working and lower class children in order to change or modify their values and early life experiences so that they can become interested in and benefit from available educational programs. Another goal is educating teachers (or training special personnel) to reach and interest lower class children in education, either academic or vocational.[42] Other solutions are *corrective*, that is, they aim to help the presently unemployed and unemployable to find and hold a job either by creating jobs (or changing the working conditions or the image of jobs where vacancies exist) or by retraining them so that they can qualify for jobs requiring specific skills.[43]

Among the preventive programs, one with great potential has been the Head Start Program for preschool children and their families. This program has been attempting to reduce the number of unskilled and uneducated by improving the intellectual, conceptual, and linguistic skills of preschool children—and to some extent the corresponding skills of their parents, although much less emphasis has been placed on this population. Teachers have been trained to be more effective with lower class children. Unfortunately, there are indications that the Head Start program, like most welfare programs, does not focus on those who most need the services. Those helped are most often the working class and the upper lower class who hold a more middle class outlook, have an intact family structure, and so forth, rather than the hard core of the lower class.

Corrective solutions, on the other hand, must cope with the present situation and alleviate the current problems of the unemployed.

One suggested solution is the creation of jobs in the public sector, since there are many jobs that need doing which would absorb the unemployed, facilitate the work of others, and provide the unemployed with an income hopefully higher than that provided by the welfare check.[44] Sometimes, of course, the issue is not the literal creation of jobs, but rather the improvement of pay (by government subsidy), public image, and working conditions of jobs such as those in the services where at present there are shortages.[45] In the case of other jobs such as teacher's aides or aides to other professionals or to homemakers, some training may be required. For example, some jobs could provide homemaking and child supervision services for working mothers in low or medium income brackets who could not otherwise work. Other jobs could provide help to a variety of professionals who would be relieved of routine work with which they are often burdened and freed to give the services for which they have special training to a greater number of people.[46]

This solution partially overlaps the very popular suggestion of upgrading the unemployed through vocational training. The latter is a preferable solution because it agrees with prevalent American values which favor the upgrading of workers through the acquisition of greater skill. While this is the solution most often suggested, the problems involved in applying it are seldom mentioned or considered. Gursslin and Roach's article is an outstanding exception. They report that training programs are faced with a basic dilemma: If they are geared toward high-skill-level training, they can train only a small percentage of the unemployed workers, but the rate of placement success will be high. If, on the contrary, training is geared at the low-skill level at which most unemployed workers would be trainable, the rate of placement success will be very low because a large number of workers compete for these jobs. The reasons for the inevitability of this dilemma are the preponderance of persons among the "hard core" unemployed with a high incidence of impairment to their intellectual functioning (particularly low IQ), deficiencies in conceptual abilities, inadequate verbal skills, cognitive restriction, defective self-system and low self-esteem, limited role repertory, and minimal motivation.[47]

London and Wenkert point out two other obstacles which prevent uneducated lower class persons from accepting (and doing well in) vocational training programs. First, these workers do not value "bookish" learning but rather learning on the job (which could be an alternative in vocational training), and they tend to be intimidated by any type of school-like activity because of the usual early disillusionment with school and their poor performance in it. Second, workers in training not only are not guaranteed a job, but training programs are not always in tune with current openings in the labor market, so that an unemployed worker who was met in the past with impossible difficulties in securing a job may be quite skeptical of investing time and effort in a strenuous project of questionable utility.[48]

It has also been pointed out that such legislative corrective acts as The Manpower Development and Training Act cannot be easily implemented or effectively reach large enough numbers of unemployed to make a real difference, because there is an insurmountable shortage of qualified instructors and program administrators.[49] On-the-job-training, however, often seems to be relatively more successful, probably because it has none of the disadvantages of formal retraining mentioned above and because it gives the worker greater assurance that he will have a job at the end.[50] But this type of training as well as all other types of training or retraining imply a built-in decision regarding the criteria according to which applicants will be screened and trainees chosen. The desire to succeed as a program and to secure continuous federal support tends to lead the personnel responsible for these programs into the usual pitfall of selecting those who have a better chance of success but who are least in need of retraining.[51] In this way corrective solutions for the elimination of the hard core unemployed create a smaller but "harder" core of unemployed who have been rejected by all programs and who become unreachable because they have accumulated frustrations and lost faith in all programs.

A different type of question is raised by the difficulty involved in training workers with low IQs who are not really trainable for jobs which require skill. What can be done with them? Michael Young in a quasi-humorous way suggests they could or should be used as servants in the homes of the brilliant in his "meritocratic" world.[52] Unless human genetics advances to the point of making it possible to manipulate genes so as to produce only intelligent human beings,

Young's solution may not be so offbeat or cruel. But even this solution may not be entirely feasible, for as Chaplin points out, there is a proportion of humans so socially incompetent that they are not even capable of being servants.[53]

Finally, some writers such as Theobald have suggested the establishment of an "economic floor" for each individual unrelated to employment or personal adequacy which would secure him a standard of living above subsistence level. Then training programs could begin to operate effectively.[54] Others like Galbraith have suggested offering an amount corresponding to their "normal" salary to all those who are unemployed through no fault of their own.[55] It is rather interesting to note that this is in a way what many of the unskilled and semiskilled workers with compensable disabilities do when they choose to remain disabled and decide to collect workmen's compensation throughout life. Some people would then raise this question: Is their unemployment in this case entirely through no fault of their own?

As things stand today, it seems that no satisfactory programs that could eliminate the social handicaps of the lower class (and sometimes of the semiskilled working class, especially when complicated by the presence of a disability) have been devised and applied. Therefore, vocational rehabilitation programs must develop techniques and methods to cope with these handicaps rather than avoid them through the rejection of a considerable number of lower class disabled persons. The rejects from federal vocational rehabilitation programs do not usually fall within the administrative jurisdiction of another governmental agency, so that vocational rehabilitation programs still bear the main responsibility for helping them even when they are classified as "unmotivated" or "uncooperative" according to middle class standards.

NOTES

1. D. C. Braun and T. D. Truan, "An Epidemiological Study of Lung Cancer in Asbestos Miners," *American Medical Association Archives of Industrial Health*, 17 (June 1958), 634–53; and Philip E. Enterline, "Mortality Rates Among Coal Miners," *American Journal of Public Health*, 54 (May 1964), 758–68; see also J. C. Wagner, C. A. Sleggs, and P. Marchand, "Diffuse Pleural Mesothelioma and Asbestos Exposure in the North-Western Cape Province," *British Journal of Industrial Medicine*, 17, 4 (October 1960), 260–71; and I. T. T. Higgins, "An Approach to the Problem of Bronchitis in Industry: Studies in Agriculture, Mining, and Foundry Communities," in E. King and C. M. Fletcher (eds.), *Industrial Pulmonary Diseases* (Boston: Little, Brown, 1960).
2. Philip E. Enterline, "The Estimation of Expected Rates in Occupational Diseases Epidemiology," *Public Health Reports*, 79, 11 (November 1964), 973–78.
3. U.S. Department of Health, Education and Welfare, *Selected Health Characteristics by Occupation, United States, July 1961– June 1963*, Public Health Service Publication, no. 1000, series 10, no. 21 (August 1965), pp. 1, 27, 49. Here it should be noted that the incidence of chronic conditions may be under-estimated for the entire labor force, since it is based only on the workers' awareness of the existence of such conditions, and the conditions quite often go undetected by the afflicted individual for a long time. However, we can safely assume that the underestimation is much greater in the case of blue collar workers (especially the semiskilled and unskilled workers), who seldom visit a physician and who may be afraid to find out that they suffer from a serious disease and therefore avoid seeking medical care despite the presence of some symptoms.
4. A. J. Jaffe and Lincoln H. Day, "Some Illustrative Tables on Seriously Disabling Work Injuries," in A. J. Jaffe (ed.), *Research Conference on Workmen's Compensation and Vocational Rehabilitation, 1960* (New York: Bureau of Applied Research, Columbia University, 1961), p. 86.
5. *Selected Health Characteristics by Occupation, op. cit.*, pp. 5–7. When age is taken into consideration, we find that 10.8% of

the white collar workers over 65 years of age have chronic limitations, but only 7.8% of farm workers under 44 years of age are similarly limited. See Philip E. Enterline, "Sick Absence for Men and Women by Marital Status," *Archives of Environmental Health*, 8 (March 1964), 466–70.

6. *Ibid.*, p. 9. Also, Doris K. Lewis, "Prevalence of Disabilities in the Work Force," *Monthly Labor Review*, 87, 9 (September 1964), 1002–8. Lewis writes that women up to 44 years of age also report higher rates of restricted activity, even when a chronic condition does not exist. See also B. L. Wells, "The Woman Worker," *Archives of Environmental Health*, 4 (April 1962), 439–45; L. E. Hinkle *et al.*, "An Examination of the Relation Between Symptoms, Disability, and Serious Illness in 2 Homogeneous Groups of Men and Women," *American Journal of Public Health*, 50 (September 1960), 1327–36; J. C. Naylor and N. L. Vincent, "Predicting Female Absenteeism," *Personnel Psychology*, 12 (Spring 1959), 81–84; and Enterline, "Sick Absence for Men and Women by Marital Status," *op. cit.*, p. 470.

7. Enterline, "Sick Absence for Men and Women by Marital Status," *op. cit.*, p. 470.

8. *Selected Health Characteristics by Occupation, op. cit.*, table 1, p. 7; table 4, p. 29; pp. 7–8.

9. Although the performance of tasks required of salespeople may be more often affected and by more types of disabilities (handicaps of communication, mobility, or appearance) than the tasks required of professional and clerical people.

10. Daniel Rosenblatt and Edward Q. Suchman, "The Underutilization of Medical Care Services by Blue-Collarites," in A. B. Shostak and W. Gomberg (eds.), *Blue Collar World* (Englewood Cliffs, N.J.: Prentice-Hall, 1964), pp. 341–49; and Irving Kenneth Zola, "Illness Behavior of the Working Class: Implications and Recommendations," in Shostak and Gomberg, *op. cit.*, pp. 350–61.

11. Lawrence D. Haber, *Prevalence of Disability Among Noninstitutionalized Adults Under Age 65: 1966 Survey of Disabled Adults*, Research and Statistics Note 4 (Washington, D.C.: U.S. Department of Health, Education and Welfare, Social Security Administration, Office of Research and Statistics, February 20, 1968).

12. Lawrence D. Haber, *Disability, Work, and Income Maintenance: Prevalence of Disability, 1966*, Report 2 (Washington, D.C.: Social Security Administration, Office of Research and Statistics, May 1968), p. 5.

13. *Selected Health Characteristics by Occupation, op. cit.*, pp. 10–11, 40.

14. Gerald Gordon, *Role Theory and Illness: A Sociological Perspective* (New Haven, Conn.: College and University Press, 1966), pp. 63–67.
15. Robin M. Williams, Jr., *American Society* (New York: Knopf, 1954), pp. 394–96.
16. In the case of women, the question of work becomes quite blurred. Married women, but increasingly only mothers of young children, are considered under no "moral" or "social" obligation to engage in any other type of work except housekeeping and mothering. Changing social norms seem to be not only increasingly approving the employment of mothers of children 12 years of age and over, but probably also expecting them to work. However, the norm to work does not seem to be imperative for any other category but single women and possibly with less force for women with grown children (18 and over). In the case of men, those possessing a large fortune are usually expected to volunteer their services without pay, their refusing to be paid—officially at least—entitling them to set their own work schedule.
17. Often, of course, even for those institutionalized (unless they belong to the "vegetable" category), some kind of "sheltered" employment is often made available, and they are expected (or made) to participate.
18. Williams, *op. cit.*; Lee Rainwater, "Work and Identity in the Lower Class" (paper presented at the Washington University Conference on Planning for the Quality of Urban Life, November 1964, revised April 1965); Robert S. Weiss and David Riesman, "Work and Automation: Problems and Prospects," in Robert K. Merton and Robert A. Nisbet (eds.), *Contemporary Social Problems* (New York: Harcourt, Brace & World, 1961), pp. 553–618; Louis A. Ferman, "Sociological Perspectives in Unemployment Research," in Shostak and Gomberg, *op. cit.*, pp. 505–9; Hyman Rodman, "Family and Social Pathology in the Ghetto," *Science*, 161, 3843 (August 23, 1968), 756–62; and Elliot Liebow, *Tally's Corner* (Boston: Little, Brown, 1967).
19. Rainwater, *op. cit.* Rainwater has reviewed the relevant literature, such as Everett C. Hughes, *Men and Their Work* (New York: Free Press, 1958); and Bennett M. Berger, "Suburbs, Subcultures, and Styles of Life: Problems of Cultural Pluralism in American Life" (paper presented at the Washington University Conference on Planning for the Quality of Urban Life, November 1964).
20. Weiss and Riesman, *op. cit.*, pp. 558, 598–602.
21. F. Herzberg, B. Mausner, and B. Snyderman, *The Motivation to Work* (New York: Wiley, 1959); and Elizabeth Lyman,

"Occupational Differences in the Value Attached to Work," *American Journal of Sociology*, 61 (September 1955), 138–44.

22. Robert K. Merton, *Social Theory and Social Structure* (New York: Free Press, 1949), pp. 134–46.

23. Of course, it is possible that some professionals disillusioned with their careers and the possibility of ever becoming successful may be returning to work ritualistically after having denied their disability partially or totally.

24. E. A. Friedman and R. J. Havighurst, "Work and Retirement," in S. Nosow and W. Form (eds.), *Man, Work and Society* (New York: Basic Books, 1962), pp. 44–45.

25. Rainwater writes that the complex value of the "good American life" and "the good provider" is the prevailing and valued life orientation of the working class, for whom "career" is not a part of the occupational world. See Rainwater, *op. cit.*; also, Lee Rainwater, Richard Coleman, and Gerald Handel, *Workingman's Wife: Her Personality, World, and Life Style* (New York: Random House, 1964); S. M. Miller and Frank Riesman, "The Working Class Subculture: A New View," in Shostak and Gomberg, *op. cit.*; Gerald Handel and Lee Rainwater, "Persistence and Change in the Workingclass Life Style," in Shostak and Gomberg, *op. cit.*; and Lee Rainwater and Gerald Handel, "Changing Family Roles in the Workingclass," in Shostak and Gomberg, *op. cit.*

26. Constantina Safilios-Rothschild, "The Reaction to Disability in Rehabilitation" (unpublished Ph.D. dissertation, Ohio State University, 1963).

27. Michael R. Malinovsky and John R. Barry, "Determinants of Work Attitudes," *Journal of Applied Psychology*, 49, 6 (1965), 446–51, especially 450; and Lyman, *op. cit.*

28. Robert Bloom and John R. Barry, "Determinants of Work Attitudes Among Negroes," *Journal of Applied Psychology*, 51, 3 (1967), 291–94.

29. An excellent discussion of the working experiences of black lower class men and of the "developmental" process which leads to their detachment from their jobs can be found in Liebow, *op. cit.*, pp. 29–71. Most of the ensuing discussion is based upon his ideas and descriptions.

30. *Ibid.*, p. 54.

31. N. C. Morse and R. S. Weiss, "The Function of Meaning of Work and the Job," in Nosow and Form, *op. cit.*, p. 34. The prevalent "American dream" is to quit the routine job and start a small business—a dream that is mostly a pleasant daydream. See also Ely Chinoy, "The Traditions of Opportunity and the Aspirations of Automobile Workers," *American Journal of Sociology*, 57, 5 (March 1952), 453–59.

32. Richard A. Cloward and Richard M. Elman, "Advocacy in the Ghetto," *Trans-action*, 4, 2 (December 1966), 27–35; Rodman, *op. cit.*; and Ferman, *op. cit.*, p. 509.
33. Rainwater, "Work and Identity," *op. cit.*
34. The author's research on urban Greek lower class families has shown that these men, even when unemployed or unable to provide for their family because of very low wages, have complete control over familial decision-making (the lower class family was actually more patriarchal than the family in the other classes), and their authority goes unchallenged. See Constantina Safilios-Rothschild, "A Comparison of Power Structure and Marital Satisfaction in Urban Greek and French Families," *The Journal of Marriage and the Family*, 29 (May 1967), 347–50.
35. It seems that lower class males are able to rationalize their marital failures (most often due to their failure in the occupational-breadwinner role) by blaming them on the "basic" masculinity that makes them "bad" and unfaithful husbands —what Liebow calls "the theory of manly flaws." See Liebow, *op. cit.*, pp. 116–26.
36. Walter B. Miller, "Lower Class Culture as a Generating Milieu of Gang Delinquency," *The Journal of Social Issues*, 14, 3 (1958), 9–10.
37. Rainwater, "Work and Identity," *op. cit.*; and Miller, *op. cit.*, pp. 9–10.
38. Rainwater, "Work and Identity," *op. cit.*; and Liebow, *op. cit.*, pp. 213–16.
39. Lee Rainwater, "The Lower Class: Health, Illness and Medical Institutions" (background paper for a study of medical facilities planning conducted by Anselm L. Strauss for the Institute of Policy Studies, March 1965); Safilios-Rothschild, "The Reactions to Disability in Rehabilitation," *op. cit.*
40. There are no statistics available on the extent to which lower class disabled are referred to vocational rehabilitation facilities. We do not know whether the lower class disabled are less or more frequently referred than are the disabled in other classes. The only available information is that the lower class disabled are very seldom self-referred in comparison to the middle class disabled. A recent survey of state vocational rehabilitation agencies showed that each year about 60,000 applicants are refused services because they were labeled "unmotivated" after they did not appear for appointments, could not be contacted, or did not respond to communications. It is highly likely that the majority of these applicants were lower class. See Martin Dishart, *A National Study of 84,699 Applicants for Services from State Vocational Rehabilitation Agencies in*

the United States (Washington, D.C.: National Rehabilitation Association, 1964).

41. Seymour L. Wolfbein, Employment and Unemployment in the United States (Chicago: Science Research Associates, 1964), pp. 194–98.

42. Rodman believes there is no need to change the values of the lower class people who have essentially middle class values but are forced to "stretch" them in order to adapt to their deprived occupational and economic conditions. Rather, he thinks that by providing them with adequate economic and occupational resources, their children will avail themselves of educational and training opportunities. Corrective techniques would thus also serve as effective preventive techniques. See Rodman, op. cit. We believe that both conditions must be fulfilled in order for the vicious circle to be broken—the change of values as well as the provision of adequately paying jobs.

43. Orville R. Gursslin and Jack L. Roach, "Some Issues in Training the Unemployed," Social Problems, 12, 1 (Summer 1964), 96–98.

44. Ibid.

45. Garth L. Mangum, Contributions and Costs of Manpower Development and Training, Policy Papers in Human Resources and Industrial Relations, no. 5 (Ann Arbor and Detroit: The Institute of Labor and Industrial Relations, December 1967), especially pp. 40–44.

46. A recent response of the American government has been the JOBS program (Jobs Opportunities in the Business Sector): federal subsidies to business to hire and train some 500,000 men and women chronically unable to find work or out of work for a long time. But some point out that the real number of the "hard core" unemployed is many times this figure and may be continuously increasing. The JOBS program should be supplemented by subsidizing business to keep these people employed and by creating federal and state jobs in the areas mentioned in our discussion. For an interesting discussion, see Alan L. Otten, "How Many Jobs," The Wall Street Journal, April 26, 1968.

47. Gursslin and Roach, op. cit., pp. 86–98.

48. Jack London and Robert Wenkert, "Obstacles to Blue-collar Participation in Adult Education," in Shostak and Gomberg, op. cit., pp. 455–56.

49. Charles C. Killingsworth, "Automation, Jobs and Manpower," in Louis A. Ferman, Joyce Kornbluh, and Alan Haber (eds.), Poverty in America (Ann Arbor, Mich.: University of Michigan Press, 1965), p. 152.

50. An interesting account of the on-job training experience of the

Chrysler Corporation with hard-core unemployed is given in Jerry M. Flint, "Jobless Training Begins With ABCs," *The New York Times*, June 16, 1968. It has also been found that workers, especially the older ones, are reluctant and tend to resist even on-the-job training. See Ira R. Hoos, *Retraining the Work Force* (Berkeley and Los Angeles: University of California Press, 1967), especially pp. 90–91.

51. Martin Rein, "The Strange Case of Public Dependency," *Transaction*, 2, 3 (March–April 1965), 20.
52. Michael Young, *The Rise of Meritocracy, 1980–2033* (New York: Penguin, 1961), p. 120.
53. David Chaplin, "Domestic Service and the Negro," in Shostak and Gomberg, *op. cit.*, p. 534.
54. As quoted in Gursslin and Roach, *op. cit.*, p. 96.
55. As quoted in Weiss and Riesman, *op. cit.*, p. 609.

CHAPTER 6

The Successful
Rehabilitant

Up to now we have followed the disabled's careers from the time they are afflicted with an accident or a chronic disease until the time they become rehabilitants. We shall now see how they "make out" at the termination of the rehabilitation program as well as the reasons accounting for success or failure. Since rehabilitation entails three major areas in the disabled's life; namely, his physical condition, his reintegration into gainful employment, and his psychosocial adjustment within the family and the larger community, we shall examine the rehabilitation outcome in each of these areas. The disabled's degree of success in becoming socially and psychologically reintegrated, however, will be dealt with in more detail in the following chapter.

Success in Physical Rehabilitation

Because the emphasis of rehabilitation services has been and to a considerable extent continues to be the vocational rehabilitation of disabled people, rehabilitation success has very often been measured on the basis of whether or not the individual returns to work. This trend has obscured the other aspects of rehabilitation in which a disabled person may have succeeded or not succeeded despite the fact that he returned to work. If a person returns to work without having diminished the degree of his disability to the fullest extent possible, can he be considered a rehabilitation success? On the other hand, if a 45-year-old, black, unskilled worker with a low IQ improves considerably or maximally in view of the type and extent of his disability but does not return to work, can he be considered a rehabilitation failure? If we postpone until the next section the examination of the return to work as an index of successful rehabilitation, we can concentrate here on other measures of rehabilitation success, their adequacies and shortcomings, as well as the social, sociopsychological, psychological, and medical factors which usually determine the degree of success on the basis of the criteria used.

Aside from return to work, degree of physical recovery is the most common measure of rehabilitation success. Physical recovery can be examined from two different points of view: (1) The extent to which the disabled improve from the time of admisison to the time of discharge in the performance of three categories of activities: (a) functional activities of daily living (ADL), including eating, dressing, personal hygiene, and transportation; (b) travel activities, that is, driving and the use of public transportation; and (c) work activities (that is, work potential). (2) Their rehabilitation achievement; that is, the extent to which the rehabilitants attained the goals set for them by the rehabilitation team on the basis of their physical potential.[1]

Both measures of physical rehabilitation success are necessary since they tap different aspects of success. For example, some disabled may improve but not attain the prognosticated goals. Others may attain the goals—which in this case refer mainly to psychosocial adjustment rather than to physical recovery—but not improve, their limitations in the different activities on admission having been categorized as "slight" or "none."[2] Of course, it must be remembered that none of these measures informs us about the actual physical and psychosocial condition of the disabled individual unless the degree of improvement and of attainment of goals is combined with the degree and the nature of remaining restrictions and limitations. For it is possible that a disabled who has both improved and attained goals (which had to be modest because of his severe disability) still may be much more limited by his disability at discharge than one who neither improved nor attained rehabilitation goals but had only slight or moderate limitations at the time of admission (and discharge).

These measures of rehabilitation success are rarely used together. Usually, the medical staff or the rehabilitation team evaluates the degree of physical improvement only. Criteria for rehabilitation success are restricted to physical recovery and ignore aspects of psychosocial adjustment that are often included in rehabilitation goals. Very rarely has the degree of physical improvement been evaluated by the rehabilitants themselves. Whenever this has been done, however, interesting and little-understood discrepancies between objective and subjective evaluations have been observed.[3] The fact that measurement of the degree of rehabilitation success relies upon the evaluation of the disabled's physical condition and ability at admission and discharge involves a number of difficulties.

First, since the time of discharge is most often determined by the rehabilitation team, it is up to this team to decide, for example, that a disabled can improve no more (or at all) and discharge him as a rehabilitation failure. It could be, however, that given sufficient time and proper motivation, he could have been counted a success. In at least one study it was found that those chronically ill who had stayed sixty days or more in the hospital had improved at discharge, while those who had stayed less than sixty days were evaluated as unchanged at the time of discharge.[4] Thus, it is possible that if the rehabilitation staff did not become discouraged with patients who show a slower or lesser response to treatment but instead gave more of their time and effort to them, they might show considerable improvement. Some evidence also points to the fact that rehabilitation staff members usually tend to concentrate their efforts on those cases that they think are most worthwhile or have the best chance of showing impressive improvement.[5] So, rehabilitation success may sometimes be an artifact, the product of a spurious relationship between the staff's desire to rehabilitate certain types of disabled individuals and the actual rehabilitation outcome.

Second, the evaluation of the degree of disability may not be accurate, and it may often vary considerably from physician to physician (within the same specialty as well as across specialties) and from the practitioner in one discipline to the practitioner in another discipline.[6] Thus, in the evaluative assessment of the rehabilitant at admission and at discharge, a different judgment of performance ability may be made by the different team members. In such cases, the physician's opinion usually predominates, and an apparently unanimous team estimate is given. It is, however, an estimate of doubtful validity that may sometimes significantly distort the dynamics of the rehabilitation process, for it is possible that a rehabilitant has developed a good relationship with a particular team member and when tested by this person may be highly motivated to perform to the utmost of his capacity in order to reward the staff member's efforts and encouragement.[7] Moreover, since the level of performance of many tasks (especially when they require considerable effort) is greatly influenced by motivational and contextual factors, a rehabilitant may be actually performing at a higher level when examined by one staff member than by another.[8] On the other hand, it may be that a staff member who has invested a great amount of time and effort on a particular patient may be less objective in his assessment of that rehabilitant's degree of improvement than a less "involved" staff member because he is anxious to see that his efforts have been rewarded.

Of course, among all types of evaluation (medical, social, psychological, and vocational), the medical one is most amenable to objective measurement. As we have seen, however, accurate and objective measures that give reliable and valid results are not available for all types of disabilities. The measurement problems multiply when one deals with social, psychological, and vocational evaluations both because the areas of evaluation can be much more easily distorted through subjective bias and because measurement techniques are not always sophisticated, reliable, or valid.

Third, because the evaluative assessment is based at least in part on the rehabilitant's behavior while in the center and on his reported ability or inability to perform certain activities, the evaluated rehabilitant can in certain cases "fake" the desirable degree of ability or disability in a particular area or task. Thus, at the initial evaluation some rehabilitants become wise to the fact that their stay at the rehabilitation center, the sustained interest of the staff, and their chance for physical improvement (in the areas they deem important) depend upon their appearing "motivated" to become physically independent and return to work as well as upon their promising to be "cooperative" in all aspects of the rehabilitation program.[9] Some are able to fake these desirable attitudes intermittently whenever their good intentions are questioned and as long as they are interested in receiving rehabilitation treatment. Others who wish to go home may purposefully show a retrogression in their physical status that may discourage the staff and lead to their discharge. And because several of the rehabilitants treated in vocational rehabilitation centers may be in the process of claiming workmen's compensation or intend to do so in the future, they may often have a vested interest in hiding their improvement from the rehabilitation team in order not to jeopardize the size of the compensation award.

Fourth, available data indicate that while there is a correlation between self-reported and medically evaluated degree of improvement, in some cases there is a considerable degree of discrepancy between the two evaluations.[10] When, therefore, a rehabilitant is medically rated as having improved more than that he himself feels he has and he is not a workmen's compensation claimant motivated to disguise his physical recovery, can we say he is a rehabilitation success if he has not been helped "to bring his perception of what he can do into closer coordination with reality?"[11] Or is it that the only "reality" is the rehabilitant's reality, and he is in fact rehabilitated only to the extent that he thinks he is? For example, in the case of low back injuries, some medical investigators maintain that objective improvement is of little value if the patient is having too much pain to return to work.[12] Some evidence, on the other hand, points to the fact that because of complex motivational factors, the disabled cannot accurately evaluate their own physical condition.[13] Obviously, more research in this area is warranted.

Fifth, the way in which improvement scores are calculated distorts the real picture of improvement. For instance, the improvement score measures the difference between an individual's status at admission and at discharge; the lesser the disability, the less the potential improvement score that may be assigned.[14] Thus, if one person's performance at admission was scored 3 on a particular activity and another's 2 on the same activity and they both perform this activity without any difficulty at discharge (and are both scored 4), the originally less disabled person will be assessed as having improved less than the originally more impaired rehabilitant.

When the attainment of set rehabilitation goals is the sole or additional criterion of rehabilitation success, a number of problems may exist. The most prominent danger is that if the rehabilitants were not consulted and could not participate in the formulation of these plans, they may not have attained them because the goals were not relevant and meaningful for their life situation.[15] This danger is real because most of the rehabilitation team members are predominantly middle class, while many rehabilitants are working or lower class. Unless a permissive philosophy permeates the rehabilitation center, there may be a tendency for the rehabilitation team to set goals for lower class patients without first discussing their relevance and desirability. Rehabilitation may sometimes become synonymous with socialization into middle class values. And we have already seen that when the disabled do not participate in the formulation of goals, they are often not motivated to do their utmost to attain them. They may instead attain those goals which they have set for themselves, goals possibly more realistic at times than those prognosticated by the rehabilitation team. Could they, then, be considered "failures" because they did not attain the goals set for them?

Since it is difficult to evaluate the degree of disability and even more so to make an accurate prognosis about potential progress and degree of return of function, the rehabilitation team may set goals higher than the actual potential of the rehabilitant. When the discrepancy is not serious, the set goals may motivate the team as well as the rehabilitant to intensify the efforts toward attainment and achieve for him a higher level of improvement. When, however, the discrepancy between set goals and actual potential is great, the rehabilitant as well as the team members may become discouraged over the small degree of improvement and progress, give up the effort, and consider the case a failure. On the other hand, a rehabilitant judged at admission to have little chance for improvement may be refused rehabilitation services on a totally or partially erroneous medical judgment.

Finally, according to most scoring systems in use, which are based on the relative achievement of rehabilitation goals, seriously impaired patients are usually rated low even when at admission they were not expected to become able to perform. In a recently developed scale, an additional category of "nonapplicable" was included and scored with the maximum score so that the seriously impaired would not be discriminated against and consistently presented as rehabilitation failures.[16]

B sides the specific shortcomings of the criteria used for the determination of rehabilitation success, let us now examine how well the studies evaluating the effectiveness of rehabilitation and the differential response to treatment meet the requirements of an evaluation program *per se*: the systematic study of two groups of disabled persons matched for a number of relevant medical, demographic, social, and sociopsychological variables. While the experimental group undergoes a planned rehabilitation program, the control group does not undergo any type of rehabilitation treatment.[17] Similarly, a specific type of rehabilitation program may be compared to an isolated rehabilitation treatment, for example, physical therapy treatments. The first type of evaluation research is practically nonexistent. The only exceptions seem to be two "controlled trial" studies conducted in England, in which patients referred for rehabilitation were randomly distributed in rehabilitation programs or in continuous care by a general practitioner. These studies—one conducted in an urban setting and the other in a semirural community—showed that a planned rehabilitation program was of value in improving patients' functional status and individual disabilities as well as in returning them to work and reducing the time off work.[18] But even in these studies we cannot be sure that at least some of the patients under the care of general practitioners did not receive some types of treatment quite similar to those received by at least some patients in rehabilitation programs and that the evaluative findings are not to some extent contaminated by this overlap.[19]

The majority of available studies are such that it is highly questionable whether or not they can truly be considered evaluative studies. Most of these studies examine the effectiveness of rehabilitation among "treated" populations, that is, the differential effectiveness of the rehabilitation program for patients with different medical, social, sociopsychological, and vocational characteristics. Usually the assumptions, the goals of the rehabilitation program, and the particular techniques used are not specified. Of course, the results of such evaluative studies have limited value. If, for example, one finds that the young, well-educated, and not severely disabled respond best to rehabilitation treatment, it is hardly a valid reason for preferential acceptance of this type of patient for the efficient use of limited staff and facilities. It is quite possible that this very type of patient (who becomes the rehabilitation success statistic) would have shown the same extent of improvement under the care of a specialist. In such a case, the limited facilities might better have been used to aid those who cannot improve without special and intensive rehabilitation treatments even when their response to these treatments is not always spectacular.

The lack of specification of treatments received in different programs does not aid the determination of the degree of efficacy of different specific rehabilitation techniques and probably interferes with the comparison of evaluative results obtained from different rehabilitation settings. Not all settings follow to the same extent the official rehabilitation philosophy or implement it by means of the same methods. There is, of course, a variability even within the same rehabilitation setting with regard to the rehabilitation plan selected and the methods used in implementing it, a variability often determined by the very characteristics of the patients who are being evaluated. So at best the evaluative studies undertaken seldom meet the requirements of good evaluative research and are beset by a number of subjective biases because of a basic difficulty in establishing objective criteria to measure disability in a reliable and valid manner.

Having in mind all the shortcomings and limitations discussed above, let us now turn to an examination of the studies concerning the differential response of patients to rehabilitation. Here again, it should be kept in mind that the majority of available studies have been conducted on the populations of rehabilitation centers, where only disabled with a working potential are accepted and where vocational rehabilitation is primarily emphasized. Only a few sporadic reports exist concerning the rehabilitation progress of physicians' private patients versus patients with compensable disabilities. For example, it has been reported that private patients with low back pain respond better to surgical intervention than do compensation and liability patients. It has also been reported that while 88.5 percent of patients with noncompensable low back injuries were rated as improved on subjective grounds, only 55.8 percent of patients treated for compensable low back injuries were rated as improved.[20] We do not know, however, whether or not these observed differences are due only to differences in social class, since most probably a much higher percentage of middle and upper middle class patients can be found among private patients and noncompensable cases than among compensable cases.

Several investigators tend to agree that "younger age" is more conducive than "older age" to rehabilitation success. While most studies agree that the disabled 20 to 40 years of age have the best chance for success, each study reports a different age ceiling beyond which the rehabilitation outcome becomes problematic.[21] Despite such evidence, it may be erroneous to conclude that advanced age in itself has an adverse effect upon rehabilitation; that is, that older disabled persons are less amenable to rehabilitation. More likely, the rehabilitation team may not be equally interested and "motivated" to intensify its efforts and rehabilitate the older disabled. This differential attitude could account at least in part for the lower rehabilitation success found among the older disabled. Furthermore, some investigators have found that age is not inversely related to rehabilitation response. As a matter of fact, Bourestom has reported that while younger disabled persons maintain "a considerably higher level of functioning in terms of absolute score," they do not improve more than the older patients from admission to discharge or followup.[22]

In addition, a fairly consistent negative relationship has been found between lack of financial concern and lack of financial resources or low income and degree of physical improvement.[23] Probably these findings might be interpreted, at least in part, in terms of the lesser motivation on the part of the rehabilitation staff to invest a lot of time and effort in lower class patients when these patients compete with middle class patients.

Some investigators have found that the degree of motivation to overcome the disability[24] and acceptance of the disability[25] are related to rehabilitation success. Such findings may once more indicate that the rehabilitation team fails to make an intensive effort unless the rehabilitant is already "highly motivated" and conforms to staff expectations. Such a picture portrays the rehabilitation process as rather static, since the staff does not particularly seem to strive to alter the level of motivation in "poorly" motivated rehabilitants, but instead prefers to work and obtain results with those already motivated.[26]

In the case of the disabled with back injuries or the paraplegics, not only was surgery found to be related to rehabilitation success,[27] but also the type of surgery. Thus, in the case of back injuries, a fusion seems to be more conducive to rehabilitation success than a laminectomy.[28] In both cases the explanation seems to be that such patients are not willing to accept the finality of their disabled status until all possible medical treatment has been tried. As long as they receive only conservative treatment, they cannot easily accept their disability in the knowledge that some people with the same condition undergo surgery which sometimes at least relieves pain and betters the physical condition. Only when they have undergone fusion, the last resort in the treatment of back pain, can they accept the finality of their status and start working diligently in the rehabilitation setting.

On the other hand, the evidence is quite inconclusive about some variables, such as lapse of time between onset of disability and admission for rehabilitation[29] and the family's reaction toward the disability.[30] But Bourestom's contribution to the understanding of the complexity of the prediction problem in rehabilitation improvement is unique.[31] His findings make us aware that it is dangerous to draw conclusions about one or the other factor being significantly related to rehabilitation success or physical improvement and on the basis of this finding to attempt predicting rehabilitation outcome. He has demonstrated that the real picture is much more complex, since six factors accounted for only 36 percent of the variance in self-care improvement of patients with cerebrovascular diseases. Many factors may not be significant predictors per se but may contribute to a number of other predictors. Thus, it seems rather conclusive that if we wish to be able to predict rehabilitation outcome, we must utilize a multivariate analysis that will unravel the interrelated effect of different factors upon such outcome.

Finally, let us examine to what extent the degree of rehabilitation success at the time of discharge from a rehabilitation facility indicates

the degree to which disabled individuals can function in everyday
life after they are "on their own." As we have already seen, there is
considerable evidence suggesting that a disabled person's level of
performance is greatly affected by such factors as the person who is
observing him, the expectations of the observer, the relationship of
the patient to the observer, and the symbolic meaning that the disability has for the patient at that particular time and place, as well
as the overall prevailing psychological atmosphere. In addition, it
has been found that the disabled who have been hospitalized for
some time in a rehabilitation center tend to experience crises when
they are about to leave the center and are making their first contacts
with the larger community.[32] If the time of transition from the rehabilitation center to the larger community is such a traumatic and
anomic situation, it is rather evident that the two settings are quite
dissimilar. Effective socialization and performance in the one setting
may not prepare the disabled for effective performance and adjustment in the other.

There are several questions that must be answered through systematic followup studies: What is the degree of carryover of improvement gained in a rehabilitation setting when it is transferred to "normal," noninstitutional life? To what extent does the "therapeutic
milieu" of a rehabilitation setting fostering independence for all the
disabled create an artificial environment conducive to a degree of
improvement that is not sustained after discharge? And are there any
differences between those who tend to improve considerably while
at the rehabilitation center and sustain the level of obtained improvement after discharge, and those who show little improvement while at
the center and much more improvement once they are on their own?

To some extent the answers to these questions may be in a
number of existing followup studies. Some studies have only examined whether or not the disabled improved, remained the same, or
regressed, and have not paid any attention to the patients' characteristics, life situations, and motivations. For example, a followup
study of 46 quadriplegics showed that 17 had improved in functional
ability, 5 were the same, 13 had regressed, and 11 had improved in
some areas and regressed in others.[33] Other studies, however, have
provided us with more information about the disabled's characteristics
and their life situations in addition to the degree of stability or change

in physical status. Thus, one study found that 72.2 percent of the disabled studied an average of 30.9 months after discharge had maintained the improvement they had gained at discharge; only 28.8 percent were rated as being below their discharge level. It is interesting to note that the self-ratings of these disabled were very similar to the ratings given by the medical consultant. The same study concluded that the patient's attitude toward his disability and, even more important, the degree of responsibility he has toward others (in terms of number of dependents, financial or homemaking responsibilities) determines the level at which he will be motivated to maintain those gains in physical status obtained during rehabilitation.[34]

Another followup study of the chronically ill discharged from a chronic disease hospital concluded that there was a relatively high rate of rehospitalization episodes (23 percent of all the cases), about half of which (47 percent) had received the services of a private physician. It was found that a single, widowed, or divorced status, the Protestant faith, and low economic status seemed to be positively related to a favorable level of functional independence. Membership in the Jewish faith and high economic status, on the contrary, were found to be related to a high rehospitalization rate.[35] Similar findings were reported in a longitudinal study of stroke patients who were receiving ordinary medical care at home: patients in lower class or anomic families tended to experience a greater degree of recovery than those in middle class, well-integrated families.[36] These data corroborate the findings of other followup studies according to which the characteristics that make for good hospital adjustment or for satisfactory response to treatment are incompatible with those required for good family or community adjustment.[37]

Despite the lack of extensive and sophisticated followup studies about different types of disabilities, we can attempt to answer our original questions. First, it is rather striking that most of the studies report a high degree of overall stability in the physical status and level of performance of the followup cases, a finding that suggests a considerable amount of carryover of the functional level achieved at discharge. Second, it seems that there are definite differences between those who are rated successful or improved at discharge and those who are rated as improved at followup. At least for some types of disabilities, especially heart disease, the lower class and those bearing most of the financial or maintenance-homemaking responsibilities are those who improve most, despite the fact that they are usually poorly rated in rehabilitation success studies.

These two main conclusions seem at first to be contradictory. One basic difficulty results from the fact that the examined followup studies have not systematically taken into account the type of disability examined. Thus we do not know for what types of illnesses and degrees of severity the second conclusion is valid and under what conditions it does not hold true or is reversed. We also do not know how valid the conclusion is regarding the high degree of carryover of rehabilitation gains. The main reason for this is the fact that in most of the studies, the disabled's physical status was judged by a medical team or a physician alone so that the assessment of the disabled's status may be biased by factors similar to those which entered into the physical evaluation at admission and discharge. And unless a medically diagnosable change has come about, probably the medical evaluation will not be different from that at discharge. Even evaluations based upon observation may not always be reliable, since we do not know in what direction the presence of an observer can influence the disabled's performance. In one study it was found, for example, that the professionals in and outside the rehabilitation institute evaluating the level of performance of ADL agreed very poorly with the patients themselves (or their spouses, who were most often in agreement with the disabled).[38] This finding suggests again that in the rehabilitation setting or outside it, professional evaluations often do not take into consideration and do not reflect the patients' motivations and hierarchy of values and therefore do not correspond to the "real" level of performance.

At this point it is quite enlightening to consider New's findings, according to which each significant other rated differentially the disabled's degree of ability and disability in performing the functional activities of everyday living (ADL), the spouses having the highest degree of agreement with the disabled's own view of the extent of his dependence or independence.[39] He also found that the degree and direction of discrepancy between the ratings of the significant other and those of the disabled has a great influence on whether or not the disabled will improve, remain stationary, or retrogress regardless of the gains achieved during rehabilitation. Depending upon the disabled's personality and his relationships with "core" significant others, he may move toward their definitions or may continue to assert his desired dependent or independent state. It seems, then, that ultimately motivational factors resulting from the disabled's own evaluation of activities and hierarchy of values as well as from the nature of his interpersonal relations with his significant others and the latter's evaluation of activities, definition of, and reaction to the disability are crucial in the determination of the level of disabled's performance in real life.

One additional question may be raised concerning the disabled's community adjustment or status in the postdischarge state. Should we consider rehospitalization rates as a valid criterion of success or failure to adjust to "normal" living and to maintain rehabilitation gains? One study indicates that medical events rather than social or psychological crises were responsible for precipitating rehospitalization.[40] And most often the precipitating medical events were expected manifestations of the illness. So it is rather difficult to consider rehospitalization as an index of physical regression and deterioration unless the precipitating medical event does not fall within the "normal" pattern of the disability or illness or unless such rehospitalization could have been easily avoided and clearly indicates a failure to become successfully integrated into the family and the community.

We will probably not have reliable and valid data about the postdischarge career of the disabled unless the following conditions are fulfilled: (a) Good comparative data about the different types of disabilities are collected in a series of research studies. (b) Besides a professional evaluation of the disabled's physical status and level of performance, the disabled themselves (as well as the significant others) are interviewed about their level of performance so that the real level of performance (as well as the dynamics that account for it) can be assessed. (c) A multivariate analysis of the different factors determining the level of performance while at home or while living in the community is conducted in order to understand the interplay of variables and the extent to which they can predict the degree of community adjustment and long-term rehabilitation.

Finally, it should be noted that some people have questioned whether or not a rehabilitation program must be administered within the setting of a special center or facility and not in the disabled's home. A home-rehabilitation program has a number of distinct advantages, such as closer touch with the patient's type of reality in terms of facilities, interpersonal relations, and everyday life. The artificial atmosphere of a rehabilitation center is avoided, the disabled's family is educated and socialized into a new type of life along with the disabled, and the problems that the rehabilitated disabled would usually encounter at the postdischarge stage can be anticipated and met. Some studies of home rehabilitation care have started to appear, and the reported success may widen this trend, especially since such programs seem to be less expensive and do help decongest crowded hospitals and rehabilitation centers.[41]

Success in Vocational Rehabilitation: Who Returns to Work

The final test that a disabled has to pass in order to be considered a good investment for rehabilitation expense and effort is the vocational one. After the termination of rehabilitation he must return to gainful employment, since this is the ultimate proof of his success in overcoming physical limitations and of his ability to fully use his remaining potential. Whenever a disabled person does not return to work, he tends to be viewed as a "failure" and as somewhat suspect for having made use of the rehabilitation facilities and opportunities offered by society without having returned to society its due. The usual argument in favor of rehabilitation in terms of dollars and cents is no longer valid—he does not return to society the money which it has spent to rehabilitate him.[42]

A configuration of factors seems to be responsible for the great emphasis in American culture upon returning to work. One is the prevalent cultural value placed upon work for all males over the age of 18; societal legitimation of nonparticipation in the active labor force is given with great difficulty and only to very severely disabled persons. And even then it is "unofficially" expected that despite their legitimate exemption from work, they will engage in some kind of remunerative activity. People who are ingenious in overcoming a total disability are greatly admired and held up as examples to others. This societal attitude suggests that *in fact* American society rarely—

if ever—exempts people from work even when they are totally disabled. The only legitimate exceptions to this rule are: (a) the already retired, who can usually establish their successful rehabilitation by becoming functionally independent and self-reliant; (b) disabled children and teenagers who, however, are expected to become employable at the termination of their schooling and/or training; and (c) disabled housewives who are considered to be successfully rehabilitated when they can resume their predisability tasks and responsibilities so that the family breadwinner is not prevented from·carrying out his occupational responsibilities.

Because of this exaggerated emphasis on and preoccupation with vocational rehabilitation, there have been several studies attempting to establish the factors that differentiate the disabled who return to work from those who do not. Table 4 presents all the factors that have been found to be significantly associated with postdisability gainful employment in at least one study (see page 233).

Of the demographic factors listed, sex is, of course, important. Even if women worked before the onset of a disability, they very seldom go back to work, especially if their disability is compensable.[43] Recent statistics for the total female population indicate than even among disabled women with secondary work limitations, only 40 percent return to full-time employment.[44] The only women who sometimes returned to work were usually single, rated as more neurotic, and with lower job skills than those who did not.[45] Probably a composite "economic pressure" variable operates in the case of women workers, but no conclusions can be drawn since they have been studied very inadequately and on the basis of very small samples.

With the exception of two studies, age has been found to be a very significant factor in vocational rehabilitation.[46] In some studies, age was specified as age at onset of disability,[47] in others as present age,[48] and in others the time reference is not specified.[49] The results concerning age at onset place the ceiling under which men have the greatest inclination or chance to return to work in some cases at 30 and in other cases at 45 (except for disability from birth).[50] This disagreement in the ceiling of age at onset for optimum vocational rehabilitation may be due to the possible relationship of age at onset to the type of disability, the latter factor also related to the rate of postdisability employment. And since each study examines different types of disabilities, the discrepancy of findings about optimum age at onset may be reflecting differences in population composition. With respect to present age, men younger than 40 (or 45) returned to work much more often than did older men. The latter finding, of course, is more a reflection of the requirements of the job market and the unwillingness of employers to hire older people than of the disposition of the disabled to work. And we do not know how age at onset as well as present age is associated with the type and degree of disability, the latter probably being intervening variables in vocational rehabilitation outcome.

Besides age and sex, education, type of occupation, and income seem to be important predictors in the vocational rehabilitation of the disabled. The higher the disabled's educational accomplishment, the better his chance to return to work, this chance already being very good if he has completed high school.[51] Similarly, those who engaged in skilled, sales or clerical, or professional jobs prior to the onset of disability have the greatest probability of returning to gainful employment and do not experience occupational downgrading, underemployment, or unemployment.[52] Finally, the level of predisability income (reflecting the individual's type of occupation as well as his social status) and the monthly income while drawing disability benefits also have been found to influence return to work.[53] Level of education and type of occupation again tend to reflect the demand for a skill in the job market rather than the disabled's disinclination to work.

Another factor that has been found to affect the disabled's employability is race, since the possession of black skin drastically diminishes his demand in the labor market.[54] Thus, the older, black, uneducated, and unskilled workers who even in the absence of physical disability are vocationally handicapped become more so when a physical or mental disability is added to their predicament. (See Chapter 5 for a discussion of the meaning of work as well as of the social reasons for unemployment.) Vocational rehabilitation services do not seem to have been able to produce any kind of significant change in the vocational outcome of these socially disadvantaged people despite the fact that such services must intervene for exactly this purpose. Supposedly vocational training should break the vicious circle in which the socially disadvantaged are caught. But despite the fact that having received vocational training is related to return to

TABLE 4.
Factors Found to Be Related to the Disabled's Return to Work

A. Demographic Variables
  1. Age (at onset of disability and present age)
  2. Race
  3. Education
  4. Marital status
  5. Number of dependents
  6. Predisability income
  7. Sex
  8. Monthly income while drawing disability benefits
  9. Source of referral
B. Sociopsychological Variables
  1. Reaction (or attitude) to disability
  2. Attitudes of significant others toward the disabled as perceived by the disabled
  3. Sexual activities
  4. Leisure activities
  5. Level of aspiration
  6. Rating of dependency
  7. Relationship with family before onset of disability
C. Vocational Variables
  1. Work stability
  2. Job skill level
  3. Predisability employment status
  4. Vocational training
  5. Union membership
  6. Work history
  7. Panel rating of attitude toward work
D. Medical Variables
  1. Degree or severity of disability
  2. Duration of disability
  3. Presence of secondary disabilities
  4. Presence of psychiatric symptoms
  5. Type of disability
  6. Capacity for functional performance
  7. Subjective evaluation of physical status and progress
E. Psychological Variables
  1. Intelligence quotient
  2. Motivation to work
  3. Adaptability to change
  4. Capacity for emotional control
  5. Better planning and more efficient methods of work
  6. Good capacity for self-criticism

work, those who are selected as vocational training candidates tend again to be white, young, better educated (have completed at least 8 to 10 years), and even sometimes more skilled than those who are rejected.[55]

Other demographic factors found to be associated with return to work are: marital status,[56] number of dependents,[57] and source of referral.[58] The first two variables, insofar as they connote the degree of responsibility (especially financial responsibility) the disabled has toward others, compel him to work (unless, of course, a redefinition of roles takes place and the wife assumes the breadwinner role). Probably more important than the disabled's marital status and number of dependents, however, is his relationship with his family before the onset of the disability.[59]

The disabled's reaction to his disability,[60] his attitude toward it,[61] and his level of aspiration[62] have also been found to be significantly related to the return to gainful employment. While those who have accepted their disability and those who have "realistic" ambitions tend to return to work, it is inconclusive whether the more dependent or the less dependent among the disabled tend to return to work more often.[63] In the case of some sociopsychological variables, such as attitudes of significant others toward the disabled as perceived by the disabled,[64] sexual activities,[65] and leisure activities[66] found to be associated with return to work, it is difficult to say what comes first. It is entirely plausible that those men who for a variety of reasons cannot return to work are rejected by their families and, feeling depressed, decrease or cease their sexual and leisure activities.[67]

In terms of vocational variables, the disabled who go back to work most often are those who were employed full-time before the onset of the disability and had experienced little unemployment,[68] had a satisfactory work history[69] and an intermediate work stability,[70] a favorable panel rating of attitude toward work[71] and, if workers, a union membership.[72]

In terms of medical variables, the successful vocational rehabilitant can be described as one with a mild or moderate disability,[73] a high degree of functional performance (or self-care),[74] no other health problems except his primary disability,[75] free of psychiatric symptoms,[76] and rated by the physicians and himself as being in as good or better physical condition than at discharge.[77] Data concerning the type of disability are incomplete, so that generalizations are not yet possible.[78] Finally, the disabled who return to work may be described as intelligent (at least above normal),[79] motivated, adaptable to change, able to control their emotions, to criticize themselves, to plan well, and to use efficient methods of work.[80]

Despite this wealth of studies, few have really been predictive studies utilizing multivariate analysis of the factors conducive to vocational rehabilitation. Most of the research motivated primarily by a wish to predict accurately the vocational (or medical) rehabilitation outcome seems to have been encouraged and even demanded by federal agencies and rehabilitation centers because the findings have a direct application: They can be used by the rehabilitation team during the evaluation stage in screening out poor rehabilitation risks. The application of these findings can increase their "efficiency" and help utilize the staff's time and the available facilities in the most "productive" way possible by making them available only to those who will benefit most and thereby improve the center's success statistics. However, a number of dangers and misconceptions are inherent in the application of the research findings.

First, in the case of success in physical rehabilitation, as we have seen, the criteria used are of questionable reliability and validity; some of the findings are inconclusive or cannot be generalized to other types of disabilities; and the interaction of the different factors and their combined impact on the rehabilitation outcome is inadequately understood. Thus, accurate prediction of the rehabilitation outcome remains problematic.

Second, there are ethical questions as to whether or not such predictive instruments, even when perfected, can or should be applied in the case of the disabled. Especially since failure in physical rehabilitation outcome may signify either a failure on the part of the rehabilitation team, or the patients' unwillingness or lack of interest (or potential) to work toward improvement, or both. Moreover, failure in vocational rehabilitation may often reflect structural occupational conditions rather than the individual disabled's motivation to work. Even when available studies indicate that the severity of the disability is negatively related to the disabled's response to rehabilitation, does this license us to bar severely disabled persons from rehabilitation services? Even if the rehabilitation resources and facilities are limited and some selection of cases must be made, is it not ethically wrong to deny rehabilitation treatment to the severely disabled because they respond less well to such treatment, in the same way that it would be ethically wrong to deny medical care to seriously ill persons because they may die or not recover completely? Is it not unjustifiable and inhuman not to offer any possible alleviation, comfort, and help to all those who need it desperately? Besides, it is not true that the cases labeled rehabilitation "failures" do not improve at all. They do improve to some extent or in some areas but relatively less than others or they do not reach the goals set for them by the rehabilitation team, goals that may have been inaccurately high or irrelevant to begin with. And in the case of vocational rehabilitation, even if the "failures" do not return to work, they may have improved in self-care so as to warrant the investment of the rehabilitation team's effort and time. Because most women do not work or are not under any pressing societal obligation to work (or to continue working), is it permissible to exclude them in most cases from vocational rehabilitation and thus deny them the benefits of physical improvement? Must their rights to rehabilitation be protected in the name of the potential interference their disability may cause to male significant others' occupational performances?

But besides the ethical questions, it seems that at the present time the construction of predictive instruments for physical and vocational rehabilitation success may be premature because of the many unknowns involved in the dynamics of the rehabilitation process and the many limitations of the rehabilitation team members in working with some types of disabilities and some types of disabled. It may be that at this time it would be more productive if the discovery of those variables significantly related to an unfavorable response to rehabilitation treatment and unemployment were to sensitize rehabilitation researchers and practitioners to the problem areas that require solutions and the invention of new methods.

Whether or not the disabled return to gainful employment after the occurrence of disability (and the intervention of rehabilitation), three related and very important questions can be asked about their vocational adjustment: (1) What type of employment do they return to compared to the predisability employment and what are their chances for advancement in it? (2) How long do they stay in this employment and why do they leave, if they leave? (3) What is their work performance and work adjustment? The answers to these questions would give us a more complete picture of the disabled's satisfactory societal integration rather than the mere information that he is no longer on some type of relief or welfare roll.

The first question includes several more specific questions. Does the rehabilitated worker return to his previous job, or just to the previous employer who gives him a different job which may or may not be at the same level of his previous job in terms of pay, chances for promotion, degree of responsibility, desirability, and prestige? Or does he accept a job, any job, often below the level of his predisability employment in one or more aspects? Does he work full-time or part-time? The issues of underemployment in terms of time, level of pay, or advancement have been overshadowed by the preoccupation of the large majority of evaluative followup studies which focus on statistics concerning the extent of employment—any type of employment.

The fragmentary information available, however, indicates that most disabled suffer some job income loss; and for a large number of disabled (at least in disabilities such as paraplegia), unless they are engaged in higher intellectual occupations, these losses may be 50 percent or more.[81] There is also evidence that loss of wages and decrease in occupational status are more often than not associated with change of firm and/or type of occupation (the majority of such changes being involuntary). Jaffe, Day, and Adams report that among those who returned to the same firm (63 percent of all disabled workers), 91 percent received the same or higher than predisability wages, while only 54 percent of those returning to a different employer did as well. A larger percentage of those who returned to the previous employer had "better" jobs and enjoyed greater steadiness of employment than those who changed jobs. Allowance, of course, must be made for a few workers who voluntarily change firm and occupation in order to ameliorate their pay and status and who succeed in doing so.[82] In the Syracuse University cardiac project, 80 percent of the rehabilitants had returned to their job and reported no change; 4 percent reported downgrading; and 12 percent were uncertain about the job.[83] Dvonch *et al.* report an increase in clerical-type jobs among those patients with spinal cord dysfunction who are employed after

discharge from rehabilitation; that they earned on the average a
10.4 percent higher mean salary prior to disability; and that their
earnings increased by 20.9 percent during the 3½-year followup
period.[84]

Other studies do not report the extent of change in the disabled's
work status or their promotion chances, but only whether or not
they work part- or full-time. Thus, McPhee reports that 55 percent
of the rehabilitants in his study were employed full-time, 19 percent
part-time, 11 percent unemployed, and 2 percent retired. Weiner
reports that 40 percent of the tuberculosis rehabilitants returned to
former employment; 14 percent, to other jobs; and the remaining 46
percent were either unemployed, retired, had moved from the area,
died, or been rehospitalized. Fallstrom reports that 41 percent of
neurologic patients were self-supporting, 20 percent had "contributory
earning capacity," and 39 percent did not earn anything. Finally,
Hastings reports an equal number of paraplegic workers employed
and unemployed, but 1 out of 5 worked part-time or a little more than
part-time.[85]

While it seems that the percentage of return to full-time gainful
employment is, on the average, around 50 percent or lower, there
are no systematic and conclusive data concerning the differential rate
of reemployment of individuals afflicted with different types of disabilities. Jaffe, Day, and Adams found that workers with injuries
to the lower extremities were more likely to be rehired by the same
firm than workers with back injuries, heart conditions, or hernia.
Similarly, there are few and inadequate data about the effect of the
type and size of the industry on policies concerning the hiring or rehiring of disabled persons. Again, Jaffe, Day, and Adams report that
the larger the size of the industry, the more favorable the hiring
policies; that the best rate of rehiring disabled workers was found in
nondurable and durable goods manufacturing (71 and 66 percent,
respectively), and the poorest rates in construction (55 percent) and
service (54 percent.)[86]

While we know that the majority of those who return to gainful
employment are reemployed by the former firm, we have only
sporadic information about whether or not the job is exactly the same
or similar in terms of pay and status to the predisability one and
whether or not the worker's chances for advancement and a regular

career are affected by his disability status. The available data show that some workers are given responsibility and/or salary increases while others are not; some of them are downgraded; others, not. The Syracuse cardiac project data suggest that the workers who were downgraded and uncertain of their jobs had the same characteristics as the usually unemployed disabled: advanced age, low education, unskilled or semiskilled jobs, and a moderate to severe degree of disability.[87] We do not know to what extent disabled workers who return to the same firm are given jobs suited to their disabilities, what necessary job adaptations are brought about, and to what extent "suitable" employment means downgrading.[88] Many more such analyses of the sociopsychological characteristics of those who return to their previous employment are needed in order to better understand the dynamics involved in the worker's return to the previous employer and the factors that determine his occupational career there.

Some data exist concerning the differences between those who return to the same job and those who change jobs. Weiner found that the latter were intermediate in terms of their sociopsychological characteristics between those who return to previous jobs and those who remain unemployed. Thus, those who change jobs had the least degree of disability of all other groups, the shortest length of hospitalization, the highest representation in the professional occupations, the highest proportion of three or more dependents, were the youngest, had the least job stability, and had a high proportion of separations and divorces.[89] Jaffe, Day, and Adams found that those who changed jobs tended to be those who had suffered a series of injuries, were older than 45, had eight years of schooling or less, and were nonwhite more often than white.[90] These data suggest that this group resembles most closely those who remain unemployed. However, no conclusive statement can be made about the characteristics which distinguish those who return to the same job from those who change jobs without further research in this area.

It is also important to understand what factors distinguish those who become self-supporting after the termination of rehabilitation and those who earn only a small amount through part-time work. McPhee's data indicate that those working part-time had the same sociopsychological characteristics as the unemployed except that they did not receive public assistance at the time of application for rehabilitation and had job aspirations in personal services instead of in the unskilled field.[91]

On the basis, then, of the very limited and inconclusive evidence that is presently available, we could tentatively conclude that those employed part-time bear a closer resemblance to the unemployed than to those employed full-time, while those changing jobs seem to be intermediate between those returning to the same job and those remaining unemployed. And it is probable that those who are downgraded or stagnant while working for their previous employer will be found to resemble those changing jobs in terms of basic sociopsychological characteristics.

As far as the second question is concerned, namely, the disabled's postdisability job stability, the available evidence tends to suggest that steady employment occurs more often among workers returning to the same firm than among those changing jobs, probably because better care is taken to adjust the job to the worker.[92] Extensive or refined data are equally lacking in this area.

Finally, the subject of level of work performance and work adjustment leads to the question of values. Why should disabled workers have to "prove" their abilities in order to be accepted? Only groups discriminated against, such as women, blacks, and members of some ethnic groups, have to prove their excellence in order to be accepted despite their possessing an unfavorable characteristic. An average performance is not considered sufficient as it would be in the case of the "normal" population. Advertising campaigns on the employment of the handicapped emphasize the fact that such workers have much better work records and higher work performance than the nondisabled so that hiring them is "good business." Apart from this moral controversy, the available evidence indicates that disabled workers are as good as the nondisabled and in some ways a little "better."[93] For example, McPhee writes that "employers of the rehabilitants stated that the quality and quantity of their work was the same as, or better than, their other employees, and that they had less absenteeism than their other employees."[94]

Evaluative studies in vocational rehabilitation should become more refined and go beyond counting numbers of working rehabilitants. They should attempt to study and assess the characteristics of: (a) those who return to the same employer and whose occupational career is unaffected by disability in contrast to those who are stagnating or downgraded; (b) those who change firms but not occupation; (c) those who change both firm and occupation; (d) those who work part-time; and (e) those who remain unemployed. Followup studies should investigate the dynamics involved in all these occupational decisions and career outcomes and pay particular attention to the extent to which the postdisability job is suited to the worker's occupational and educational background and the extent to which the injury has handicapped him on the job, since both variables indicate the degree of the disabled's vocational adjustment. Rehabilitation studies should free themselves from condescending "philanthropic" values and biases according to which the disabled and the poor have the moral obligation to be hard-working and should consider themselves fortunate to be able to work regardless of the type of employment available to them. An objective look at vocational rehabilitation may also indicate the reasons why some disabled do not work and whether or not some kind of intervention could change their motivation and/or structural conditions. If the final purpose of rehabilitation is the successful societal integration of the disabled, it is not enough that they work, they should work in satisfactory types of occupations where they can best use their talents and abilities and in which they have the same chance for advancement and success as the nondisabled.

Let us now study more in depth the situation of a disabled after he has undergone rehabilitation and tries to make a new niche for himself in the world. A number of powerful and influential "agents" intervene at various stages of his disability career, and their impact shapes to a considerable degree the extent and the type of postdisability adjustment. Let us see how each "agent" separately as well as in combination influences and even often determines the disabled's mode of adaptation to and integration into the "normal" society.

NOTES

1. Constantina Safilios-Rothschild, "The Reaction to Disability in Rehabilitation (unpublished Ph.D. dissertation, Ohio State University, 1963).
2. Saad Z. Nagi, Richard D. Burk, and Harry R. Potter, "Back Disorders and Rehabilitation Achievement," *Journal of Chronic Diseases,* 18 (February 1965), 181–97.
3. *A Study of the Integration of Services of Industrial Medical Departments and a Rehabilitation Center: Final Report* (Special Project Grant Rd 221, Pittsburgh, Harmarville Rehabilitation Center, June 1963), p. 26; and David J. Kallen, "The Socio-economic Correlates of Rehabilitation" (paper read at the Cleveland Symposium on Behavioral Research in Rehabilitation, Cleveland, November 4, 1959).
4. George J. Vlasak and Harry T. Phillips, *What Comes After Discharge* (Boston: Bureau of Chronic Disease Control, Massachusetts Department of Public Health, 1967), p. 21.
5. Julius A. Roth and Elizabeth M. Eddy, *Rehabilitation for the Unwanted* (New York: Atherton, 1967).
6. Jonas N. Muller, "Rehabilitation Evaluation—Some Social and Clinical Problems," *American Journal of Public Health,* 51, 3 (March 1961), 403–8; F. Miles Skultety, "The Doctor's Role in Disability Evaluation," *Nebraska State Medical Journal,* 50 (June 1965), 309–12; Saad Z. Nagi, "A Study in the Evaluation of Disability and Rehabilitation Potential," *American Journal of Public Health,* 54, 9 (September 1964), 1568–79; Henry Kessler and George G. Manning, Jr., "The Effect of Personal Opinion on Disability Evaluation," *Journal of Occupational Medicine,* 5, 9 (September 1963), 411–17; and Howard R. Kelman and Arthur Wilner, "Problems in Measurement and Evaluation of Rehabilitation," *Archives of Physical Medicine and Rehabilitation,* 43 (April 1962), 174–80.
7. Kelman and Wilner, *op. cit.*
8. *Ibid.*
9. *Ibid.*
10. The Harmarville data show that 72% of the patients thought they had received some or a great deal of help, while the staff rated 68% of them as having improved. There were considerable differences, however, since 20% of the patients thought they had not improved at all, while the staff rated 14% in this way; 8% of the patients thought they had improved a

little, while the staff rated 18% in this category of improvement, and so on. See *A Study of the Integration of Services of Industrial Medical Departments and a Rehabilitation Center: Final Report, op. cit.,* pp. 26–27. Kallen found that the correlation between general rehabilitation and self-report was +.48, but there was a considerable discrepancy between individual scores (standard deviation was 47.04). See Kallen, *op. cit.*

11. Kallen, *op. cit.*
12. E. M. Krusen and Dorothy E. Ford, "Compensation Factor in Low Back Injuries," *The Journal of the American Medical Association,* 166, 10 (March 8, 1958), 1129.
13. Commission on Chronic Illness, *Chronic Illness in a Large City,* vol. 4 (Cambridge, Mass.: Harvard University Press, 1957).
14. Aaron M. Rosenthal *et al.,* "Correlation of Perceptual Factors With Rehabilitation of Hemiplegic Patients," *Archives of Physical Medicine,* 46 (July 1965), 464–65.
15. "Behavioral Research in Rehabilitation" (report on the Cleveland Symposium, Highland View Hospital, November 4–6, 1959), p. 22.
16. Wilbur I. Hoff and Sedgwick Mead, "Evaluation of Rehabilitation Outcome: An Objective Assessment of the Physically Disabled," *American Journal of Physical Medicine,* 44, 3 (1964), 116.
17. The best source concerning evaluative research is undoubtedly Edward A. Suchman, *Evaluative Research: Principles and Practice in Public Service and Social Action Programs* (New York: Russell Sage Foundation, 1967). For discussions on evaluative research in rehabilitation, see Edward A. Suchman, "A Model for Research and Evaluation on Rehabilitation," in Marvin B. Sussman (ed.), *Sociology and Rehabilitation* (Washington, D.C.: American Sociological Association, 1965), pp. 52–70; and Howard R. Kelman, "Evaluation of Rehabilitation for the Long-term Ill and Disabled Patient: Some Persistent Research Problems," *Journal of Chronic Diseases,* 17 (July 1964), 631–39.
18. E. P. Copp, "A Controlled Trial of Rehabilitation," *Annals of Physical Medicine,* 8, 5 (1965–66), 151–67; and E. P. Copp and R. Harris, "A Further Controlled Trial of Rehabilitation," *Annals of Physical Medicine,* 8, 6 (1965–66), 220–23.
19. Kelman, *op. cit.,* pp. 634–35.
20. R. K. Diveley, R. H. Kiene, and P. W. Meyer, "Low Back Pain," *The Journal of the American Medical Association,* 160, 9 (March 3, 1956), 731; and Krusen and Ford, *op. cit.,* pp. 1129–30.

21. G. F. McCoy and H. Rusk, *An Evaluation of Rehabilitation*, Rehabilitation Monograph I (New York: New York University, Bellevue Medical Center, 1953); K. Keeler, "Appraisal of Patient Goals in a Community Rehabilitation Center," *Archives of Physical Medicine*, 37 (1956), 293–96; A. L. Anderson, L. J. Hanvik, and J. R. Brown, "A Statistical Analysis of Rehabilitation in Hemiplegia," *Geriatrics*, 5, 4 (1950), 214; Nagi, Burk, and Potter, *op. cit.*, p. 185; Kallen, *op. cit.*; John E. F. Hastings, "A Study of the Paraplegic Patient" (study sponsored by The Workmen's Compensation Board, Ontario, 1959); Jeanne K. Smith, Edwin N. Rise, and David E. Gralnek, "Speech Recovery in Laryngectomized Patients," *Laryngoscope*, 76 (September 1966), 1542–44; and Roth and Eddy, *op. cit.*, pp. 168–93.

22. Theodor J. Litman, "Influence of Age on Physical Rehabilitation," *Geriatrics*, 19, 3 (March 1964), 202–7; and Norman C. Bourestom, "Predictors of Long-term Recovery in Cerebrovascular Disease," *Archives of Physical Medicine and Rehabilitation*, 48 (August 1967), 417–18.

23. Theodor J. Litman, "The Influence of Self-conception and Life Orientation Factors in the Rehabilitation of the Orthopedically Disabled," *Journal of Health and Human Behavior*, 3 (Winter 1962), 253–56; Kallen, *op. cit;* Nagi *et al.*, *op. cit.*, p. 191; Roth and Eddy, *op. cit.*, pp. 168–93; Smith *et al.*, *op. cit.*, p. 1542.

24. Nagi *et al.*, *op. cit.*, pp. 194–95; Safilios-Rothschild, *op. cit.*; Roth and Eddy, *op. cit.*, pp. 168–93.

25. Litman, "The Influence of Self-conception and Life Orientation Factors in the Rehabilitation of the Orthopedically Disabled," *op. cit.*; and Safilios-Rothschild, *op. cit.*

26. Roth and Eddy point out that early in the rehabilitation process some patients grasp the importance of persuading the rehabilitation staff that they are "highly motivated" in order to receive attention and good care. See Roth and Eddy, *op. cit.*, p. 192.

27. Hastings, *op. cit.*, p. 18.

28. Safilios-Rothschild, *op. cit.*; and Nagi *et al.*, *op. cit.*, pp. 187–88.

29. Bourestom found that time since onset of the disability had little intrinsic validity for prognostic purposes in rehabilitation success; it contributes significantly only to other predictors. See Bourestom, *op. cit.* On the other hand, Nagi's less sophisticated analysis of data showed that an early referral (less than two years) was negatively related to rehabilitation success and physical disability improvement, while referral after two to four years from the onset of disability seemed to be optimum. See Nagi *et al.*, *op. cit.*, p. 188.

30. Theodor J. Litman, "The Family and Physical Rehabilitation," *Journal of Chronic Diseases*, 19 (February 1966), 211–17; and Roth and Eddy, *op. cit.*, pp. 168–93.
31. Bourestom, *op. cit.*, pp. 415–19.
32. Elliot A. Krause, "On the Time and Place of Crises," *Human Organization*, 27, 2 (Summer 1968), 110–16.
33. Lucy V. McDaniel, "Rehabilitation: Then What? Quadriplegia Follow-up," *Journal of the American Physical Therapy Association*, 45, 11 (November 1965), 1044.
34. Edward Scull, David Komisar, Harry L. Leonhardt, and Anne S. Weitz, "A Follow-up Study of Patients Discharged From a Community Rehabilitation Center," *Journal of Chronic Diseases*, 15 (February 1962), 207–13.
35. Vlasak and Phillips, *op. cit.*, pp. 18, 27–29. The Jews had the lowest proportion of independent individuals in self-care capacity (52%), while the Catholics were between the Jews and the Protestants (73% of them independent).
36. Jane C. Kronick, "The Rehabilitation of Stroke Patients: An Experimental Analysis of the Effects of Physical and Social Factors in Determining Recovery" (mimeographed, Bryn Mawr, Pa.: Bryn Mawr College, Department of Social Work and Social Research, 1962).
37. Claire M. Vernier *et al.*, "Psychosocial Study of the Patient With Pulmonary Tuberculosis: A Cooperative Research Approach," *Psychological Monographs*, 75, 6, whole no. 510 (1961), 27–28; and Rose L. Coser, "A Home Away From Home," *Social Problems*, 4, 1 (July 1956), 3–17.
38. Peter Kong-Ming New, Linda A. George, and Anthony T. Ruscio, "Hope and Reality: A Study of Patients' Pathways Through the World of Rehabilitation" (mimeographed, Boston: School of Medicine, Tufts University, October 1968).
39. *Ibid.*
40. Howard R. Kelman, Jonas N. Muller, and Milton Lowenthal, "Post-hospital Adaptation of a Chronically Ill and Disabled Rehabilitation Population," *Journal of Health and Human Behavior*, 5, 2–3 (Summer–Fall 1964).
41. Kronick, *op. cit.*; and Joseph B. Rogoff, Donald V. Cooney, and Bernard Kutner, "Hemiplegia: A Study of Home Rehabilitation," *Journal of Chronic Diseases*, 17 (June 1964), 539–50; Christine McArthur, "Rehabilitation Nursing in the Home," *Health Newsletter* (Saskatchewan Department of Public Health, March 15, 1960); J. L. Russ and H. Grigsby, "Home Care Program for an Outpatient Clinic," *Journal of American Physical Therapy*, 42 (1962), 299–302; and I. Rossman, M. Clarke, and B. Rudnick, "Total Rehabilitation in a Home Care

Setting," *New York State Journal of Medicine*, 62, 8 (April 15, 1962), 1215–19.

42. Robert Strauss, "Social Change and the Rehabilitation Concept," in Sussman, *op. cit.*, pp. 14–23.

43. Krusen and Ford, *op. cit.*, p. 133; Douglas Allen Fenderson, *A Study of the Vocational Rehabilitation Potential of Applicants for Social Security Disability Benefits Whose Claims Have Been Denied* (Ann Arbor, Mich.: University Microfilms, 1966), pp. 103–4; William Kir-Stimon, *Discards on Trial* (Chicago: Rehabilitation Institute of Chicago, June 1963).

44. Lawrence D. Haber, *Disability, Work, and Income Maintenance: Prevalence of Disability, 1966*, Report 2 (Washington, D.C.: Social Security Administration, Office of Research and Statistics, May 1968), p. 5.

45. Fenderson, *op. cit.*

46. F. A. Sneath, "Forecasting Success in the Vocational Training of the Disabled," in *Industrial Society and Rehabilitation— Problems and Solutions, Proceedings of the Tenth World Congress, International Society for Rehabilitation of the Disabled* (Stuttgart: Georg Thieme Verlag, 1967), pp. 196–99; and Charles E. Lewis, "Factors Influencing the Return to Work of Men With Congestive Heart Failure," *Journal of Chronic Diseases*, 19 (November–December 1966), 1193–1209. In the Syracuse study they found there was a curvilinear relationship between age and rate of employment, probably because their sample included several highly skilled and well-educated persons whose employment status would be little affected by advanced age (over 50) and disability. See *Final Report of the Cardiac Rehabilitation Project* (New York: Syracuse University and Upstate Medical Center, April 1966).

47. Hastings, *op. cit.*, p. 41; V. M. Schletzer, R. V. Davis, G. W. England, and L. H. Lofquist, *Minnesota Studies in Vocational Rehabilitation: VII. Factors Related to Employment Success* (Minneapolis, Minn.: University of Minnesota Press, 1959); Michael M. De Mann, "A Predictive Study of Rehabilitation Counseling Outcome," *Journal of Counseling Psychology*, 10, 4 (1963), 340–43; Jean Spencer Felton and Myra Litman, "Study of Employment of 222 Men With Spinal Cord Injury," *Archives of Physical Medicine*, 46 (December 1965), 809–14; and Marion S. Lesser and Robert C. Darling, "Factors Prognostic for Vocational Rehabilitation Among the Physically Handicapped," in A. J. Jaffe (ed), *Research Conference on Workmen's Compensation and Vocational Rehabilitation* (New York: Bureau of Applied Social Research, Columbia University, March 1961), p. 101.

48. Frank H. Echols, "Medical, Social, and Rehabilitation Factors

in the Employment of Discharges From Tuberculosis Hospitals," *Personnel and Guidance Journal*, 42, 5 (January 1964), 495– 96 (referring to age at admission); Hubert Weiner, "Characteristics Associated With Rehabilitation Success," *Personnel and Guidance Journal*, 42, 7 (March 1964), 687–94; Carl Eric Fallstrom, "Study on Working Capacity of Persons Physically Disabled by Neurologic Disease or Injury," *Acta Neurologica Scandinavia,* supp. 6, vol. 40 (1964), 40–89; William M. McPhee, Kenneth A. Griffiths, and F. LeGrande Magleby, *Adjustment of Vocational Rehabilitation Clients* (Washington, D.C.: U.S. Department of Health, Education and Welfare, Vocational Rehabilitation Administration, September 1963), pp. 18–19; Felton and Litman, *op. cit.*; Patricia Dvonch, Lawrence I. Kaplan, Bruce B. Grynbaum, and Howard A. Rusk, "Vocational Findings in Post-disability Employment of Patients With Spinal Cord Dysfunction," *Archives of Physical Medicine*, 46 (November 1965), 761–66; A. J. Jaffe, Lincoln H. Day, and Walter Adams, *Disabled Workers in the Labor Market* (Totowa, N.J.: Bedminster, 1964), pp. 19–44; and *Final Report of the Cardiac Rehabilitation Project, op. cit.,* pp. 90–91.

49. Fenderson, *op. cit.*

50. For example, Lesser and Darling, *op. cit.*, found 30 years of age as the ceiling of successful vocational rehabilitation, and Schletzer *et al., op. cit.*, found 45 years of age to be the ceiling.

51. Hastings, *op. cit.*, p. 54; Schletzer *et al., op. cit.*; Felton and Litman, *op. cit.*; Dvonch *et. al., op. cit.*; Jaffe *et al., op. cit.*; McPhee *et al., op. cit.*; *Final Report of the Cardiac Rehabilitation Project, op. cit.*; Lesser and Darling, *op. cit.*; Lewis, *op. cit.*, pp. 1198–99; Fred A. Novak, *Program for Serving the More Severely Disabled Individuals In Nebraska* (Lincoln, Neb.: Division of Rehabilitation Service, April 1965); and A. G. Garris, *Rehabilitation Service for Severely Disabled OASDI Recipients* (Sacramento: California State Department of Rehabilitation, 1965). However, the level of education was not found to be significantly related to the rate of postdisability employment in Sneath, *op. cit.*

52. Weiner, *op. cit.*; Fallstrom, *op. cit.*; Felton and Litman, *op. cit.*; Dvonch *et al., op. cit.*; Jaffe *et al., op. cit.*; McPhee *et al., op. cit.*; and *Final Report of the Cardiac Rehabilitation Project, op. cit.* One study found that the level of skill was not related to the rate of the postdisability employment: see Sneath, *op. cit.*

53. Weiner, *op. cit.*; Felton and Litman, *op. cit.*; Lewis, *op. cit.*, p. 1207; De Mann, *op cit.*; Schletzer *et al., op. cit.*; Garris,

op. cit. Kir-Stimon found that the monthly income while drawing disability benefits was negatively related to vocational re-
54. Weiner, *op. cit.*; and Jaffe *et al., op. cit.*
    habilitation. See Kir-Stimon, *op. cit.*
55. Felton and Litman, *op. cit.*; Dvonch *et al., op. cit.*; and McPhee
    et al., op. cit.
56. Weiner, *op. cit.*; Schletzer *et al., op. cit.*; Novak, *op. cit.*; and
    Jaffe *et al., op. cit.* In one study marital status was not related
    to vocational rehabilitation. See Garris, *op. cit.*
57. Weiner, *op. cit.*; Garris, *op. cit.*; Novak, *op. cit.* In one study,
    however, the number of dependents was found to be inversely
    related to vocational rehabilitation. See Kir-Stimon, *op. cit.*
58. De Mann, *op. cit.*
59. Fenderson, *op. cit.*; and McPhee *et al., op. cit.*
60. Safilios-Rothschild, *op. cit.*
61. *Ibid.*; Kir-Stimon, *op. cit.*
62. Kir-Stimon, *op. cit.*
63. While Kir-Stimon found that the less dependent the disabled,
    the more they tended to return to work, Novak found that the
    more dependent the disabled, the more they tended to return
    to work. See *ibid.*; Novak, *op. cit.*, and Garris found no relation-
    ship between dependency and rate of postdisability employ-
    ment. See Garris, *op. cit.*
64. Novak, *op. cit.*; Garris, *op. cit.*; Kir-Stimon, *op. cit.*; Lewis,
    op. cit., pp. 1203–4.
65. Lewis, *op. cit.*, p. 1204.
66. *Ibid.*
67. Lewis found that most of the nonworking disabled were 45 to
    49 years old and were laid off. *Ibid.*, p. 1202.
68. Weiner, *op. cit.*; Jaffe *et al., op. cit.*; and McPhee *et al., op. cit.*
69. Sneath, *op. cit.*; Novak, *op. cit.*; Garris, *op. cit.*; and De Mann,
    op. cit.
70. Some studies found a linear relationship between work stability
    and the rate of postdisability employment. See Weiner, *op. cit.*;
    Dvonch *et al., op. cit.*; and *Final Report of the Cardiac Re-
    habilitation Project, op. cit.* Others found a curvilinear relation-
    ship. See Fenderson, *op. cit.*
71. Fenderson, *op. cit.*; and Safilios-Rothschild, *op. cit.*
72. Lewis, *op. cit.*, p. 1198. All these variables fit in the typology
    developed in Chapter 5.
73. Weiner, *op. cit.*; Fallstrom, *op. cit.*; McPhee *et al., op. cit.*;
    Echols, *op. cit.*; Lesser and Darling, *op. cit.*; Sneath, *op. cit.*;
    and *Final Report of the Cardiac Rehabilitation Project, op. cit.*
74. Hastings, *op. cit.*, pp. 42 and 48; and Lesser and Darling, *op.
    cit.*
75. Weiner, *op. cit.*; Lewis, *op. cit.*, p. 1200; and Kir-Stimon, *op.
    cit.*

76. Kir-Stimon, *op. cit.*; Fallstrom, *op. cit.*; and Jaffe *et al., op. cit.* One study, however, found no significant relationship between psychiatric history and the rate of postdisability employment. See Garris, *op. cit.*
77. Lewis, *op. cit.*, p. 1203; and Jaffe *et al., op. cit.*
78. In at least two studies a relationship was found between the type of disability and the rate of postdisability employment. See G. C. Krantz, "Screening Out Failure in Vocational Rehabilitation" (unpublished M.A. thesis, University of Minnesota, 1953). But in one study, no such relationship was found. See Sneath, *op. cit.*
79. Novak, *op. cit.*; Lesser and Darling, *op. cit.*; and Hastings, *op. cit.*, p. 53.
80. Murray Z. Safian, *A Study of Certain Psychological Factors in the Rehabilitation of Potentially Employable Homebound Adults* (Ann Arbor, Mich.: University Microfilms, Inc., 1958).
81. Hastings, *op. cit.*, p. 66.
82. Jaffe *et al., op. cit.*, pp. 65, 71.
83. *Final Report of the Cardiac Rehabilitation Project, op. cit.*
84. Dvonch *et al., op. cit.*, pp. 763–65.
85. McPhee *et al., op. cit.*; Weiner, *op. cit.*; Fallstrom, *op. cit.*; Hastings, *op. cit.*, p. 56.
86. Jaffe *et al., op. cit.*, pp. 100–12.
87. *Final Report of the Cardiac Rehabilitation Project, op. cit.*
88. It is interesting to note that in countries with obligatory quota legislation for the employment of the disabled, some authors believe that one of the most serious problems is the fact that employers do not adapt the jobs to the disabled's abilities and disabilities. See Roux, "Les handicapés dans la vie professionnelle," in Bloch-Lainé, *Etude du problème général de l'inadaptation des personnes handicapées* (Paris, December 1967), p. 74.
89. Weiner, *op. cit.*
90. Jaffe *et al., op. cit.*, p. 65.
91. McPhee *et al., op. cit.*
92. Jaffe *et al., op. cit.*, p. 69.
93. Allan has reviewed a number of relevant studies in W. Scott Allan, "Successful Placement of Handicapped Workers," *Archives of Environmental Health*, 7 (November 1963), 621–24.
94. McPhee *et al., op. cit.*

CHAPTER 7

After Rehabilitation

The disabled's problems do not end with and
are not solved by rehabilitation. Often some of
their serious psychosocial problems become
accentuated after the completion of rehabilitation when they have to cope with the nondisabled world "on their own." The "rehabilitated"
disabled can no longer focus primarily upon
improving or developing physical abilities and
skills but must now find a place for themselves
in society. They may have specific dreams,
aspirations, and desires concerning the direction their lives ought to take in order to find
the optimum equilibrium. But in addition to
friends and family, a multitude of professionals
with whom they have come into contact since

the onset of their disability may have coinciding or diverging suggestions, ideas, and plans about the "best" way to organize their lives.
The question to which we will address ourselves in this chapter refers
to the degree of self-determination left to the disabled after rehabilitation and after all the "interested" others have decided what he should
do and what his place in society ought to be.

However, since not all the disabled are accepted or even considered for rehabilitation, a considerable number have to cope with
the nondisabled without the benefit of rehabilitation services. And of
course, not all the disabled accepted for rehabilitation have a successful rehabilitation stay and outcome. In a sense, we shall be examining
all those disabled who attempted to avail themselves of rehabilitation
services regardless of their success in obtaining them or of making
use of them.

All disabled must cope with the activities of everyday living,
with the performance of their usual roles, and with the difficulties
involved in interacting with the nondisabled, whether significant
others or not. While theoretically they have several choices, the
predominant cultural values delineate quite clearly what is expected
of them. If they are male, they must return to gainful employment
(unless they are below 18 or above 65); if female, they have a choice
between working and not working, but they must at least coordinate
the household activities if they are physically unable to perform
them. Beyond these overall cultural values, however, the values and
preferences of a number of people (including the disabled themselves)
complicate the decision-making process. These intervening "others,"
often with conflicting interests and beliefs, may not only influence
the disabled's decision outcome, but may sometimes more or less
determine it.

The social system of interested others, in which the disabled
is caught before, during, and after rehabilitation, is made up of
physicians (specialists, family, and industrial physicians), lawyers,
employers, insurance representatives, labor unions, administrators of
a variety of state and federal programs of vocational rehabilitation,
officials of special disability organizations and agencies, family
members, friends, and the rehabilitation staff (vocational counselors
in particular), as well as the other disabled with whom he comes into
contact. We shall see that some of these decision agents push the dis-

abled toward reintegration within the larger society while others impede him from doing so by encouraging him to stay apart from the mainstream of social life, identify primarily with other disabled, and avoid living a "normal" life which includes a productive, regular working role. Under the influence of conflicting and powerful points of view, the disabled may at times or even perpetually feel "alienated" in every way possible.[1] That is, he may feel a sense of "powerlessness" because he may realize that he has little control over what is happening to his life; a sense of "normlessness" because although there are no clear-cut societal norms regulating the behavior of disabled persons, he is expected by different persons to behave in different ways; a sense of "meaninglessness" because different interested others may have set goals for him and/or made decisions for him which he considers irrelevant; a sense of "self-estrangement" because he may be forced according to the occasion and the desired effect to play up the role of the "invalid" who is seriously incapacitated for life or to hide his disability and try to pass as "normal." In the end it is difficult to know which of these many selves is genuine, and the disabled may be feeling inwardly uneasy with his many impersonations.

While the structural and psychological conditions of the disabled's lives can easily produce alienation, it does not necessarily follow that all disabled experience alienation, or any type of it. It is even conceivable that some disabled under some conditions may enjoy the fact that some of life's important decisions are out of their hands. Let us now examine the role that different types of agents play in the lives of the disabled, particularly during their efforts to become rehabilitated or reintegrated into "normal" society or to find an idiosyncratically suitable mode of coping with their disability.

The Physician: Beyond the Treating Role

From the moment a person defines himself as sick and in need of medical attention, the role of the physician becomes paramount. During the treatment phase physicians are of course much more at ease, since they are performing the tasks and role for which they have been trained. However, even during this period the pitfalls are many, for the science of medicine is by no means exact. Wrong, uncertain, or conflicting diagnoses; disagreements as to the appropriate treatment method (for example, surgery versus conservative treatment in the case of back injuries); and conflicting or fluctuating prognoses may already have set the psychological climate for alienation since the patients feel uncertain about the nature and extent of their disability as well as about what they ought to do.[2] These experiences are not uniform and may be extreme in some cases and altogether lacking in others. The feeling of alienation may be reinforced by the fact that doctors discuss and explain little to their patients (especially their lower class patients), but expect them to follow all their directions and recommendations with "no questions asked." Besides the fact that patients tend to feel powerless, it may also be that in some cases they have little faith in following a particular treatment or set of instructions because of the contradictory diagnoses and prescriptions given by different physicians. During this stage, feelings of alienation seem to be more pronounced among lower than among middle class patients.

If later the disabled person enters a rehabilitation center, depending upon the type of center he selects or is sent to, he may either find that he is still supposed to fill the sick role expectations (with the same psychological consequences for his morale as described in the previous paragraph) or that he is now, with very little preparation for the new role, expected to think and behave like an autonomous, creative individual. Although the prevailing rehabilitation philosophy encourages him to play the latter role, all team members do not always completely agree about the degree of autonomy and initiative that should be granted. Rehabilitants may be treated by some team members more like "patients" and by others more like "clients." Such contradictions in behavioral expectations can occasionally further alienate the disabled.

Even during the treatment and rehabilitation phases, the nature of the patient-physician relationship and the physician's medical behavior may sometimes be alienative, but the most serious problems arise when the physician is called upon as an expert to give his opinion about the extent of permanent disability present. This may be done for at least two reasons: (1) in order to determine the amount of compensation due the disabled person for a compensable disability and (2) in order to assess whether or not the disabled individual can work and what type of work he can perform. In the first instance, although the physician is asked to make a medical evaluation, this evaluation is by no means easy to achieve. Even when an opinion will not be used for compensation purposes, it is often extremely difficult to evaluate disabilities which are justified mainly on the basis of subjective symptoms and incapacitating pain rather than on the basis of objective medical findings.[3] The amount of experienced pain, for example, cannot be checked; it may vary with the sociocultural characteristics of the disabled individual as well as with his psychological makeup, including conscious or subconscious motivations.

It is also very difficult for a physician to evaluate the extent to which different individuals afflicted with exactly the same degree of physical disability will make use of their remaining abilities, because the differential use of the remaining abilities depends again upon the influence of different motivational forces, values, and self-definitions as well as upon basic socioeconomic characteristics. Exactly because extramedical factors—psychological, sociopsychological and sociological—play an important role in determining the extent to which an individual will finally overcome his disability or will be impaired by it, physicians often are not adequately equipped to make accurate prognoses and evaluations. Physiatrists, of course, are better equipped than other physicians to make such evaluations, but even they often meet with great difficulties in the case of disabilities involving subjective symptomatology, for example, back injuries.

When the subject of compensation enters the picture, the whole process of evaluation becomes complicated. Sometimes the crucial question that the physician must answer is whether or not the incurred disability is compensable. This is true of some types of back disorders and is especially common with disabilities due to heart disease, because in both cases it is not clear or demonstrable that there is a "causal" relationship between work or work episodes and heart attacks or back pain.[4] The average practitioner or even internist is not prepared by training to make such judgments with complete confidence; family physicians may often tend to lean toward affirmation of the causal relationship out of sympathy for the patient or out of fear of the potential loss of this patient, his family, and his friends if they flatly denied the existence of any causal bond.[5] Furthermore, the espousal of a particular medical theory may lead even heart specialists to support or reject a causal relationship between work and heart disease regardless of "objective" medical and work-related factors. For example, those who espouse White's theory, that heart disease is not caused by hard work, consistently deny that such a causal relationship may exist, advise employers that heart disease is not compensable, and enter into emotional polemics with those specialists who do not accept this theory and are willing to testify that their patient's illness is compensable.[6]

It is interesting to note the fact that the pro-White specialists (who in a sense can be considered anticlient) often seem to be the most eminent and successful, while the opposite is true for the anti-White and proclient physicians.[7] The implications of this finding may be quite serious if we also consider the available evidence which indicates that only a few physicians regularly accept compensation cases. Those who more often treat compensation patients are predominantly in occupational medicine or orthopedic surgery.[8] There is some evidence that members of prestigious medical specialties reported they do not like to treat compensation cases because there is too much paperwork, the patients are not motivated to improve, and the fees received are inadequate.[9] Of course, compensable patients (especially through workmen's compensation) are often lower or working class and may be shunned by prestigious physicians for this reason as well as because of the red tape connected with compensation. It is also possible that in some cases the espousal of a particular medical theory (that favors the employers and insurance carriers) may spring from self-interest, since association with powerful employers and well-known insurance companies may bring the physician equal prominence.[10]

It must be noted, however, that there is a considerable number of physicians in all specialties who are most willing to treat the disabled and defend their "rights" as they define them. But because the medical field is split, especially in the case of some compensable disabilities, both sides must be studied and understood. For it is exactly this split into "pro-disabled" and "pro-employer" or "pro-insurance" that produces structural conditions for alienation in the disabled.[11]

The second major area of consultation in which physicians are asked to serve as experts is the evaluation of the extent to which a physical disability constitutes a vocational handicap. This judgment often enters into and is probably the most important element upon which the decision on amount of compensation is based. However, physicians are not always well equipped to make this judgment. Unless they have specialized in occupational medicine, they have only a very general knowledge of different types of occupations and their specific requirements in terms of physical ability, stamina, rhythm of work, or emotional stress and know very little—if anything— about the possibilities of job redesign, through which many jobs could be adapted to the potential of disabled persons. Many physicians have a stereotypic knowledge about jobs similar to that of the general lay public. Thus, all construction work is heavy labor and all office work requires light physical effort. And they are not always aware or do not always sufficiently understand the influence of a variety of familial, socioeconomic, sociopsychological, and psychological factors that may restrict or extend an individual's work potentialities.[12]

Despite these shortcomings in physicians' evaluations of vocational disability, they are consulted by employers, by insurance companies, by lawyers, and by judges in a court of law. If they are industrial or insurance physicians, they usually have more specialized knowledge. Industrial physicians in particular generally have a better knowledge of the physical requirements of most industrial jobs than do other physicians and are usually in a position to evaluate with relative accuracy the work potential of some categories of disabled workers. Their judgment, however, may not be totally objective since they are employed by an industrial firm whose set policies about hiring disabled workers significantly influence their recommendations. Existing evidence suggests that they tend to be unnecessarily conservative and in favor of the company's not taking risks.[13]

General practitioners and specialists are either directly consulted about a patient's work potential (as, for example, in court as part of the overall disability evaluation) or indirectly influence employers' decisions by their reports, or by recommending or not recommending the rehiring or hiring of a disabled person. The family physician, because he understands to some extent the disabled individual's sociopsychological condition, may be in a fairly good position to estimate the degree to which remaining abilities will be used and, conversely, the degree to which the physical disability constitutes a handicap. However, he may know little about the occupational requirements of a particular job and may be biased toward presenting his patient's degree of vocational ability according to his own wishes rather than his best judgment. Specialists, on the other hand, usually have a very sketchy knowledge of their patients' sociopsychological condition so that they can even less accurately estimate the extent of the social or vocational handicap resulting from physical disability. They tend to be more concerned with its accurate medical evaluation, and their final specific recommendations may be dictated more by their adherence to one school of medical thought about the particular disability than upon the idiosyncratic sociopsychological makeup of the disabled individual. If they are involved in a litigation case, their judgment may be obscured by whether their prime loyalties lie with the patient or with the insurance carrier or employer.

The physician who has not clearly taken sides often is caught in a series of related moral and ethical dilemmas. Should he or should he not testify for a disabled patient so that he will then receive some kind of compensation for his disability? Sometimes this dilemma may be simply because he is not entirely sure that this activity is a necessary part of his role as a physician and because he does not particularly like to lay open existing medical ambiguities in court.[14]

How much medical information should the physician provide to the employer so that he neither compromises his professional ethics nor unnecessarily harms the disabled worker's chance of becoming reemployed? There is a danger that by including in his medical report some valid doubts or observations concerning possible limitations created by the worker's disability or disease, he may implant not always warranted fears in the employer's mind that could lead to the worker being rejected from employment or downgraded in his reemployment. Should he recommend return to the previous job, to full-time work with some special adaptations to be made in the working conditions, to a different type of work—or should he recommend that the disabled person work only part-time or not at all? This is probably the most crucial but also the most difficult question about which physicians are consulted. Different physicians solve this critical consultation problem in different ways. Some physicians avoid making an evaluation of vocational ability and potential altogether by relying entirely upon the patient's judgment and wishes. If patients say they want and plan to work, they are not evaluated as disabled (unless it is temporarily disabled), while those who say that they do not want or plan to work are evaluated as permanently disabled. Because of physicians' lack of knowledge about the requirements of different jobs, it is easy for a patient, sometimes with the collaboration of an employer or potential employer, to fool a physician if he wishes to do so. A patient can rather easily convince his doctor that he is able, or not able, to carry out a particular job, because the physician usually does not have a basis for challenging or contradicting the statement.[15]

Some physicians may feel that in many cases they can best serve their patient by recommending a return to the previous job. They probably assume that if some minor adaptations are needed in the setup of the job, the employer will be willing to make them. However, if the worker does not readjust to his previous job because of the limitations resulting from his injury or disease, he will tend to give a below-average performance. As a result, he will stagnate, be downgraded, or even be fired, and experience feelings of dissatisfaction and demoralization. In contrast, some physicians tend to feel overprotective toward their patients and either forbid them to work altogether (because they do not like to assume any responsibility for advising them to work in case their disease should show signs of aggravation) or keep them from working for such a long period that it is virtually impossible for them to return to the previous job (or sometimes even the previous firm). Still others lightheartedly make recommendations of "change of job" or "can work only part-time" or "light work" whenever they are not 100 percent sure the worker could function in his previous job without any complication or aggravation of his condition, and thus seriously compromise the worker's chance of being placed in any type of gainful employment.[16] Finally, if the physician is going to testify for the worker in his compensation claim, he often tends to overdramatize the work limitations and unemployability of the worker. But after the closure of the claim, when the worker may be interested in working, the physician's pessimistic evaluation will be a block to his vocational placement.

If a disabled person saw one physician throughout his disability and only this physician was called upon to evaluate the extent of the disability, the situation would not be as frustrating, baffling, and alienating to the disabled person as it is in reality. Unfortunately, in practically all cases, the disabled person has—partially by necessity and partially by choice—consulted a variety of physicians and specialists. He has heard a number of sometimes contradictory diagnoses, recommendations, prognoses, and evaluations. Even in the absence of compensation, one physician may tell him that he can return to his previous job, another that he must change the nature of his work to a "lighter" one, and possibly another that he must stop working altogether for at least a year or two. Since the disabled person has no objective rationale for disregarding the opinion of any physician, he has two major modes of conflict resolution. Either he can pick the medical opinion that agrees with his preference, or he will experience some type of self-estrangement if he cannot conclude whether or not he is an invalid and, if so, to what extent. If the disability is compensable, he then has a much higher probability of feeling alienated and self-estranged during the different medicolegal stages, for he is presented by "his" doctors as a total invalid and by the company or the insurance doctor as minimally disabled. He will often witness heated, emotional battles between disagreeing physicians as well as between lawyers and physicians, the subject always being his degree of invalidism.[17] Finally, the disabled may substitute his own feelings and judgment as to how disabled he really is for the court decision or his doctor's evaluation. He may then become totally estranged and the victim of incomprehensible complex systems. In the case of some disabled, their self-estrangement may lead to schizophrenic-like behavior. They may undergo rehabilitation and benefit considerably by these services but pretend that they have a lot of pain and discomfort in order to be able to uphold their disabled image in court (see Chapter 6).

Probably the only way to diminish somewhat the often incapacitating and alienating effect of differential disability evaluations upon the disabled would be the establishment of an "objective" medical committee paid equally by all interested parties so that no client-oriented allegiances could develop.[18] Of course, this proposal would not solve all the problems—even if the court would not then accept the testimony of any other physician. But such a solution would tend to diminish the incapacitating effect that medicolegal controversies can have upon the disabled.

The Lawyer: Villain or Hero?

The position of the lawyer is often intimately related to that of the physician. He cooperates with some physicians and is supported by them, fights vehemently against others in trying to prove that their consultation is not valid or substantiated. Actually, since most physicians are not legally sophisticated, it is relatively easy for a skilled lawyer by means of "word play" and cross-examination to make their testimony appear weak. Besides, physicians do not like to publicize professional disagreements and conflicts in order not to weaken their professional image. The publicity that such disagreements receive during a court trial is threatening and shakes their self-image as experts—and lawyers, of course, capitalize upon such psychological confusion and emotionalism.[19]

In most rehabilitation literature, the lawyer is represented as a villain who, because he benefits from other people's disabilities, tends to nurture and emphasize them.[20] Because the lawyer has a vested interest (the size of his fee) in presenting his client's disability as maximum, he is often portrayed as being preoccupied with his client's being labeled considerably or totally and permanently disabled. The worker is coaxed into not cooperating with the rehabilitation effort so that even when he is accepted for such services, he refuses much of the treatment or refuses to acknowledge that he has improved in any way. Thus, at the end of the rehabilitation process, the physicians do not have any objective evidence that would permit them to alter their evaluation and classify him at a lower level of disability.[21] The worker is also advised not to come in contact with his employer and of course not to respond to offers about returning to his old job. The worker may then get a high claim settlement, but he may have jeopardized not only his chance to return to his job, but his chance to return to gainful employment as well. The reasons usually given for the latter are: (1) his developed attitude that "the world owes him a living" and his disinclination to meet the requirements of a regular job, especially after a long period of unemployment;

and (2) the employers' negative attitude toward hiring a disabled worker who has been involved in litigation. And at the end of all this, even when the amount of compensation granted is large, a significant percentage (up to 25 percent) goes to the lawyer and to pay the expenses incurred during the period of unemployment.[22]

While the procedures usually described and deplored in rehabilitation literature are sometimes accurate for lump sum settlements, they are not necessarily accurate or true when the lawyer really fights the case. Some authors have observed that lawyers soon find out that fighting compensation cases is too time-consuming and unprofitable. The "unscrupulous lawyer makes his profit, not from fighting a case, but from settling it. . . ."[23] Available studies have shown that lump sum settlements are usually sought in ambiguous cases, such as back injuries, in which the seriousness of the disability and the prognosis are notoriously difficult to establish. But in order to achieve a settlement through negotiation, there must be a relative congruence of medical opinion on both sides. In these cases, the patient does not have to submit himself to medicolegal battles concerning the degree of his disability, but this does not seem to affect the probability of his returning to work. However, it is not clear to what extent such lump sum settlements are from a financial point of view more advantageous for the lawyer than for the disabled person —especially since there is evidence that workers who accept lump sum settlements do so not by choice but by economic necessity or ignorance of existing options.[24] They may have been high-pressured by insurance agents, employers, and their lawyer to accept a settlement because each of these agents has a definite vested interest in their doing so. In terms of the often small settlements and their primary use for paying off accumulated debts, the worker may have been better off had he continued on small weekly payments.

When a disabled's case is fought in court, the lawyer may often have the client's interest foremost in mind, an interest defined in terms of legal and economic principles which to him seem to be worth fighting for even at the expense of other important considerations. Some lawyers see themselves as the disabled's advocate who must counter the lawyer retained by the employer. These lawyers justify a legal battle on the basis of the variety of opinions, disability evaluations, and work recommendations given by various consulted physicians and specialists in different fields (or even specialists in the same field). Such a wide range of expert medical opinions often makes the lawyer feel that if he is to protect his client's legal rights, it might be safer to base the case on the most pessimistic medical opinion and evaluation rather than on the more optimistic one in order to safeguard him from future unpleasant developments in case the optimistic report is wrong.[25] But while the lawyer is trying to do what he thinks is best for the disabled person, the latter may be involved in endless, frustrating, often incomprehensible (to him) medicolegal controversies that may cause him to develop a traumatic neurosis or other psychological complications.[26] The employer meanwhile would have become hostile to this worker, and other potential employers may refuse to hire him because he was involved in litigation.[27] So at the end of these procedures, the disabled person may be thoroughly confused and uncertain about what he can do and what he cannot do, who he is, and what his prospects for the future are, and may finally become—unnecessarily—a true invalid, psychologically and physically.

The Employer: Prejudice and Fact

Despite the optimistic figure of 2 million disabled people reported by the Vocational Rehabilitation Administration as having been prepared for and placed in almost any kind of job since the establishment of vocational rehabilitation programs in 1920 and the advertising and educational campaigns aimed at increasing the rate of employment of the physically handicapped, no substantial changes have occurred in the degree of true acceptance of the disabled in industry. The percentages of disabled who return to work reported in the different studies vary considerably. This variability is primarily due to the fact that the followup studies are done after a differential length of time ranging from three months to five years after the injury or the termination of rehabilitation. But a host of other factors—some related to the disability, some to the social and sociopsychological characteristics of the disabled, some to the type of employer and union membership, and some to the socioeconomic conditions at the time of the study— significantly affect the rate of the disabled's employment.

Specifically, some of these factors are: the degree of disability; the type of disability; the disabled's age, sex, race, level of education, and occupational skill; his work history, length of employment, type and size of firm, union membership; and the level of overall unemployment and national prosperity (see Chapter 6). Thus, unless disability-specific, age-specific, education-specific, and so forth, rates of employment are calculated, the percentages reported are neither meaningful nor valid. The reported employment rates are also distorted because the admission and acceptance policies of vocational rehabilitation programs eliminate those who have little probability of returning to competitive employment. As we have already seen, vocational rehabilitation counselors further select those who can be placed relatively easily. Therefore, the reported employment rates are of a very select population made up of disabled who are on the average less severely afflicted and better educated than the total population of disabled. But even with such limitations in reporting, it is interesting to note that seldom are more than one-half of the disabled found to be employed at some time after discharge from rehabilitation.

Probably the most important issue of all and the one that is least studied is the type of work the disabled perform when employed and how it compares with their former job in terms of prestige, income, and promotion chances. Because it has been assumed that the disabled are lucky just to get a job, there has been little concern with the type of job they are usually able to obtain. There is evidence indicating that at least among some of the reemployed disabled, the chances for promotion were reduced. And these instances of downward occupational mobility or occupational uncertainty were much more frequent among semi- and unskilled workers than among all other occupational categories.[28] However, available data about the degree of downward occupational mobility are so spotty and unsystematic that no definite conclusion can be drawn about the pattern followed by disabled with differing types of disabilities and sociopsychological characteristics.

The issue of downward occupational mobility is very important because there is evidence that it may produce an alienative effect equal to that of forced unemployment after multiple rejections from employers who are reluctant to hire the disabled.[29] In some cases it may be even more self-devaluing and belittling for the disabled man to work at a lower level than not to work at all. It must not be forgotten that even if a disabled is rehired without any humiliating experiences and procrastinations, he is always made to understand (by personnel officers, supervisors, fellow workers, researchers, and rehabilitation workers) that he is "different" from the other workers and therefore under perennial observation and evaluation. He is made to feel "deviant" just because he is too much studied and evaluated. Job performance, absenteeism, and job safety are carefully evaluated and advertised when above average because the disabled must still prove that they are "better" in order to be acceptable (see Chapter 6).

But why are the disabled not truly acceptable to employers even after extensive advertising and educational campaigns to change the image of the handicapped from that of a helpless person to one of an above-average worker? Employers in general and industrial concerns in particular have profit as a major goal and not the solution of social problems. They become sensitive to the problem of the handicapped whenever their refusal to hire them could adversely affect their image in the community. Then, they may agree to hire some visibly handicapped who create much more sensational publicity than do the nonvisibly disabled.[30] Probably because this is their "weak spot," employers report that they greatly resent "selling" on an emotional basis, that is, arousing the employer's pity, sympathy, humanitarianism or sense of "community service." They claim (probably justly) that placement of the disabled under such pressures tends to be short-lived and "leads to concepts of charity and 'shelf jobs.' "[31]

There is, however, general agreement in the available literature that most employers are much more willing to rehire disabled workers who worked for them prior to their disability than new workers with a partial disability.[32] The rationale offered by the employers is that workers who have already been with their firm may have been very good workers so that there is less of an element of risk involved in their being rehired. And probably rejection of these workers would have had more serious consequences for their public image than a refusal to hire new disabled workers. A more plausible explanation may be a vested interest in rehiring their own disabled workers as soon as they are judged employable in order to stop compensation payments. Usually, their willingness to give lump sum settlements to some disabled workers has represented a "sugared pill," that is, a legal way to

get rid of undesirable workers. A definite process of selectivity operates, the selection generally resting on past performance, need for the
disabled's skills, length of employment (seniority rights), membership in a labor union (and therefore the protection and degree of
pressure exerted by the union), whether or not the disability is work-
connected, and the nature of workmen's compensation procedures.
In addition, legal trials as well as the degree and nature of the disability may or may not dictate some accommodation in work conditions and setting. This severe selective process in the rehiring of
disabled workers as well as the necessity for many workers to change
occupation because of disability-imposed limitations can explain the
large numbers of unemployed disabled seeking jobs.

Why are employers unwilling to hire new employees who are
disabled? There seems to be a controversy over whether employers are
prejudiced toward disabled applicants or are guided by occupational
stereotypes and traditional thinking, according to which the disabled
are not able to give a satisfactory work performance due to a high
rate of absenteeism or due to an aggravation of their disability.[33]
According to the latter explanation, employers are afraid that in
the long run disabled workers will either directly increase the cost
of production (through additional and excessive compensation or
through increased insurance rates) or at least indirectly lower the
level of profit. A survey study of a nonrandom sample of employers
in California showed that many of them were not aware of the legislation concerning compensation for second injuries and claimed that
they discouraged the employment of the disabled because they were
preoccupied with the possibility of paying excessive compensation for
highly probable work-connected injuries or illnesses. Whether this is
only a cover for more deep-seated prejudices or simple ignorance of
the law which could be easily corrected through education cannot
be demonstrated without appropriate empirical data. Only a very
small percentage of these employers (5 percent) had some knowledge
about the actual level of performance of disabled workers in work
settings.[34] The possible implication of these findings is that all such
misconceptions could be changed through education and familiarity
with the actual work performance of disabled workers. It seems,
however, that educational campaigns have failed to substantially
change employers' attitudes toward hiring the disabled; only past

experience with disabled workers seems to be associated with favorable hiring policies.[35]

Another standard complaint and justification for negative attitudes toward hiring the disabled on the part of surveyed employers, managers, and personnel officers has been the rigid seniority rules set by unions. These, employers claim, are one of the most difficult barriers to employing the disab'ed because jobs that could be comfortably and safely performed by disabled workers are often above the common labor category and either must be filled by workers with seniority or are already occupied by able-bodied workers with seniority who cannot be transferred to other jobs.[36] Here again, it is difficult to assess the degree to which this justification is a handy means of transferring blame to the unions. Nevertheless, some degree of reported difficulty may be due to rigid seniority rules—although in certain cases adherence to the same rules may work to the advantage of the disabled worker if he happens to have seniority. Since many of the serious vocational placement problems arise with older workers (who often have seniority), it may be that seniority rights protect rather than impede the employment of the disabled. An objective study of the actual effects of seniority rules upon the employment of the disabled is necessary in order to conclude whether or not recommendations for some kind of modification in the seniority rules should be made to the unions.

It is necessary to go beyond the controversy concerning employer prejudice and look at some of the facts that face an employer. It should not be forgotten that the information that reaches the employer with regard to the disabled's status is not always clear, specific, or consistent. Often he receives a variety of contradictory messages from different sources. The fund-raising campaigns of different health agencies tend to overdramatize the helplessness of the disabled, the gravity of the disability, and its ensuing limitations. Physicians may offer contradictory or vague recommendations pertaining to the exact extent of disability residue and to the kinds of jobs that could be adequately performed without being hazardous to the health of the disabled.[37] Differences in opinion, as we have already seen, exist not only between general practitioners and specialists, but also among specialists who follow different schools of medical philosophy. Finally, job descriptions are not very specific regarding exact requirements in terms of physical effort and psychological stress. In view of the amount of ambiguity facing employers, their decision not to hire the disabled may in some cases represent a rational choice on their part, since they cannot always afford to take risks and reduce profit. Granted that these risks may more often be imaginary than real, due to the Second Injury Law and the often uneventful work performance of the disabled, the employer is still not obliged to take any risk or to make any special accommodation in terms of job adaptation for the sake of the disabled as long as there is an abundant supply of non-disabled workers. Only a shortage in the labor force (for example, wartime) could force them to take risks and make special concessions.

Thus employers, frustrated by contradictory expert medical opinions and by the experience of long, costly, and ambiguous compensation trials, very often choose not to hire the disabled. Unfortunately, they may be adding the final straw to a disabled worker's psychological resistance, for he may have already had to wage a battle against his own (and/or his family's) reluctance to have him regain employment and against confusing medical recommendations and legal admonitions to stay away from work.

The Vocational Counselor: The Go-between

The vocational counselor, caught by contradictory philosophies, bureaucratic demands, and realistic considerations, may adapt and cope with this stressful situation in a variety of ways. These have been organized in a typology by Krause. As discussed earlier, the usual problems of the vocational counselors are the heavy workload, the pressure to present vocational rehabilitation success statistics, professional ethics which demand that they help as many disabled as possible, the reluctance of employers to hire the disabled, and the disabled's own complex motivational ambivalences toward work in general or some types of work in particular. Under the influence of these conflicts and pressures, the vocational counselor may become aggressive toward his clients and reject as "not feasible" or "unmotivated" all marginal cases or all those who do not show a great deal of interest in returning to work. He may conform strictly to formal rules and regulations, according to which only those who can reasonably be expected to benefit from vocational rehabilitation services need be provided with such services, and thus avoid even seeing clients who might in some way be problematic.[38]

Most of the mechanisms vocational counselors use to solve their professional conflicts aim at obtaining "tangible" proof of their having rendered an important and socially useful service—namely, the return to gainful employment of as many of the disabled as they can include in their "active" files.[39] This central aim serves an important psychological function for the vocational counselor, who belongs to an "emerging" profession and who feels that he ". . . can command little attention unless there is a demand—genuine or artificially contrived—for the service."[40] However, a considerable number of socially and physically disabled individuals get squeezed out of vocational rehabilitation at least partially because of the vocational counselor's professional problems and dilemmas. Because they do not enhance the counselor's professional status but instead may impede the advancement of his career, these "poor" cases are eliminated from the rolls although they more than any other category of disabled need effective vocational rehabilitation services.[41]

Whether a rehabilitant will be granted vocational training or not depends again upon the vocational counselor who, according to stereotypic thinking, rejects all those who need it most, that is, those who are socially disabled—particularly in terms of age and education. There is, however, some evidence that on-the-job training may have excellent results with socially disabled people because it is more concrete than scholastic training, has a built-in monetary reinforcement, and some reassurance of a job.[42] Furthermore, vocational counselors are often accused of not offering the disabled the types of vocational training that are in demand because vocational courses are not adjusted to current and actual market needs.[43] Thus a rehabilitant may successfully complete a six- or twelve-month training program only to discover that all this time and effort cannot help him find a job.

While the role of the vocational counselor is restricted to the rehabilitation center, his decisions considerably influence the disabled's mode of adjustment when he returns to the community. The disabled may be given vocational training that is useless or he may be sent to potential employers without much research on the part of the vocational counselor and collect rejections that completely break down his morale and finally cause him to lose interest in seeking a job.[44] The vocational counselor anxious to see "success"—that is, the gainful employment of his client—may place him in a job much lower than his predisability one in terms of prestige and/or financial reward (a deadend job) or one that is not appropriate for his physical condition. In the former case, the disabled worker may soon become alienated from his job; his performance may become poor; and he may be fired at the first adverse business cycle. In the latter case, the physical (and/or emotional) strains of the job may cause an aggravation of the disabled worker's physical condition resulting in high absenteeism, eventual firing, and a fear to work again.

The Insurance Carrier: The "Enemy"

The insurance carrier seems to hinder the return of disabled workers to gainful employment either directly or indirectly. Although employers often mention the insurance problem as a reason for not hiring the handicapped, there are indications that it constitutes a rationalization rather than a real reason. This is evidenced by the fact that the frequency of its mention depends largely upon whether or not the employer is reminded of compensation costs. The direct intervention of compensation in the disabled workers' rehabilitation has been discussed in detail elsewhere in this book. The indirect effects of insurance, however, merit at least a brief mention. The policy of "retrospective insurance coverage" may often motivate the personnel and/or medical departments of a firm to refuse employment to old or new disabled workers so that a portion of the prepaid insurance premium is returned. Despite the fact that insurance carriers do not dictate hiring policies, they may issue "warnings" about "high claim risk" workers that can be very effective barriers to the hiring (or keeping on) of several categories of disabled workers. Finally, through insurance an employer can prematurely "retire" a disabled worker who is capable of returning to work because he is labeled a "high risk" in terms of future claims.[45]

Besides the direct influence of insurance upon reemployment, the disabled may have experienced extremely bad treatment at the hands of insurance company representatives, who may have handled him as if his disability were not *bona fide* and he was trying to cheat. There may have been delays in paying the compensation wages upon which the worker relies for providing for himself and his family, and the negative nature of this relationship may have rendered him uncooperative and distrustful.[46] The insurance representatives may have exerted pressure upon the disabled to accept a settlement by threatening to discontinue (or actually discontinuing) his weekly payments. In such cases the disabled, out of an extreme need for money, may have accepted the settlement and felt "cheated out of his rights."[47]

The Unions: Are They Interested in the Disabled Worker?

The role of the unions in the disabled worker's return to work seems to be ambivalent and at times contradictory. Some investigators have suggested that the disabled worker may be viewed as a pawn in the endless power struggle between union and management. In the case of a disabled worker with many years of stable work and a record of good performance who has been certified by physicians as being able to return to his previous work, the union fights vehemently for his reinstatement and seniority rights. If, however, the individual's work record does not look good, the union will not intervene on his behalf, and he will most probably be rejected and forced to look for a new job with all the odds against him.[48]

A survey study conducted among representative large firms in Atlanta, Georgia, showed that of the eleven unions involved, only one union's attitude was judged by management as favorable toward the employment of physically handicapped workers. Three unions were indifferent, and two were indifferent unless there was interference with seniority provisions. Five unions were said to want the disabled workers kept on the payroll but did not support the idea of their being reemployed. As a union representative said: "Handicapped people cause trouble, and we would rather not have them."[49] Another study of five industrial plants in New Jersey, in which industrial physicians, management, union leaders, and workers were interviewed about the role of the unions in safety, health matters, and compensation cases, showed considerable variation from union to union.[50] While all unions were more or less concerned about safety, the quality of medical care received by workers, the amount of weekly payments to injured workers, and their education concerning their right to compensation, few were actively involved in further compensation issues. The physicians and management in some of these industries were under the impression that unions try to help workers prove that every pain and ache is occupationally caused, and there is evidence that union leaders perceive management and physicians as exploitative and hostile toward the disabled worker.[51] However, the collected data are not nearly complete enough to permit us to assess clearly the role of the unions.

It also seems that the much-defended seniority rights which may work for a disabled worker who is physically able to return to his previous job may become a stumbling block in the reemployment of those who must change job categories or departments within the same firm because of disability. In the case of such transfers, union rules require them to start at the bottom of the seniority ladder in terms of pay, pension prospects, and degree of assurance of continued employment. This is reported by the employed disabled workers themselves and always by surveyed employers or managers, but is usually denied by union leaders.[52] An objective study of the actual role played by different types of unions is needed before any definite conclusions can be drawn.

The Family: Stimulus or Hindrance?

The role of the family in the disability and rehabilitation odyssey has not always been studied in depth; many studies have gone only so far as to examine the disabled's marital status and the number of his dependents. But even these descriptive family variables have provided some interesting findings, especially when combined with the sex of the disabled person. For example, there is evidence that married women with young or adolescent children, even if seriously disabled, are taken back by their families at the end of treatment or rehabilitation. They are thus aided in getting reintegrated into their family so that they can best perform their wife and mother roles. In contrast, men who have families in the same stage of the family cycle are not usually welcome back unless they can still perform the breadwinner role (either by working or by having independent means to support the family in a style close to the predisability one). These findings tend to indicate that when the woman's primary role is that of mother and housekeeper, the basic tasks involved in this role can be satisfactorily performed even in the presence of a serious physical or mental disability. On the contrary, the husband's breadwinner role has tasks and requirements which are often profoundly disturbed by the onset of a physical or mental disability. It is possible that in the case of men, the sexual role tends to be more disturbed by disabilities than in the case of women and that dependence is less tolerated by their wives. Thus, the frequency of wives divorcing or deserting their husbands in this case (probably in order to replace them with gainfully employed and sexually potent husbands) is high, while no incidence of husbands deserting their disabled wives has been reported in the literature.[53]

Among the unmarried young adult disabled, women again fare much better than men since they are usually taken back by their families while men are not. Among children the sex differential does not operate since they can all return to their families. Of course, the obvious questions which have been raised but not answered are:[54] (a) What happens to married women after their mothering role is over? Probably, at this point the degree of the husband's satisfaction with the marriage may be the determining factor as to whether the wife can still function successfully or whether she will be abandoned to a hospital or nursing home. (b) What happens to seriously disabled male children when they become young adults? Do all parents give them up to a hospital or some other type of institution? Or here again, does the type of parent-child relationship determine the outcome? The most satisfactory answers to these questions can come only from more longitudinal research. Of course, it must be remembered that all these findings are based on seriously disabled persons; the trends may be very different when the degree of disability is slighter.

It is known, however, that women 65 years of age and over have less chance of returning to their homes than do men in the same age group because of the greater probability that they are already widowed. But these women are more welcomed by their relatives than are men.[55] There is also some evidence that older married men are more readily welcomed back to their families because their wives, having raised the children, are in a position (and may be willing) to take over the breadwinner role.[56]

Marital status seems to be related in a seemingly surprising way to the disabled individual's rate of recovery and rehabilitation. Whenever married and unmarried disabled who have left the hospital are examined, it is found that single, widowed, divorced, and separated disabled tend to be more independent in daily functional activities (ADL) than the married disabled in the same sample.[57] The explanation for this probably lies in the fact that the absence of someone very close, emotionally and affectively, on whom an individual depends to a large extent for the performance of the activities of daily living, forces the disabled to use all their abilities and skills and therefore to become as independent as their disability permits. There is also some evidence that the poor improvement rate among the married disabled may be due to anxiety-ridden or overprotective families who prevent them from recovering to the fullest extent possible or in some cases from even making use of rehabilitation services.[58]

But it has also been found that among the married disabled pressing role demands and high level of expectation on the part of other family members are conducive to the successful rehabilitation of the disabled member. For example, resumption of the working role by male disabled was much higher when there were young children or young adult children in the family than at any other stage of the family cycle, because at these two stages the pressure for the successful performance of the instrumental role is the highest. In the case of working married women (even those who are predisposed to work during all stages of the family cycle), whenever the mothering role is important because of the young age of the children, they opt for this role—which, as we have seen, is more compatible with the presence of disabilities.[59]

We could summarize these findings as follows: *In the case of the noninstitutionalized disabled, the greater the necessity to perform tasks and roles, the greater the probability that they will use all their abilities to do so.* This conclusion can also explain some of the contradictory findings of studies investigating the effects of family solidarity, cohesion, or organization upon the disabled's rehabilitation.[60] Of course, it must be noted that some of these studies examined the relationship among these variables during the disabled's stay at a rehabilitation center rather than after he had been discharged and was living at home. As would be expected, the influence of the family in the two settings is very different, being considerably weaker while the disabled is in any type of institutional setting, including a rehabilitation center.[61] Still, Litman found that the existence of close family ties and the willingness of significant others to take care of the disabled often discouraged the individual from undergoing the rigors of rehabilitative treatment.[62] There was, however, a significant relationship between family reinforcement and rehabilitation success.

One detailed study of the disabled's return to their families has shown that there is seldom a complete congruency between the disabled and his significant others about the degree to which he is dependent or independent in the activities of everyday living (ADL). The degree of such agreement, however, is higher between the disabled and their spouses than between the disabled and their children or the disabled and their friends or rehabilitation professionals when the spouses tend to think that the disabled spouse is dependent. The authors of this study have assumed that agreement in the perceptions of the disabled and their significant others about the extent of independence or dependence is most conducive to the disabled's maintaining rehabilitation gains and further improving their physical condition.[63] All the literature examined above, however, points out that successful improvement in ADL is achieved when spouses and other significant others think the disabled person is more independent than he thinks he is or wishes the others to believe and urge him to behave according to their expectations.

The worst combination for the disabled's rehabilitation outcome is most probably that in which the significant others (especially the spouse) perceive the disabled as more dependent than he himself thinks he is, since this is usually the portrait of an overprotective family thwarting the disabled's efforts toward independence. But agreement between the disabled and his spouse that he is dependent may often have similarly unfavorable results for the disabled's long-range adjustment, since it will most probably lead to a gradual deterioration in his physical status and the gradual loss of gains during active rehabilitation treatment.

To complicate things, significant others do not agree among themselves about the degree to which the disabled person is dependent or independent, and their expectations as well as their behavior toward him are shaped by their perceptions. Thus, most often the disabled is caught in the "cross-fire" of his differing significant others. A spouse may think he is more independent than the disabled himself thinks he is and expect him to behave accordingly. His children may think he is more dependent than he himself thinks he is (as has often been found to be the case)[64] and prevent him from conforming to his spouse's expectations by doing things for him. Like his wife, his friends may also think he is more independent than he himself thinks he is. The disabled may then experience frustration and a sense of powerlessness because everybody around him is deciding the things he can and cannot do. He may be pervaded with a sense of meaninglessness and self-estrangement since he will have difficulty in deciding who he is, how disabled he is, and why. The effect of being subject to a variety of often contradictory expectations and demands may give him a feeling of normlessness.

It is, however, possible that all the significant others' perceptions agree with those of the disabled in that he is quite dependent or quite independent in ADL. The congruence of perceptions toward independence could be hypothesized as being the most conducive to successful long-range rehabilitation outcome, since the significant others will continuously reinforce the disabled's efforts toward greater independence.

Let us now see briefly how the disability may affect significant others, particularly those involved in the marital relationship. There is some evidence that spouses of chronically ill (or mentally ill) persons develop symptoms such as nervousness, feelings of fatigue, symptoms of role tension (getting jumpy or jittery, easily angry or easily depressed), and report reduction in their work activities during illness.[65] And since the symptoms and role tension experienced by some spouses are equal or greater than those experienced by the "sick" spouse, it is sometimes quite possible that he or she falls sick when the patient returns home after treatment or rehabilitation.[66] It is this possibility which sometimes prevents the return home of the disabled person and renders his rehabilitation chances slim.[67]

There is also evidence that a spouse's degree of marital satisfaction does not vary directly with the degree of disability afflicting the other spouse. Actually it seems that in the case of clear-cut serious disabilities severely affecting physical mobility, there is little ambiguity in role definitions and expectations. This favors the marital relationship despite the fact that the spouse's companionship satisfaction may be decreased. In the case of moderate disabilities with ambiguous and often variable prognoses, role definitions and expectations on the part of the spouses may be so ambiguous and inconsistent that marital interaction and satisfaction are affected in a way that is not much different from when the spouse is seriously disabled. It is also interesting to note that sexual relations are not linearly affected by the degree of disability. In one study the great majority of seriously disabled women living with their husbands reported "normal" sexual relations and some had borne children since their disablement.[68] Among a group of men with heart disease, return to normal sexual activity was related to return to gainful employment.[69] But as marital status was not considered in this study, we cannot be sure whether this relationship holds equally for married and unmarried men.

After having separately examined the different agents that legitimately enter into a disabled's life and determine much of it, let us take a synthetic look at their total interactive effect upon one disabled individual. He usually becomes the victim of all these "interested" parties, some ostensibly working for him and concerned about some particular aspect of his welfare, others clearly attempting to protect their proper interests against him. But even in the case of those agents on the side of the disabled, personal and professional interests and beliefs predominate or at best considerably color their recommendations. And they hardly ever take the wishes and needs of the disabled into consideration. In their view they are more skilled than he so that their judgment about what is "best" for him is necessarily more "valid."

There are some differences between the compensable and non-compensable disabled since the former have more "hostile" agents added to their list and only two to some extent "favorable" ones (at least according to their value systems): the lawyer and the "pro-disabled" physician. The overall picture is not very different, although the compensable disabled has even less chance of being permitted to find his own way and realize his own plans and decisions. Most disabled are caught in a situation in which the structural conditions for experiencing acute and multiple alienation are many. Their disability having rendered them socially deviant, each "interested" agent has a different prescription as to how they ought to cope with their deviance—that is, to what extent they should stay deviant and make the best of it or to what extent they ought to try to escape the deviance stigma and get reintegrated in the nondisabled society. Thus, they are continuously pulled and pushed between the two poles of social deviance and societal reintegration regardless of physical disability or personal preference. Eventually, having experienced all forms of alienation in all degrees of intensity, they may live their lives like marionettes whose strings are being moved by a number of uncoordinated puppeteers. At this point they may even become psychologically deviant and by withdrawing completely in order to find some kind of emotional equilibrium, may experience intense feelings of isolation.

Those disabled who in addition to their physical disability have a number of social disabilities are the ones who are faced with an even greater number of potentially alienative life situations. Thus, older disabled persons with a low level of education and occupational skills may have felt alienated since the early stages of their disability careers because of the type of medical care received as well as the mode of its being delivered to them. During the different stages of rehabilitation, from the initial evaluation period to the discharge, they are again the people who have a higher probability than others of being rejected altogether or of being discharged before any substantial improvement has come about. They also more often than others may be denied vocational training and may encounter extremely difficult problems when seeking employment. Most often they are the ones who at followups are found to be unemployed, working part-time, or working in stagnant or downgraded jobs, all these employment statuses having been found as highly alienative to those bearing them. Thus, the physically and socially disabled seem to combine in the postrehabilitation stage (if they ever got rehabilitated) much more acutely all alienative structural conditions. This pattern of alienation is even more exaggerated in the case of those physically and socially disabled who are afflicted with a rather severe disability which requires a careful and complicated medical regime that they are not always able to maintain. Then, a further vicious circle may be set between their physical and social disabilities and their feelings of alienation, which may be aggravated by and aggravate further both types of disabilities.

It is quite disheartening to find that the lives of the disabled, especially those doubly disabled at the end of intensive treatment, provide a vivid, nonfiction illustration of the total alienation described by Kafka in *The Trial*. It is a perfect example of a complex network of institutions and high-prestige professions, not necessarily interrelated and each for different reasons and out of different motivations, imposing upon a single individual conditions and decisions that will profoundly and irreversibly affect the course of his entire life. In addition, the bewildered individual has very little recourse for fighting back and asserting his own individuality and power to make decisions. He is crushed by too many heterogeneous and warring influences which usually end up dominating the mode and outcome of his disabled life because at a very early point they were successful in taking away his sense of autonomy and self-determination.

NOTES

1. For a typology of alienation, see Melvin Seeman, "On the Meaning of Alienation," *American Sociological Review*, 24 (December 1959), 783–91.
2. Such examples abound throughout Raymond Duff and August B. Hollingshead, *Sickness and Society* (New York: Harper & Row, 1968), especially pp. 107–216. See also D. C. Riedel, R. L. Eichorn, and W. H. M. Morris, "Information and Beliefs Concerning Health and Heart Disease," *Proceedings of the Purdue Farm Cardiac Seminar* (Lafayette, Ind., September 10–11, 1958). The latter presents a good example of the kind of erroneous diagnosis which can shape people's lives as if they were disabled. See also H. Kessler and G. C. Manning, Jr., "The Effect of Personal Opinion on Disability Evaluation," *Journal of Occupational Medicine*, 5, 9 (September 1963), 411–17; G. C. Manning, Jr., "Estimation of Disability Following Injury," *Journal of International College of Surgery*, 33 (April 1960), 471–81; and G. C. Manning, Jr., *Disability and the Law* (Baltimore: Williams and Wilkins, 1962).

3. J. N. Muller, "Rehabilitation Evaluation—Some Social and Clinical Problems," *American Journal of Public Health,* 51, 3 (March 1961), 403–8; Leonard Policoff, "Diagnostic Challenge of Back Pain," *Archives of Physical Medicine and Rehabilitation,* 41 (October 1960), 441–45; Earl D. McBride, "Disability Evaluation Suggestions for the Solution of Some Irksome Medicolegal Perplexities," *The Journal of Bone and Joint Surgery,* 44A, 7 (October 1962), 1441–49; and Alan M. Mann and Ellen M. Gold, "Psychological Sequelae of Accidental Injury: A Medico-legal Quagmire," *The Canadian Medical Association Journal,* 95 (December 1966), 1359–63.

4. Gordon G. Bergy and Donald R. Sparkman, "Analysis of Experience in Workman's Compensation for Heart Cases," *Circulation,* 33 (March 1966), 461–73; and Chester C. Schneider, "Industrial Compensation for Low Back Injuries: Special Problems," *Journal of International College of Surgeons,* 35, 1 (January 1961), 105–10.

5. *Ibid.*; also *Final Report of the Cardiac Rehabilitation Project* (New York: Syracuse University, Upstate Medical Center, April 1966), especially p. 57.

6. Paul D. White *et al., Cardiovascular Rehabilitation* (New York: McGraw-Hill, 1957); "Report of the Committee on the Effect of Strain and Trauma on the Heart and Great Vessels," *Circulation,* 26 (October 1962), 612–21; and *Final Report of the Cardiac Rehabilitation Project, op. cit.,* pp. 51–54.

7. *Final Report of the Cardiac Rehabilitation Project, op. cit.,* pp. 34–41, 51–57.

8. *The California Workmen's Compensation System: Attitudes and Experiences of a Cross-section of California Physicians* (San Francisco: California Medical Association, Bureau of Research and Planning, July 1964), pp. 2–3, 12–13.

9. *Ibid.*; and Leo Price, "The Dilemma of Disability," *Journal of Occupational Medicine,* 7, 4 (April 1965), 148–49.

10. *Final Report of the Cardiac Rehabilitation Project, op. cit.,* pp. 34–35, 51–57. The implications of the indication that the most reputable doctors may not always welcome compensation patients are many in addition to the fact that such patients are not always able to avail themselves of the best medical care. There is some evidence that prominent physicians who do not believe that a particular type of illness or injury is compensable may be quite influential and contribute to the employers' distrust of the disabled.

11. We do not know the nature of the dynamics involved. Does sympathy for disabled persons or the identification with an employer (or insurance company) come first and then a medical rationalization that consistently favors the disabled or

the employers? Or does the espousal of medical theories that
are more favorable to the disabled or to the employers come
first? In any case, we also know little about the characteristics
that distinguish the "pro-disabled" from the "pro-employer"
physicians. See Mann and Gold, *op. cit.*, p. 1362.
12. There are, of course, exceptions to this. Some physicians are
exceptionally aware and sensitive to the role played by a vast
number of such variables. For example, see Leon J. Warshaw,
"Chronic Disease and Employability: The Physician's Role,"
Journal of American Medical Women's Association, 20, 12
(December 1965), 1120–25.
13. Rhoda L. Goldstein and Bernard Goldstein, *Doctors and Nurses
in Industry* (New Brunswick, N.J.: Rutgers University Press,
1967), pp. 35–53.
14. Bergy and Sparkman, *op. cit.,* p. 470; and *Final Report of the
Cardiac Rehabilitation Project, op. cit.,* p. 53.
15. Private communication of Julius A. Roth at the University of
California, Davis, included in his written comments on this
chapter.
16. Lindsay Thompson, "The Doctor," in the symposium, "The
Return of the Injured Worker to Work," *The Medical Journal
of Australia,* 2, 22 (November 26, 1966), 1063.
17. Marc H. Hollender *et al.,* "The Compensation Problem," *Inter-
national Psychiatry Clinics,* 2 (July 1965), 594; Gordon J.
Samuels, "The Lawyer's Point of View," in the symposium,
"The Return of the Injured Worker to Work," *The Medical
Journal of Australia,* 2, 22 (November 26, 1966), 1064–66;
Wilbur J. Lawrence, "The Legal Aspects of Employment of
Impaired Workers," *Industrial Medicine and Surgery,* 26
(November 1957), 512–15; and Douglass A. Campbell, "Heart
Disease and Compensability Under Workmen's Compensation,"
Journal of Occupational Medicine, 3 (February 1961), 73.
18. Some authors have mentioned this possibility but without
specification as to how such an objective medical committee
would be financed in order to guarantee its objectivity. See
Howard J. Scott, "Employment Problems of the Cardiac,"
Industrial Medicine and Surgery, 23 (October 1954), 451;
and Bergy and Sparkman, *op. cit.,* p. 471.
19. *Final Report of the Cardiac Rehabilitation Project, op. cit.,* pp.
38–41, 53; Lawrence, *op. cit.,* pp. 512–14.
20. Z. L. Gulledge, "Summary Statement: Vocational Rehabilitation
of Industrially Injured Covered by California Workmen's
Compensation Laws," in A. J. Jaffe (ed.), *Research Conference
on Workmen's Compensation and Vocational Rehabilitation*
(New York: Bureau of Applied Social Research, Columbia
University, March 1961), p. 118; Monroe Berkowitz, "Sum-

mary Statement: Workmen's Compensation: The New Jersey Experience," in *ibid.*, p. 132; Earl F. Cheit, *Injury and Recovery in the Course of Employment* (New York: Wiley, 1961), p. 8; W. Scott Allan, "One or One Hundred Rehabilitation Agencies," *Rhode Island Medical Journal*, 46, 7 (July 1963), 364–67.

21. Allan, *op. cit.*, p. 366. Theodor J. Litman provided the following interesting case study in a personal communication included in the comments to the second draft of this chapter: "A 45-year-old welder was injured when his torch set off an explosion in a railroad roundhouse. During his course of treatment at the rehabilitation center, his lawyer refused to have him seen by a psychiatrist, a clinical psychologist, a research sociologist (Litman) or anyone other than his physician. Moreover, he was told how important it was for his case to appear as sick as possible when he went to court. As a result, throughout the 3-month period of rehabilitation, he refused to cooperate with the rehabilitation therapists and became a self-accentuated invalid even though his prognosis was considered at least fair to good. His lack of motivation and cooperation was periodically reinforced by his attorney. Ultimately, it appeared to pay off with a $500,000 settlement, the largest in the state's history—which was later reduced to $150,000 by an appellate court. He was subsequently released from the rehabilitation center, $150,000 in hand, and a pitifully invalidated man."

22. James N. Morgan, Marvin Snider, and Marion G. Sobol, *Lump Sum Redemption Settlements and Rehabilitation* (Ann Arbor, Mich.: Survey Research Center, Institute for Social Research, 1959), p. 97.

23. Samuels, *op. cit.*, p. 1064; and William Schwarz, " 'Compensable' Trauma," *Medical Trial Technique Quarterly*, 9 (1962–1963), p. 43.

24. Samuels, *op. cit.*; Morgan *et al.*, *op. cit.*, pp. 105–16. When, however, the injuries were distinguished into ambiguous and clear-cut (with obvious clinical symptoms), workers who had received lump sum settlements were more likely to return to work than those compensated weekly. The contrary was true in the case of clear-cut injuries. Since, however, the degree of disability was not taken into consideration, the evidence is not conclusive as to whether the observed difference is due to the system of compensation or to the differential distribution of severe disabilities in the two groups of injuries. The entire discussion on lump sum settlements is based upon the findings of the Morgan *et al.* study.

25. *Ibid.*

26. Dawson, quoted in Lawrence, *op. cit.*, p. 515.

27. Morgan *et al., op. cit.*, p. 62; Lawrence, *op. cit.*, p. 511; and W. Scott Allen, "Successful Placement of Handicapped Workers," *Archives of Environmental Health*, 7 (November 1963), 623; Earl D. McBride, "Trauma, Rehabilitation, and Permanent Disability," *Industrial Medicine and Surgery*, 29 (May 1960), 199.
28. *Final Report of the Cardiac Rehabilitation Project, op. cit.*, pp. 83–99; and *A Study of the Integration of Services of Industrial Medical Departments and a Rehabilitation Center: Final Report* (Special Project Grant RD 221, Pittsburgh, Harmarville Rehabilitation Center, June 1963), p. 29.
29. Harold L. Sheppard, "Unemployment Experiences of Older Workers," *Geriatrics*, 15, 6 (June 1960), 430–33; and L. Myrton Gaines *et al.*, "Vocational Evaluation of the Handicapped," *Maryland State Medical Journal*, 15 (March 1966), 124.
30. *Final Report of the Cardiac Rehabilitation Project, op. cit.*, pp. 67, 70–72.
31. Jack Pockrass, "Selective Placement in Hiring the Handicapped," *Public Personnel Review*, 20, 1 (January 1959), 25–32; E. H. Barton, Arthur P. Coladarci, and Karl E. Carlson, "The Employability and Job-seeking Behavior of the Physically Handicapped: Employers' Views," *Archives of Physical Medicine and Rehabilitation*, 35 (December 1954), 763–64.
32. *Final Report of the Cardiac Rehabilitation Project, op. cit.*, pp. 66–72; E. T. Eggers, "Employment of the Physically Handicapped," *Industrial Medicine and Surgery*, 29 (September 1960), 428–29; and Simon Olshansky *et al.*, "A Survey of Employment Policies as Related to Cardiac Patients in Greater Boston," *The New England Journal of Medicine*, 253, 12 (September 22, 1955), 507.
33. At least one study concluded that employers are prejudiced against disabled applicants. See Thomas E. Rickard, H. C. Triandis, and C. H. Patterson, "Indices of Employer Prejudice Toward Disabled Applicants," *Journal of Applied Psychology*, 47, 1 (February 1963), 52–55.
34. Barton *et al., op. cit.*, pp. 763–64.
35. Ronald Baxt, "Selections From Survey of Employers' Practices and Policies in the Hiring of Physically Impaired Workers," in Jaffe, *op. cit.*, pp. 71–72.
36. Barton *et al., op. cit.*, p. 764; Earl R. Bramblett, "Problems of Management in the Placement of Handicapped Workers," *Archives of Physical Medicine and Rehabilitation*, 37 (September 1956), 548–49; Eggers, *op. cit.*, p. 433; Warshaw, *op. cit.*, p. 1124; and *Final Report of the Cardiac Rehabilitation Project, op. cit.*, pp. 68–69.

37. Cheit, *op. cit.*, pp. 156–59.
38. Elliot A. Krause, "Structured Strain in a Marginal Profession: Rehabilitation Counseling," *Journal of Health and Human Behavior*, 6, 1 (Spring 1965), 59–61.
39. Henry Lenard, "Issues for the Rehabilitation Counselor," *Journal of Rehabilitation*, 24 (September–October 1963), 12–13.
40. Marvin B. Sussman, "Occupational Sociology and Rehabilitation," in Marvin B. Sussman (ed.), *Sociology and Rehabilitation* (Washington, D.C.: American Sociological Association, 1965), p. 196.
41. Lenard, *op. cit.*
42. See Milton Friedman, "The Use of Training-on-the-Job (TOJ) Opportunities in Rehabilitation Services," *Rehabilitation in Canada* (Fall–Winter 1962–63); and Orville R. Gursslin and Jack L. Roach, "Some Issues in Training the Unemployed," *Social Problems*, 12, 1 (Summer 1964), 86–98.
43. Gursslin and Roach, *op. cit.*
44. Gaines *et al.*, *op. cit.*, p. 124.
45. *Final Report of the Cardiac Rehabilitation Project*, *op. cit.*, pp. 45–47.
46. Thompson, *op. cit.*, pp. 1063–64.
47. Morgan *et al.*, *op. cit.*
48. *Final Report of the Cardiac Rehabilitation Project*, *op. cit.*, pp. 74–76.
49. Eggers, *op. cit.*, pp. 430, 432. The fact that all these judgments concerning the unions' attitudes were made by management may also mean that management may not have correct information. However, since employment of the disabled is determined by management, what management regards as the unions' attitudes will greatly influence their hiring practices.
50. Goldstein and Goldstein, *op. cit.*, pp. 79–87.
51. *Final Report of the Cardiac Rehabilitation Project*, *op. cit.*, pp. 75–76.
52. Employees have been reported to complain about the difficulties created by seniority rules in *A Study of the Integration of Services of Industrial Medical Departments and a Rehabilitation Center*, *op. cit.*, p. 36. There is a vast literature reporting that employers, managers, or professionals taking management's side complain about seniority rules. Finally, the denial of serious difficulties for the employment of handicapped workers as a direct result of established seniority rules can be seen in the data presented in the *Final Report of the Cardiac Rehabilitation Project*, *op. cit.*, pp. 72–76.
53. Cynthia P. Deutch and Judith A. Goldston, "Family Factors in Home Adjustment of the Severely Disabled," *Marriage and Family Living*, 22, 4 (November 1960), 313.

54. *Ibid.*, p. 315.
55. George J. Vlasak and Harry T. Phillips, *What Comes After Discharge* (Boston: Bureau of Chronic Disease Control, Department of Public Health, 1967), p. 24.
56. Lawrence D. Haber, *The Disabled Worker Under OASDI*, Research Report 6 (Washington, D.C.: U.S. Department of Health, Education, and Welfare, Social Security Administration, Division of Research and Statistics, October 1964), pp. 45–59; and Geoffrey Gibson and Edward G. Ludwig, "Family Structure in a Disabled Population," *Journal of Marriage and the Family*, 30, 1 (February 1968), 56–57.
57. *Ibid.*, pp. 62–63.
58. Joseph B. Rogoff, Donald V. Cooney, and Bernard Kutner, "Hemiplegia: A Study of Home Rehabilitation," *Journal of Chronic Diseases*, 17 (June 1964), 539–50.
59. Geoffrey Gibson and Edward G. Ludwig, "Family Role Demands and Disability Behavior" (paper presented at the Ohio Valley Sociological Society meetings, Detroit, May 1968). Other findings indicate that retention of rehabilitation gains was also related to the degree of responsibility for others with which the disabled was burdened. See Edward Scull *et al.*, "A Follow-up Study of Patients Discharged From a Community Rehabilitation Center," *Journal of Chronic Diseases*, 15 (February 1962), 207–13.
60. Theodor J. Litman, "The Family and Physical Rehabilitation," *Journal of Chronic Diseases*, 19 (February 1966), 211–17; E. Z. Dager and D. L. Brewer, "Family Integration and the Response to Heart Disease," in *Proceedings of the Purdue Farm Cardiac Seminar, op. cit.*, pp. 62–64; and Castro De la Mata, R. G. Gingras, and E. D. Wittkower, "Impact of Sudden, Severe Disablement of the Father Upon the Family," *The Canadian Medical Association Journal*, 82 (May 1960), 1015–20; Jane C. Kronick, "The Rehabilitation of Stroke Patients: An Experimental Analysis of the Effects of Physical and Social Factors in Determining Recovery" (mimeographed, Bryn Mawr, Pa.: Bryn Mawr College, Department of Social Work and Social Research, 1962).
61. Litman, "The Family and Physical Rehabilitation," *op. cit.*; and Leon Lewis and Rose Coser, "The Dangers of Hospitalization" (part of "Observations on Patient, Response III," unpublished manuscript, Waltham, Mass., 1959–1960), pp. 307–8.
62. Litman, "The Family and Physical Rehabilitation," *op. cit.*
63. Peter Kong-Ming New *et al.*, "The Support Structure of Heart and Stroke Patients: A Study of Significant Others in Patient Rehabilitation," *Social Science and Medicine*, 2, 2 (June 1968), 185–200.

64. *Ibid.*
65. Robert F. Klein, Alfred Dean, and Morton D. Bogdonoff, "The Impact of Illness Upon the Spouse," *Journal of Chronic Diseases,* 20 (April 1967), 241–48; and Gerassimos Alivisatos and George Lyketsos, "A Preliminary Report of Research Into the Attitude of the Families of Hospitalized Mental Patients," *World Mental Health,* 14, 1 (February 1962), 20–30.
66. Klein *et al., op. cit.,* p. 247.
67. Alivisatos and Lyketsos, *op. cit.*
68. Stephen L. Fink, James K. Skipper, Jr., and Phyllis N. Hallenbeck, "Physical Disability and Problems in Marriage," *Journal of Marriage and the Family,* 30, 1 (February 1968), 64–73.
69. Charles E. Lewis, "Factors Influencing the Return to Work of Men With Congestive Heart Failure," *Journal of Chronic Diseases,* 19 (November–December 1966), 1193–1209.

CHAPTER 8

Recommendations and Projections About Disability and Rehabilitation in the Future

Despite some tentative beginnings, the most significant questions concerning rehabilitation research either have not yet been raised or have not yet been adequately answered. A number of assumptions can be found in the rehabilitation literature of the various disciplines as to factors which facilitate or impede the therapeutic or "social-integration" aspects of the rehabilitation process. However, very few of these assumptions have been adequately researched and evaluated and thus are useful only as hypotheses to be rigorously and repeatedly tested in a variety of settings.

At this point, there are few recommendations for necessary changes in the institution of rehabilitation that one could suggest on the basis of solid evidence. Most recommendations would be based on moral convictions and humanitarian concerns (or vested interest in some type of change), rather than irrefutable evidence. The only strong recommendation that an "uninvolved" scientist could make at this point would be that extensive research programs be developed in all rehabilitation centers, workmen's compensation boards, and other disability program administrations. Hopefully, extensive research would provide objective and pragmatic guidelines for effective therapy on the part of rehabilitation personnel, for a more successful integration of the disabled into "normal" society, and for policy changes in rehabilitation legislation as well as in all legislation involving disability. Throughout this book we have encountered a considerable number of research "blanks," shortcomings, and biases. We shall attempt now to delineate those research questions and areas that are crucial for therapy or policy changes.

1. What features of a disability program are most conducive to the disabled individual regardless of his socioeconomic status? (a) Receiving high-quality medical care so that he can physically improve as much as possible; (b) becoming successfully reintegrated into "normal" society as a full-fledged and "equal" member not only in terms of gainful employment, but in terms of social and emotional acceptance as well; and (c) avoiding financial and psychological suffering during his treatment. At the present time there is a great variety of disability programs in the United States and abroad. A well-controlled evaluative study comparing the different disability programs in operation, conducted on an international scale by competent sociologists and social psychologists—with the consultative services of lawyers, physicians, and insurance personnel—could be expected to yield valuable information for those who wish to establish new disability programs or to ameliorate existing ones.

2. How do the disabled perceive the "disabled" and "rehabilitant" roles according to their type and severity of disability and their social and sociopsychological makeup? We know how physicians and most rehabilitation personnel define these roles and how they expect the disabled to behave if they wish to be the recipients of rehabilitation services.[1] What we do not know is the extent to which the medical definitions of the "disabled" and "rehabilitant" roles are conducive to

the rehabilitants' physical improvement and reintegration into normal
society. It is possible that the definitions of these roles by some
categories of the disabled or some aspects of these roles as defined by
all disabled are more conducive to all aspects of rehabilitation than
the medical definitions. Therefore, empirical validation studies of these
roles should be conducted on a variety of populations—rehabilitation
personnel, disabled people with a variety of disabilities, significant
others in the lives of the disabled, and a random sample of the general
population. In addition, controlled experiments could be carried out
in which rehabilitants would be permitted to function according to
their own definitions of the "disabled" and "rehabilitant" roles while
the rehabilitation personnel would have been educated to accept and
go along with these definitions. On the other side of the experiment,
rehabilitants would be educated and socialized according to the
medical definitions of these roles and would have to function according to those operational obligations. Through a careful assessment
of the rehabilitation process and the postdischarge degree of societal
integration, we would be able to discover which role definitions were
most functional for long-range rehabilitation and, correspondingly,
whether we must "educate" the rehabilitation staff or some categories
of disabled or both.

　　　3. We do not have any good sociological study of the rehabilitation personnel as a social system, especially of the rehabilitation team
in operation, that sheds light upon the types of conflicts, problems,
and rivalries that may be handicapping efficient and coordinated
efforts. Yet it is necessary for us to know the effects, if any, of these
conflicts upon the rehabilitants' degree of cooperation with the entire
program, with particular staff member's suggestions, or with required
tasks. Such a study would indicate the problem areas as well as the
kinds of accommodations or programs which have in some instances
facilitated better communications, better coordination of effort, and
better relationships among staff members and between staff members and rehabilitants. Then, different types of accommodations
and programs could be tested out in rehabilitation settings and
evaluated for the types of changes they bring about in staff-to-staff
and in staff-to-rehabilitant interaction. The findings from this study
would clarify some questions in the area of motivation and would
indicate how the rehabilitants can develop better relationships with

the staff and become more consistently interested in working with them toward their rehabilitation. Such research would also indicate the policy that would best promote beneficial staff-to-staff and staff-to-rehabilitant interaction.

4. A related series of needed studies are those on the different rehabilitation professions. With the exception of vocational counseling, almost nothing has been done in this area. We do not know, for example, what the image of physiatry is among medical students or among other physicians and what the specific areas of friction are between physiatrists and medical practitioners, between physiatrists and physical therapists, between orthopedists and physical therapists. We also need to know the occupational problems of physical therapists, occupational therapists, speech therapists, and social workers working in rehabilitation centers. What is the extent of turnover in the occupations in which women dominate, and what is the effect of this turnover upon the occupation's prestige, power, and search for a unique identity? How do the members of the rehabilitation staff who are themselves disabled compare with those who are not, in terms of types of interaction and relationships established with the rehabilitants? Do they have an empathy with the disabled that permits them to be more effective therapists and to delineate more relevant rehabilitation goals? Does a positive relationship between a staff member's disabled status and his efficacy as a therapist hold true for all types of disabled staff and disabled rehabilitants or are there disability-specific relationships? These and other significant questions about the rehabilitation professions and their professional rivalries must be thoroughly investigated before we can start understanding the institution of rehabilitation and recommending changes.

5. What is the process that leads the disabled and his significant others to label a condition as a disability? Only a few research studies have dealt with the various aspects of the disabled's career leading from a state of relative health to the temporary acceptance of illness, to seeking rehabilitation, to the permanent acceptance of the disability label. Some theoretical typologies exist about the disabled's predisability personality and life experiences and the degree of incorporation of the disability into the self-concept (such as the one presented in Chapter 3), but very few empirical studies have tested this theoretical typology.

In the case of mental illness, some research findings are available about the definitional process followed by significant others. Data on the consequences of the type of label given to the afflicted person's condition and its effect on their relationship and the rehabilitant's chance for societal reintegration have been collected for the mentally ill, but there is hardly anything comparable for the physically disabled. We do not know, for example, what type of predisability husband-wife relationship leads to what type of disability labeling on the part of the nondisabled spouse. And once a disability label is given, we do not know what the consequences of such a label are for the marital relationship in couples with different types of husband-wife relationship, for the disabled's chance of returning to gainful employment, for being emotionally accepted as before by the nondisabled spouse, and for retaining the level of physical improvement gained during rehabilitation. The knowledge of types of marital relationships problematic for the disabled's rehabilitation could guide the efforts of rehabilitation personnel by signaling that some families need special help and counseling if they are to overcome the crisis of disability and facilitate instead of impeding the disabled's long-range acceptance in society.

6. While we have some good studies about the return of the mentally ill to their families and communities, we know very little about the adult physically disabled (rehabilitated or not) after their return to their families and communities.[2] The sporadic studies available have usually examined the employment status of the disabled and, more rarely, their physical status and progress and the type of care they receive. We have very little—and inconclusive—information about the social and emotional adjustment of the disabled, the amount and significance of the acceptance he receives from his family, his circle of friends, relatives, and co-workers, and the larger community. We also need to know more about the nature of the changes that have come about in the disabled's relationships with a number of significant others or acquaintances and the nature of the changes in life goals that he made in order to achieve a certain level of societal reintegration. Other important questions are: How has disability affected the different roles played by the other family members? How have such changes affected family equilibrium and family dynamics, such as power structure, level of marital satisfaction, degree of emotional attachment, esteem, and admiration?

Up to now, the societal concern (but also the researcher's interest) has most often stopped short of the time of discharge from a rehabilitation program, despite the fact that the real test of whether or not rehabilitation has helped the disabled reintegrate himself into the society comes after he returns home.[3] There is also a need for controlled research studies of disabled who do not receive rehabilitation services, of disabled who have failed in rehabilitation according to the rehabilitation personnel's criteria, and of disabled who have successfully completed their rehabilitation program. Controlled studies would compare these three groups of disabled in terms of their long-range rehabilitation outcome; that is, in terms of their integration into societal and familial structures as well as in terms of the familial readjustments and adaptations to their disability. Only then will we be able to evaluate the selection criteria used in rehabilitation screening, the principles and techniques used in rehabilitation, and the overall effectiveness of the rehabilitation programs even for those who successfully complete such programs.

A general research recommendation is that longitudinal research projects which would combine several of the significant areas of research already mentioned be encouraged and financed. Such longitudinal studies could begin at the time of the first consultation with a physician for an illness which will be diagnosed as chronic or for an accident that has a high probability of leaving a disability residual.[4] The afflicted person could subsequently be followed through periods of medical treatment and/or hospitalizations (and operations), rehabilitation, and his attempts to find an acceptable position in society— socially, emotionally, and financially. Such studies should cover at least five years and in some cases five to ten years if diseases or conditions requiring long periods of care and rehabilitation are to be considered.

The advantages of longitudinal studies starting at the first visit to the physician are the following: (a) the possibility of assessing the disabled's predisability personality, marital relationship, and relationships with significant others with a greater degree of accuracy than at later stages; (b) the possibility of studying gradual changes in the disabled's self-concept as well as in his relationships with significant others (on his part or on the part of the significant others) and thus obtaining a dynamic picture of on-going processes rather than static images of situations at the particular time that the research is carried out; (c) the possibility of inspecting the complex interrelations that may exist among different factors affecting different stages of the disabled's career as well as the interrelations between the different stages. It will be possible, for example, to examine for which types of disabled and at which stages of the disabled career the spouse's definition of and advice concerning the nature and extent of the disability or the type of treatment needed is more crucial than that of the physician or of different significant others. Similarly, it is important to discover at which stages in the disability career (and for which disabled) the recommendations of different significant others or of experts outweigh those of the spouse. It will be possible to assess the extent and the way in which the choices made by the disabled at one stage of his "career" necessarily influence those he will make at subsequent stages. The knowledge of the relative importance of influential factors and choices made at different levels would aid those interested in intervening and modifying "undesirable" disability careers to do so at the right time, by influencing the right factors. Finally, longitudinal studies would give the whole dynamic picture of the on-going processes and would enable practitioners, therapists, and administrators to better understand the dynamics of rehabilitation, the problem areas, and the strategic points at which appropriate intervention could bring about significant results.

In addition to those already mentioned, more research should be carried out in the following areas:

1. *Job adaptations that would permit all persons, disabled or not, to continue working.* Particularly crucial would be the investigation of adaptations of certain categories of jobs whose tasks could be performed by disabled in the major disability categories. In this way most of the disabled could continue working after the occurrence of the disability without ever being labeled "vocationally disabled" or requiring special efforts in order to cope with their problem.[5] Campaigns to persuade employers to hire the handicapped would be unnecessary, since the disabled would no longer be vocationally handicapped. Of course, this could not happen until the physical limitations resulting from disabilities as well as the degree and nature of remaining abilities were accurately evaluated. This is another area of research where interdisciplinary projects involving physiatrists, occupational physicians, psychologists, and sociologists must be en-

couraged. When such adaptations have become technically feasible and relatively inexpensive, employers could be educated to use them, since firms would soon realize that they would be less costly than paying workmen's compensation. Government subsidies (or tax exemptions) could also be employed in order to facilitate the hiring of disabled workers.

2. *Research focused on educating the nondisabled to accept the disabled socially and emotionally—in other words, research aimed at finding ways to diminish the psychological barriers that inhibit the disabled from becoming integrated into the "normal" society.* New areas of investigation should be explored, such as the possibility of intervening with sterotyped beliefs and values about the disabled through the use of such entertainment media as television, movies, magazine articles, children's books, and the like.[6] The enactment of humanitarian legislation will never solve the problems of the disabled unless it is accompanied by drastic changes in the nondisabled's (and the nonvisible disabled's) values and attitudes concerning health and beauty.

3. *Research concerning the prevention of accidents, congenital diseases, and chronic illnesses.* Such research is by necessity multidisciplinary. Sociologists and social psychologists, in particular, should not only focus upon the investigation of the social and sociopsychological factors that contribute to accidents and disabling illnesses, but also upon the ways in which such factors could be manipulated and altered so as to diminish the disability rates.

4. *Cross-cultural studies of the different subjects concerning disability and rehabilitation already mentioned.* At present hardly any truly cross-cultural study exists. Such studies are essential for determining which values, attitudes, and behavioral choices are universal and which are culturally determined. Besides its purely scientific worth, such information is important for the understanding of cultural differences among disabled of different cultural backgrounds.

In addition to research, there are other recommendations that could be made, based partly upon changing societal values and realities and partly upon the author's values. They are: (1) The present emphasis on vocational rehabilitation (leading to the exclusion of those who cannot be placed in gainful employment or who are not interested in working) should be eliminated so that everyone in need of physical rehabilitation can obtain it. Since increasingly fewer jobs will be available (even if many new jobs are created), society will have to find other ways of maintaining the unemployed disabled without placing a moral stigma upon them. (2) Some kind of reward system will have to be devised for those therapists who are most effective in improving the physical and psychological status of the "undesirable" disabled—those who are severely disabled, in low educational and socioeconomic status levels, aged, "uncooperative" and "unmotivated."[7] If special rewards existed for effectiveness with the undesirable disabled, all disabled might have a chance of being treated more or less equally during rehabilitation and would probably have similar chances of improving. Since the "desirable" disabled would still be chosen anyway, there would be no fear of their ever being neglected. (3) Rehabilitation regulations should not only allow but encourage the disabled to actively participate in decision-making processes regarding the determination of rehabilitation goals and recommended changes in their program. They would then feel part of the rehabilitation undertaking, and be inclined to do the required tasks and make an effort to improve. (4) Whenever the needed rehabilitation services (physical, psychological, social or vocational) for any person are not covered by a particular insurance scheme, such services should be available free from the government (preferably not under the auspices of welfare). Similarly, whenever living expenses for the rehabilitant (in any category) and his dependents during any phase of rehabilitation are not provided by insurance, the government again should provide adequate coverage. (5) As long as the current workmen's compensation laws remain unchanged, an "objective" medical committee should be established, paid partly by workers and partly by employers. Some of the medicolegal battles between the "employers" physicians and the "disabled's" physicians could be then avoided as well as their alienative effect upon the disabled worker.

It is interesting to note at this point that the historical development of rehabilitation discussed in Chapter 1 shows a major thrust after each of the two world wars. There are already indications that the Vietnam war is responsible for biomedical and bio-engineering research focusing upon different aspects of physical rehabilitation. It is possible that this war may bring about an even greater concentration of effort and interest, not only in medical but also in vocational and social rehabilitation, because of the longer time period, the possible higher total number of disabled soldiers returning, and the questionable social and moral basis for the war. The stimulus provided by this war might result in spectacular advances in all aspects of rehabilitation: the available knowledge in the biological, engineering, and social sciences—as well as future research potentialities—could revolutionize the rehabilitation field.[8]

And now let's take a look at the future. What kinds of trends and social changes can be anticipated, what kinds of medical and technological innovations can reasonably be expected to take place within the next few decades? How could these changes affect the status of the disabled and the nature of the rehabilitation services offered to them? If we first look at the important medical innovations relevant to the questions discussed in this book, we could probably predict the following:

1. Possibly medical science will be able to control a greater number of chronic diseases (such as heart diseases, cancer), so that instead of dying, many more afflicted people will be able to live under proper medical care with varying degrees of disabilities. For example, the heart attack deaths are expected to be cut down considerably, if not eliminated entirely, and the present cure rate for cancer of about one-third of the cases is expected to double by 2000. Medical progress may provide increasingly effective means of controlling most chronic diseases so that the afflicted can live with minimum inconvenience and can successfully perform all their "normal" social roles and tasks. For example, improved chemical control of some mental illnesses has been forecast for the last third of this century, an advance that would permit a considerable number of presently chronically ill to function in society.[9]

It is, on the other hand, doubtful that chronic diseases will have been totally eliminated through prevention, even if the mechanism and the variety of etiologic factors are clearly designated and understood. Since a number of the etiologic factors are social and sociopsychological, it is extremely difficult to intervene and change them in the desired direction, for we neither have the necessary skills to change people's values and personalities nor can we easily overcome the ethical problems entailed in such types of preventive programs. It is not inconceivable, however, that social scientists will learn how to effectively influence people's values and behavior in desirable directions and that government agencies will wish to apply this knowledge. There are also some promising public health developments, such as the plan for mass physical examinations using computers and automated techniques which would cost little (estimated $25–30) but which would be thorough enough to detect the presence of most chronic diseases.[10] Similarly, diagnostic techniques are improving, and new tests have been developed. Again, with the use of computers and automated techniques, they could become more uniform, comprehensive, and accurate. In cases in which medical treatment cannot cure or successfully control a disease, there is a hope that effective prevention may preclude the development of the disease or allow it to be arrested at a very early stage.

2. Possibly advances in surgery, biochemistry, and related biomedical specialties will permit the survival of even more persons suffering serious acidents, but again with more or less serious disabilities. Some accident-prevention devices and regulations (such as seat belts and other possible car safety features)[11] may also decrease the number of fatalities but add to the number of surviving disabled persons. Medical progress may lead to the possibility of rejoining severed limbs, an achievement that would considerably reduce, if not eliminate, amputations. Also advances in surgery, particularly plastic surgery, could reduce disabilities caused by deformities, especially facial deformities.[12]

3. Despite some discouraging results in genetics research, it is conceivable that some of the present difficulties could be overcome and that the genetic makeup of unborn babies could be modified in such a manner as to eliminate mental retardation and all other congenital illnesses and conditions.[13] Such prospects, however, seem still quite remote, and it may take fifty years or more before concrete results are obtained.

4. Biomedical and biochemical advances may lead to the development of artificial limbs and organs that can function "normally" and almost as efficiently (in some cases more efficiently) than physiological limbs and organs. An entirely new field, that of bio-engineering, has important applications for the medical field, such as the development of plastic organs (blood vessels and heart valves), the

development of artificial limbs operated on electric impulses, and the development of miniature artificial kidneys or heart-lung machines that could be implanted in the human body.[14] There are predictions that the replacement of tissues and organs by artificial ones will have become widespread within the next two decades.[15] This prediction may not be too far-fetched, since there are already over 15,000 Americans walking around with artificial heart pacemakers and about 50,000 people using blood vessels made of nylon and dacron,[16] Transplantation of live organs, although sensational, does not seem to be very practical and may create serious ethical problems even if it could be perfected, so that most of the on-going research may well continue to concentrate on the perfection of artificial organs which would be cheap, easy to replace, and efficient. With the development of compact power sources, artificial limbs could be activated by other healthy muscles of the body and made to function as "normal" limbs.[17] Already some progress has been made in creating a myo-electric arm (first constructed in the Soviet Union) which is not yet very practical or very efficient, but which represents a significant step in this direction.[18] In the case of the blind, scientists have been working on the development of electronic devices sensitive to different colors, to the different shades of light and dark, and to other environmental changes that could help the blind to "see" and feel environmental changes and texture.

What do these possible future medical and technological advances mean and what are their probable consequences? The first two medical trends we discussed indicate that the total number of disabled individuals will increase because of a decrease in deaths due to chronic disease and serious accidents. However, some relative decrease in the number of the disabled may be expected in some categories, such as amputees, the facially deformed, and some chronically ill through prevention or total cure. But more important than sheer numbers is the fact that if the last type of biomedical and engineering innovative changes come about, it will become increasingly more difficult to distinguish the disabled from the nondisabled. For example, could one call "disabled" a person living with an efficiently running artificial heart implanted in his body when the hearts of the nondisabled may have a number of imperfections and deficiencies? Such a person will not be incapacitated for any type of work or recreational activity, and his disability will not even be visibly discernible. In this way the greater majority of disabled (who according to the statistics suffer from chronic diseases) could be restored to a 100 percent level of ability without any esthetic inconvenience. Similarly, those with paralyzed or missing extremities might be restored to a 100 percent level of activity. Even when the prostheses have become quite cosmetic, however, and these people no longer meet vocational or social barriers, they may encounter discrimination at the emotional level. Many of the nondisabled may still be reluctant to fall in love with and marry a person with myoelectric arms, even perfectly functioning ones. Besides, we do not know what types of sociopsychological problems the disabled would meet in adjusting to "artificiality" and to reliance upon electronic gadgetry. We also do not know how such disabled would be able to incorporate their artificial organs in their self-concept and how necessary modifications in their self-concept would influence their behavior and interpersonal relations.[19]

Other technological and social changes may take place that will also help to integrate the disabled into the larger society. First, it is conceivable that technological progress will permit a much greater degree of control over the physical environment so that all its aspects can be significantly modified according to an individual's needs and wishes. In order, however, to take advantage of technological advances offering maximum physical comfort, speed, and efficiency, we may have to rely increasingly upon all kinds of more or less complicated gadgets and artificial devices. It is possible that in the near future human reliance upon artificial devices—some of them attached to the body—may reach such an extent that it becomes quite acceptable and "normal" for a human being to function at a maximum with artificial devices constituting extensions of the body (and at that, extensions more functional than some of the natural parts of the body). At such a point in societal development, it may be easier for the nondisabled to accept the disabled emotionally, thus enabling them to achieve the desired perfect societal integration, because there would be a definitional blur between the disabled and the nondisabled. Both will rely upon gadgets, machinery, and artificial devices in order to live, work, and generally adapt to the new conditions of living. The new image of man would be that of a man plus necessary gadgetry, an image that would facilitate the societal (and perhaps even the emotional) acceptance of the disabled. We could even envision the possibility that those with some organs, extremities, or systems impaired might be able to cope with and adapt better to the mechanical-electrical apparatus that would be necessary for everyday living and for maximum comfort and efficiency.[20]

Second, technological progress through automation may change most industrial and service jobs in such a way that a high level of muscular strength and energy are not required for their performance and they can be performed comfortably by persons at various points on the ability-disability continuum. Finally, the disabled may eventually organize into a "miliant" group and create a real social movement which will attempt to impose another image of man, that of a man with a disability, on an equal basis with all other acceptable images of man. If such a social movement comes about demanding the real (that is, the social and emotional) integration of the disabled into normal society, it could precipitate further medical, biochemical, and engineering innovations that would permit the complete and nonvisible restoration of ability in the most "physiologic" way.

Some other interrelated societal and medical changes may also profoundly affect the nature of medical care and rehabilitation. One such change may be mostly motivated by the ever-present health manpower shortage and by the fact that the overwhelming majority of the disabled are afflicted with chronic diseases.[21] Moreover, the chronically ill do not necessarily require highly skilled medical care (except during acute episodes), but rather have to become socialized into living with their disability.[22] Since there are some indications that the latter may be quite successfully accomplished while the disabled are participating in some kind of home rehabilitation program, it may be that much of the medical care and rehabilitation services to the chronically ill will be taken out of hospitals and relegated instead to special home-care programs.[23] Although the health manpower shortage could be also solved through a greater reliance on technological innovations that permit a smaller therapist-to-patient ratio,[24] the trend toward home-care programs is already evident in several hospitals across the country, and it may soon become the prevalent one.[25]

Such a development would be largely beneficial to the chronically ill who would be helped in adapting to their real environment and in coping with problematical situations in their lives instead of being aided to perform well within the artificial atmosphere of a rehabilitation center or a hospital for chronic illnesses. Such programs can also take into consideration the significant others' opinions and definitions of the situation as well as the dynamics of the disabled's relationships with his "core" significant others. Finally, the disabled do not have to undergo the stressful transition from the rehabilitation center or the hospital to their home setting and the sometimes resulting adjustment crises. Besides the benefit for the chronically ill, this solution also prevents the greater impersonalization of hospital care, since it would then be restricted to acute cases that could receive much more personal and comprehensive treatment. For this reason, the solution of home medical care rehabilitation programs may be more acceptable in terms of the present values attached to personalized medical treatment.

Another set of societal changes partly responsible for projected health manpower shortages may also lead to a decrease in the differential medical treatment received by low-income patients. For example, increasing coverage of medical and rehabilitation care by government subsidized insurance schemes (such as Medicare, Medicaid, comprehensive rehabilitation plans secured by state legislation, and so forth) may not only make medical care and rehabilitation more accessible to low-income persons, but may also decrease their undesirability as patients as the distinction between private and "public" patients becomes blurred. Continuous uplifting of the lower classes through education and rising income may also tend to restrict the observable differential in medical and rehabilitation treatment to a small persisting "core" lower class group.

But even if most jobs are adapted so that through medical and engineering innovations the disabled can be made fit for most types of work, the knotty question then becomes: Will there be jobs for all those capable of and interested in working? For example, as mothering and child-bearing lessen in importance and some married women either of their own volition or encouraged by others opt for childlessness, and as mechanical devices take over most of the housekeeping chores (since the "robot" housekeepers of science fiction are not fiction anymore), more and more women will be trained for specific occupations and jobs to which they will be greatly committed.[26] Present trends indicate that an increasing number of women enter the labor force and stay considerably longer than in former years. But if the disabled never become vocationally handicapped—and there is already a considerable degree of structural unemployment—where will the necessary number of jobs be found?[27] There are some indications that the rate of unemployment for some occupational categories may be increasing because of increasing automation as well as because of a number of other structural reasons.[28] How many new jobs, then, can be created to absorb all those potentially employable people who may be motivated to work? In view of these future trends, is it a desirable goal to urge everyone to work and to make it a necessary condition—as do vocational rehabilitation programs—for rendering services to the disabled?

A popular answer to the job dilemma is to motivate people to work in service jobs (especially domestic work) after those jobs have been upgraded in terms of pay and prestige. (See Chapter 5 for a detailed discussion.) But even if such a proposal is feasible and practical, it may only solve a present problem and do nothing to solve the same problem in the future. Since automation and all kinds of mechanical devices tend more often to replace repetitive, routine jobs requiring a low level of skill and since the highest rates of unemployment at present (and according to predictions increasingly in the future) are found among those with the lowest level of skill, how will we ever manage to handle the problem of unemployment? How can we compete with technological progress which is fast replacing unskilled people?

A problem already in evidence may soon become aggravated: What does one do with those persons who are unable to learn a skilled or supervisory job, not because they lack the motivation to learn, but because their intellectual endowment does not permit them to learn above a certain level of conceptual complexity? As the required minimum level of skill will increasingly become higher and higher, a much larger portion of the population will become vocationally "handicapped," the major disability or handicap being their relatively low IQ. Thus, rehabilitation may have to serve a more broadly defined population of "mentally retarded" persons whose vocational rehabilitation may be impossible but who need to be helped to live and function in a highly mechanized society.[29] Therefore, it seems that even under

optimum conditions, there may still be a "core" unemployable group
of people. Unless of course, science-fiction-like biochemical and
genetic research permits us to interfere with and manipulate genes in
such a way that no one is born with an IQ below a mimimum level.[30]
Or, even those born with a relatively low potential to learn could
be helped through chemical methods to learn and remember better
and to develop better analytic ability.[31]

Some people are predicting that it will not be possible or meaningful or practical to continuously create jobs—sometimes artificial
or superfluous jobs—in order to employ everyone full-time throughout his life span. They think that an alternative (or a supplementary
solution) to creating new jobs is to restrict the number of hours
that one has a right to work (for example, to lower full-time from 40
hours per week to 30 hours per week) or to lower the retirement
age to 55 or 50 years. The latter alternative would permit people
to use their knowledge, skill, and experience in a productive but
nonstressful, noncompetitive manner. They would have an adequate
income and thus be free of financial difficulties and the taxing pace of
the "rat race." If they wish and are able, they would have the time
to think, to evaluate, to create, and to invent without having to sell
their ideas and their work in order to get a promotion or a higher
salary. The higher degree of disability occurring after age 50 would
no longer represent a vocational handicap. Those above 40 who
suffer from the limitations of a disabling condition would receive
physical rehabilitation to permit them to be autonomous and to carry
on their normal activities to the fullest extent possible. There would
be no "good risks" and "bad risks" in terms of vocational placement,
since people in this age category would not work. There would therefore be fewer malingerers or persons receiving secondary gains from
disability.

Another alternative is suggested by Theobald's idea of a guaranteed income for everyone, which most probably would encourage
some people not to work, even able-bodied people of all ages. Under
his plan, anyone could, for periods of time, elect to live on the
minimum guaranteed income while engaged in activities other than
earning a livelihood. If this option were open to anyone regardless of
physical condition, age, level of skill, education or income, some
profound changes would have to come about in the present puritanical

notion so prevalent in the American middle class concerning the meaning and value of work not only as a mode of supporting oneself and one's dependents, but also as the only "right" way to live. This occasional voluntary unemployment could result in lesser stigmatization of those disabled who could not find suitable employment. If a person did not have to hold down a job to maintain a respectable place in society, rehabilitation programs might be in a better position to develop other goals and other criteria of success which may be more meaningful for human happiness.[32]

A pessimist might ask: What will happen to society if no one wants to work? In ancient Greece and Rome, work was considered demeaning and was done by slaves. Will robots be the slaves of tomorrow? And will man be successful in reaching high levels of intelligence and creativity or will acute boredom resulting from abundant leisure time and an uninterrupted sense of well-being lead to destruction?

Without being excessively optimistic, we could conclude that the future, with its promise of medical, biochemical, and technological innovations, together with its prospects of increasing societal awareness and responsibility as well as humanitarianism and tolerance, holds out hope for the integration of the disabled into the normal, non-disabled society. This integration may be realized both by blurring the distinctions between the disabled and the able-bodied as well as by modifying the physical, social, and emotional environment of the disabled so that they can be accepted equally with all other human beings.

NOTES

1. We also do not know to what extent the definitions of the "disabled" and "rehabilitant" roles differ among the rehabilitation team members, nor the effect of such possible contradictions upon the disabled's own definitions and his rehabilitation behavior. This question could be the subject of an extremely interesting study.

304 DISABILITY AND REHABILITATION

2. Interestingly enough, there are many studies concerning disabled children's return to their families and the impact of the disability upon family relations. See Fred Davis, *Passage Through Crisis* (Indianapolis: Bobbs-Merrill, 1963); Bernard Farber, "Effects of a Severely Mentally Retarded Child on Family Integration," *Monographs of the Society for Research in Child Development,* 24, 2, serial no. 71 (1959); Bernard Farber, "Family and Crisis: Maintenance of Integration in Families With a Severely Mentally Retarded Child," *Monographs of the Society for Research in Child Development,* 25, 1, serial no. 75 (1960); Joseph H. Meyerowitz and Howard B. Kaplan, "Familial Responses to Stress: The Case of Cystic Fibrosis" (mimeographed, Houston: Department of Psychiatry, Baylor University College of Medicine and Houston State Psychiatric Institute, n.d.).
3. And for those who were denied rehabilitation services because they were judged as not being able to benefit from such services, the interest stops at the time of the denial. For a review of the few followup studies available, see Chapter 7, especially the section on the family.
4. The author, acting as research consultant, has recommended such a longitudinal study (including the research areas outlined in items 2, 5, and 6 at the beginning of the chapter) at the Vocational Rehabilitation Center of Morgantown, West Virginia.
5. Lawrence D. Haber, Director, Division of Disability Studies, Social Security Administration, suggested this area in a personal communication. See also Stephen Griew, "Aménagement des postes de travail," a summary included in *Problèmes du reemploi des travailleurs agés ou handicapés* (Luxemburg: Communauté Européenne du Charbon et de l'Acier, December 1967), pp. 126–52.
6. See Constantina Safilios-Rothschild, "Prejudice Against the Disabled and Some Means to Combat It," *The International Rehabilitation Review,* 19, 4 (October 1968), 8–10, 15.
7. At present at the Vocational Rehabilitation Research Division at Morgantown, West Virginia, a scheme is being developed according to which vocational rehabilitation counselors will be rewarded for having successfully rehabilitated "difficult" cases that normally would have been excluded from rehabilitation.
8. Howard A. Rusk, "Care for Wounded G.I.'s," *The New York Times,* June 16, 1968. It is interesting to note that a greater percentage of Vietnam veterans than veterans of any other war use the G.I. Bill educational and training provisions to go to college (70%, while only 51% of the Korean War veterans and 30% of the World War II veterans did so). We do not know, however, whether or not the disabled Vietnam veterans follow the same trend and whether these trends reflect a change

in the educational aspirations of the male population or a change on the part of counselors' attitudes. See Murray Seeger, "When G.I. Joe Comes Marching Home: Will His Needs Be Met?" *The Philadelphia Inquirer,* June 2, 1968.

9. Herman Kahn and Anthony J. Weiner, *The Year 2000: A Framework for Speculation on the Next Thirty-three Years* (New York: Macmillan, 1967), pp. 54, 106–7.

10. U.S. Department of Labor, Manpower Administration, *Technology and Manpower in the Health Service Industry, 1965–75,* Manpower Research Bulletin no. 14, May 1967, p. 32.

11. For example, the use of seat belts definitely reduces fatalities but not disabilities, so that more people now survive automobile accidents and have to live with some degree of disability. See Donald F. Huelke and Paul W. Gikas, "Causes of Death in Automobile Accidents," *The Journal of the American Medical Association,* 203, 13 (March 25, 1968), 1100–07.

12. Kahn and Weiner, *op. cit.,* pp. 53, 107.

13. G. H. Beale, "Changing Cell Heredity," in Nigel Calder (ed.), *The World in 1984,* vol. 1 (Baltimore: Penguin Books, 1965), pp. 199–201.

14. R. M. Kennedi, "Bio-engineering: Opportunity Without Limit," in Calder, *op. cit.,* pp. 202–4.

15. *Ibid.,* p. 204.

16. Kahn and Weiner, *op. cit.,* 106–7.

17. R. E. Gilpin, "The Contribution of Research to Prosthetic Services," *Medical Services Journal, Canada,* 19 (October 1963), 727–46.

18. E. D. Sherman, A. L. Lippay, and G. Gingras, "Prosthesis Given New Perspectives by External Power," *Hospital Management,* 100 (November 1965), 44–49; Yves Lozac'h, A. L. Lippay, E. D. Sherman, and G. Gingras, "Helping Hands," *Electronics,* 40, 16 (August 7, 1967), 125–31; G. Gingras *et al.,* "Bio-electric Upper Extremity Prosthesis Developed in the Soviet Union: Preliminary Report," *Archives of Physical Medicine and Rehabilitation,* 47 (April 1966), 232–37; G. Gingras, "Canadian Experience With the Soviet Myoelectric Upper Extremity Prosthesis," *Orthopedic and Prosthetic Appliance Journal,* 20 (December 1966), 294–97; and Peter B. Nichols, "A Canadian Electric-arm Prosthesis for Children," *The Canadian Medical Association Journal,* 96 (April 22, 1967), 1135–40.

19. This idea was suggested by Theodor J. Litman in a personal communication on reading the second draft of this chapter.

20. It has actually been said that technological progress has already brought about such changes in living conditions that some organs and parts of the human body are no longer instrumental.

306 DISABILITY AND REHABILITATION

21. W. Scott Allan, "The Need for Rehabilitation in Industry," *The Physical Therapy Review*, 40, 11 (November 1960), 810–15. According to the statistics quoted by Allan, chronic diseases are the cause of 88% of disabilities, the most frequent being mental and emotional disorders, diseases of the heart and circulation, and arthritis and rheumatic diseases.

22. Betty E. Cogswell, "Self-socialization: Readjustment of Paraplegics in the Community," *Journal of Rehabilitation*, 34, 3 (May–June 1968), 11–13, 35; Erving Goffman, *Stigma: Notes on the Management of Spoiled Identity* (Englewood Cliffs, N.J.: Prentice-Hall, 1963); Herbert S. Rabinowitz and Spiro B. Mitsos, "Rehabilitation as Planned Social Change: A Conceptual Framework," *Journal of Health and Human Behavior*, 5, 1 (Spring 1964), 2–14; Gene G. Kassebaum and Barbara O. Baumann, "Dimensions of the Sick Role in Chronic Illness," *Journal of Health and Human Behavior*, 6, 1 (Spring 1965), 18–19; and Edwin J. Thomas, "Problems of Disability From the Perspective of Role Theory," *Journal of Health and Human Behavior*, 7, 1 (Spring 1966), 2–9.

23. Jane C. Kronick, "The Rehabilitation of Stroke Patients: An Experimental Analysis of the Effects of Physical and Social Factors in Determining Recovery" (mimeographed, Bryn Mawr, Pa.: Bryn Mawr College, Department of Social Work and Social Research, 1962); I. Rossman, M. Clarke, and B. Rudnick, "Total Rehabilitation in a Home Care Setting," *New York State Journal of Medicine*, 62, 8 (April 1962), 1215–19; Joseph B. Rogoff, Donald V. Cooney, and Bernard Kutner, "Hemiplegia: A Study of Home Rehabilitants," *Journal of Chronic Diseases*, 17 (June 1964), 539–50; E. F. Delagi *et al.*, "Rehabilitation of the Homebound in a Semirural Area," *Journal of Chronic Diseases*, 12, 5 (November 1960), 568–76; I. Rossman, S. D. Eger, and M. Cherkasky, "The Treatment of Cardiac Patients in a Home Care Program," *Mod. Conc. of Cardiovascular Diseases*, 19, 7 (July 1950), 71–72; D. Littauer, "Hospital Care at Home," *Hospitals*, 28, 11 (November 1954), 74–77; P. Rogatz and G. Crocetti, "Home Care Programs—Their Impact on the Hospital's Role in Medical Care," *American Journal of Public Health*, 48, 9 (September 1958), 1125; I. Rossman, "Treatment of Cancer in a Home Care Program," *The Journal of the American Medical Association*, 156, 9 (October 1954), 827–30.

24. Anne R. Somers, "Some Basic Determinants of Medical Care and Health Policy," *The Milbank Memorial Fund Quarterly*, 46, 1, part 2 (January 1968), 13–31; William Kissick, "Health Manpower in Transition," *The Milbank Memorial Fund Quarterly*, 46, 1, part 2 (January 1968), 53–90; and

Technology and Manpower in the Health Industry, 1965–1975 (Washington, D.C.: U.S. Department of Labor, Office of Manpower Policy, Evaluation and Research, 1967).

25. Milton I. Roemer, "Changing Patterns of Health Service: Their Dependence on a Changing World," *The Annals of the American Academy of Political and Social Science,* 436 (March 1963), 49–50. See also references in Note 23.

26. M. W. Thring, "A Robot About the House," in Calder, *op. cit.,* vol. 2, pp. 39–42.

27. Allan L. Otten, "Politics and People," *The Wall Street Journal,* April 26, 1968.

28. Opinions seem to be divided as to the extent to which automation produces unemployment. Probably the divergence of opinions is due to the fact that some authors examine the short-range effects, which are very negative for workers in the occupational groups replaced most easily by automation. Other authors tend to see the eventual societal adjustments that will have to be made in order to offset the negative effects of automation. They see no serious problems created by automation, but, on the contrary, possible benefits for all working people. For a variety of opinions, see Edward D. Kalachek, "Automation and Full Employment," *Trans-action,* 4, 4 (March 1967), 24–29; Charles C. Killingsworth, "Automation, Jobs, and Manpower," in Louis A. Ferman, Joyce Kornbluh, and Alan Haber (eds.), *Poverty in America* (Ann Arbor, Mich.: University of Michigan Press, 1965), pp. 139–52; Morris Philipson (ed.), *Automation: Implications for the Future* (New York: Vintage, 1962); Frederick Herzberg, Bernard Mausner, and Barbara Bloch Snyderman, *The Motivation to Work* (New York: Wiley, 1959), pp. 132–33; Harold L. Wilensky, "Work as a Social Problem," in Howard S. Becker (ed.), *Social Problems: A Modern Approach* (New York: Wiley, 1966), pp. 157–64; and *International Conference on Automation, Full Employment, and a Balanced Economy* (New York: The American Foundation on Automation and Employment, Inc., 1967).

29. Of course, it is also possible that in the image of the Brave New World only a few intelligent people would be necessary to regulate and control the world while all the others would need only a minimum level of competence for an easy, mechanical, nonchallenging, and thoroughly predictable life.

30. Beale, *op. cit.*

31. Kahn and Weiner, *op. cit.,* p. 54.

32. Acknowledgment for the ideas expressed in this paragraph must be given to Julius A. Roth, who suggested them in his written commentary on the manuscript.

Author Index

316   *Author Index*

Thompson, Lindsay, 258, 270, 280n,
 283n
Thoreson, Richard W., 122, 123–24,
 125, 137n
Thring, M. W., 300–1, 307n
Thume, Lee, 132n
Thumen, Judith, 118, 135–36n
Titmuss, Richard M., 157, 183n
Townsend, Peter, 126, 127, 139n
Triandis, H. C., 265, 282n
Truan, T. D., 189, 209n

Veil, Claude, 118, 120, 135n, 137n,
 173, 186n
Vernier, Claire M., 227, 245n
Vinvent, N. L., 190, 210n
Vlasak, George J., 218, 227, 242n,
 272, 284n
Volkart, Edmund H., 61, 66, 85n,
 86n, 87n
Von Slazer, C. F., 74, 90n

Wagner, J. C., 189, 209n
Walsh, James Leo, 70, 89n, 90n, 165,
 184n
Warshaw, Leon, 256, 266, 280n
Weinberg, Martin S., 119, 120, 136n
Weiner, Anthony J., 295, 296, 297,
 302, 305n
Weiner, Hubert, 231, 232, 234, 238,
 239, 247n, 248n
Weir, Donald, 159, 183n
Weiss, E., 133n
Weiss, Robert S., 194, 195, 198–99,
 208, 211n, 212n
Weissman, S., 95, 131n
Weitz, Anne S., 227, 245n

Wells, B. L., 190, 210n
Wenkert, Robert, 206–7, 214n
Wershow, Harold J., 99, 132n
Wessen, Albert, x–xi, 169, 185n
Westie, Frank R., 113, 134n
White, Paul D., 255, 279n
Whiteman, Martin, 128, 139–40n
Whittemore, Ruth, 147–48, 179n
Wilensky, Harold L., 301, 307n
Williams, Robin M., Jr., 185n, 194,
 211n
Wilner, Arthur, 219, 220, 242n
Wittkower, E. D., 41, 52n, 273, 284n
Wolfbein, Seymour, 204, 214n
Wolff, Harold G., 133n
Woolsey, Theodore D., 37, 51n
Wright, Beatrice A., ix, xiii, 7, 43n,
 74, 90n, 96, 97, 98, 108, 110, 111,
 123, 131–32n, 134n
Wright, Robert D., 91n, 185–86n

Yoder, Norman M., 106, 133n
York, Richard H., 148, 180n
Young, Michael, 207–8, 215n
Younng, Janet H., 113, 129, 130, 135n,
 140n
Yuker, Harold E., 113, 129, 130, 135n,
 140n

Zanc, Manuel D., 142, 144, 176n,
 177n
Zinker, Joseph, 137n, 143, 144, 147,
 176–77n, 178n, 179n
Zola, Irving Kenneth, 56, 58, 65, 66,
 82n, 83n, 84n, 88n, 144, 147, 177n,
 178n, 192, 210n
Zucker, M. W., 48n

Subject Index

Accident prevention, research needed on, 293
Administrative mechanisms, rehabilitation affected by, 34
Age
and chronic disabilities, 39–40, 190, 209–10n
and disability acceptance, 113
and disabled-nondisabled interaction, 124
and identity, 200
and rehabilitation success, 224
self-concept affected by, 108, 133–134n
and vocational rehabilitation success, 231–32, 246n, 247n
Age continuum, disability-nondisability continuum and, 112
Aged, as minority group, 110, 112, 113–14

Alienation, 252, 278n
created by litigation, 260–62
and life pattern of disabled, 276–78
and medical treatment differences, 252–60
and occupational mobility, 263–64
and others, significant, 274–75
Amalgamated Clothing Workers of America, rehabilitation program of, 36
American Medical Association, opposed to rehabilitation, 169, 185n
Amputation, self-concept affected by, 96
Anxiety, illness behavior affected by, 63
Architectural barriers to disabled, 9–10
Armed Forces Disability Retirement, 23

Farewell Hospital, 153, 155
Federal Disability Insurance Act (Switzerland), 24
Federal Employers' Liability Act, 19
Federal-state conflicts, and workmen's compensation, 19
Fees, medical, as factor in treatment, 32–33
Financial resources, physical improvement and, 224

General Law of Negligence, 15
Genetic research, 296
Goals, rehabilitation
  and family, 145
  and motivation, 147, 221
  patient-selected *vs.* rehabilitation-personnel-selected, 154–55
  as rehabilitation success criteria, 221–22
  and setting, 147
  and socioeconomic class, 154, 221

Harmarville Rehabilitation Center, 153–55, 242–43*n*
Head Start Program, 205
Health
  definition of, 54–68, 112
  in developing countries, 59
  by patient, 57–68
  by physician, 54–57
  and social role, 60
  and social stigma, 60–61
  to illness, 54–68
  mechanical view of, 58–59
  mental, *see* Mental health
Health legislation, and Industrial Revolution, 13–15
Home rehabilitation, 229–30, 299–300

Identity
  and age, 200
  and masculinity, 200
  and self-concept, 101–2
  and smartness, 201
  and work, 193–204 *passim*
Ideology, workmen's compensation and, 18
Illness
  chronic, 293
  definition of

in developing countries, 59
factors in, 190–93
by patient, 57–68
by physician, 54–57
and social role, 60
and social stigma, 60–61
to disability, 68–73
from health to, 54–68
mechanical view of, 58–59
see also Disability
Illness behavior, 61–68
Illness careers, typology of, 66–68
Immigrants, workmen's compensation laws and, 18
Improvement score calculation, 220–222
Income, guaranteed minimum, 208, 302–3
Income level
  and illness behavior, 85–86*n*
  in rehabilitant employment, 236–238
  and vocational rehabilitation, 232
Income maintenance level, and rehabilitation, 29–30
Industrial medicine, 160–61
Industrial Revolution
  and deviancy, tolerable range of, 127
  and health legislation, 13–15
Injury *vs.* disability, 30–31
In-service job training, 207, 214–15*n*, 268
Institutionalization
  and motivation, 146–51
  and rehabilitation, 80–81, 91–92*n*
Insurance carrier, role of, 269–70
Insurance programs, commercial, 22–23
Intelligence
  and job requirements, 301–2, 307*n*
  and job training, 207–8
  and socioeconomic development, 127
  see also Smartness
Integration, of disabled, 120
Intermarriage, 118–20, 136*n*
Invalidism, 75
Invalids' Cooperatives, 25

Job adaptations, 292–93

About the Author

Constantina Safilios-Rothschild is Senior Research Associate at the Merrill-Palmer Institute, Adjunct Professor of Sociology at Wayne State University, and Research Associate at the Harvard Center for Population Studies. In the past she has served as a Research Consultant to the Athens Center for Mental Health and Research. She has also been a Visiting Professor of Medical Sociology at the University of Montreal and a Visiting Professor of Comparative Family Sociology at Case Western Reserve University. She has presented many papers at International Family and Rehabilitation meetings and has published chapters in several books. She is Associate Editor of *The Journal of Marriage and the Family* and is a frequent contributor to a number of other journals, including the *International Rehabilitation Review*, the *International Journal of Social Psychiatry*, the *Journal of Marriage and the Family*, *Social Forces*, *Family Process*, and *Sociologie et Sociétés*.